BLOOD TRANSFUSION AND PROBLEMS OF BLEEDING

DEVELOPMENTS IN HEMATOLOGY AND IMMUNOLOGY

VOLUME 5

1. Lijnen HR, Collen D and Verstraete M, eds: Synthetic Substrates in Clinical Blood Coagulation Assays. 1980. ISBN 90-247-2409-0

2. Smit Sibinga C Th, Das PC and Forfar JO, eds: Paediatrics and Blood Transfusion. 1982. ISBN 90-247-2619-0

3. Fabris N, ed: Immunology and Ageing. 1982. ISBN 90-247-2640-9

4. Hornstra G: Dietary Fats, Prostanoids, and Arterial Thrombosis. 1982. ISBN 90-247-2667-0

Bloodtransfusion and Problems of Bleeding

edited by

C Th Smit Sibinga, P C Das and
J J van Loghem

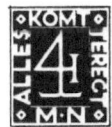

1982

Springer-Science+Business Media, B.V.

Distributors:

for the United States and Canada

Kluwer Boston, Inc.
190 Old Derby Street
Hingham, MA 02043
USA

for all other countries

Kluwer Academic Publishers Group
Distribution Center
P.O. Box 322
3300 AH Dordrecht
The Netherlands

Library of Congress Cataloging in Publication Data   CIP

Symposium on Blood Transfusion (6th : 1981 :
   Groningen, Netherlands)
   Blood transfusion and problems of bleeding.

   (Developments in hematology and immunology ;
v. 5)
   1. Blood--Transfusion--Congresses. 2. Hemophilia--
Patients--Home care--Congresses. 3. Hemorrhagic shock--
Congresses. I. Smit Sibinga, C. Th. II. Loghem, J. J.
van (Johannes Jacobus van) III. Das, P. C. IV. Stichting
Rode Kruis Bloedbank Groningen/Drente. V. Title.
VI. Series. [DNLM: 1. Blood transfusion--Congresses.
2. Blood coagulation disorders--Congresses. 3. Hemophilia
--Congresses. WI DE997VZK v. 5 / WH 322 S989 1981b]
   RM171.S946 1981   616.1'5706   82-14128
   ISBN-13:978-94-009-7694-8

ISBN 978-94-009-7694-8   ISBN 978-94-009-7692-4 (eBook)
DOI 10.1007/978-94-009-7692-4

Copyright © 1982 by Springer Science+Business Media Dordrecht
Originally published by *Martinus Nijhoff Publishers, The Hague 1982*
Softcover reprint of the hardcover 1st edition 1982

Acknowledgement

This publication has been made possible through the support of

Travenol, which is gratefully acknowledged.

CONTENTS

FOREWORD

J.J. Van Loghem

Previously to this symposium, five others have taken place in Groningen. The first one in 1976. This yearly scientific happening has continued. It has greatly stimulated the interest in blood transfusion and all allied disciplines in our country.

It is clear that these meetings are organized not only by a good scientist, but at the same time by a gifted organizer who, as director of the Red Cross Blood Bank Groningen-Drenthe, has shown that the heavy load of daily routine work can very well be combined with a large amount of experimental and clinical research in blood component therapy, coagulation disorders, blood group genetics and serology, the latter in cooperation with the Blood Group laboratory of the University Hospital Groningen under the directorship of Dr. Van Dijk.

All these activities show how much a well-organized blood bank can contribute to a national blood transfusion organization.

It should be stressed that national and international cooperation in the field of blood transfusion is essential for a good practice, based on the principles of the World Health Organization, the League of Red Cross Societies and the International Society of Blood Transfusion, which adopted the resolutions that non-profit blood transfusion services should seek to obtain sufficient blood and plasma from volunteer donors, to cover the medical needs for all blood products, including red blood cells, other cellular elements and all medical needed plasma derivates and, of course, especially F-VIII concentrates (the anti-hemophilic factor); the latter has surpassed the demands of albumin and other blood products.

Dr. Vermijlen from Leuven, Belgium, has developed a system by which the national needs of coagulation factors and the needs of other plasma derivates are completely covered. I hope that the blood banks in our country, together with the Central Laboratory of the Netherlands' Red Cross Blood Transfusion Service, will make every effort to follow this example.

Dr. Anthony Britten, director of the Northeastern New York Red Cross Blood Center in Albany, will present the opening address on behalf of the World Federation of Hemophilia.

Dr. Anthony Britten has contributed tremendously to the development of the World Federation of Hemophilia. For many years he has been the vice-president. He is still active in this organization in a.o. the Hemophilia Action Group and Task Force II.

He is an old friend of the Netherlands and worked in the Central Laboratory in the years 1964-1965, although on quite a different subject: cytotoxic antibodies against lymphocytes. Later on he specialized in HLA genetics and serology and then followed his interest in congenital blood coagulation disorders.

I hope, with Dr. Anthony Britten, that it will become possible in the future to produce factor VIII by DNA recombinant techniques in sufficient quantities to cover the increasing needs. One step further would be that we could cure hemophilia and other congenital bleeding disorders by gene therapy. But that will take, I suppose, a rather long time.

OPENING ADDRESS

A.F.H. Britten

I am delighted to be here to help celebrate the 10th an-
niversary of the Nederlandse Vereniging van Hemophilie-
Patiënten. Your organization deserves our congratulations.
You have created a model for how patients may work together with physicians, scientists, and blood transfusion
services in the consideration of mutual problems. Your
model is an excellent one for others to emulate. You are
not a pressure group; you are a group of participants.
I believe you can be very proud of what you have accomplished in this country.

The speaker that was meant to be before you at this
moment, is Mr. Frank Schnabel, president of the World Federation of Hemophilia (WFH). Frank is not able to be here
today and asked me to fill in for him.

I plan to talk to you as an outsider looking in upon
the World Federation of Hemophilia. I was part of WFH for
many years, in the 1960's and early 1970's, but I am on
the periphery now and it is with that perspective that I
am speaking now.

The World Federation is an organization which has the
ideals and the hopes of hemophilic patients as its essential concern. It comprises the national hemophilia organizations of member countries. It was formed in 1963 and has
now almost 60 member countries. WFH has developed an international network of extraordinarily motivated people. It
has formal affiliation with other international organizations such as the World Health Organization, Rehabilitation International and the International Society of Thrombosis and Hemostasis. The World Federation has established
the remarkable and unique tradition of holding international meeting attended by scientists together with patients.
All of this has happened under the leadership of Frank
Schnabel. You will appreciate my ambivalence about representing him today.

I am reminded of a little story that was told by professor Marx of Munich, after a 1980 Hemophilia Conference
in Bonn. He told of advice he had received when he was a
young medical graduate. 'If you wish your talk to be successful, you must see that one third of it is well-known
to everybody present, one third is quite original (if possible), and one third should be completely incomprehensible

I invite you to judge the success of my application of that advice.

Factor VIII is a problem area. Many parts of the world have difficulty meeting the demand for factor VIII. The task I have set myself is to bring together the needs of the World Federation of Hemophilia and my professional activity in blood banking. How can effective provision of anti-hemophilic plasma derivatives be achieved?

I have been asked by WFH to serve as co-chairman of a Task Force, charged with 'The mobilization of support for hemophilia care, world-wide'. This boils down to promoting the availability of antihemophilic plasma products and the money to pay for them. Working with me on this Task Force are Franz Etzel (Bonn), Fereydoun Ala (Birmingham), Charles Carman (President of the National Hemophilia Foundation in the USA) and your own special friend, Cees Smit Sibinga of Groningen.

TABLE I. Plasma derived from whole blood donations[*]

Plasma usage	Number of donations
Transfusion as whole blood	20,000
Transfusion as plasma	10,000
Fractionation - Factor VIII depleted	15,000[**]
- Fresh frozen	5,000[***]
Total	50,000

[*] Hypothetical usage per million population
[**] 20,000 units plasma produces 100 kg albumin
[***] 5,000 units fresh frozen plasma produces 200,000 iu factor VIII (equivalent to 0.2 iu per person or 4,000 iu per hemophilia patient).

Table I illustrates a hypothetical situation where there is a region or a country with 1 million people. The blood transfusion services are collecting sufficient blood to treat all the needs for red blood cells. This means collecting 50,000 whole blood donations each year. 50,000 is a very important figure because it seems to hold true throughout those parts of the world where medical services are fully developed. The importance of this fact to our discussion this morning is that every one of these 50,000 units also contains plasma, which contains factor VIII. What can happen to that plasma?

1. It may be left in the blood which is transfused as whole blood. There are two ways of doing this: It may be left intact or it may be separated, cryoprecipitate removed, and the plasma returned to the red cells as modified whole blood. In either event that plasma is not available for fractionation, but in the one case it is available for factor VIII production. This is a political area

as you know, an area of conflict. The surgeons and anesthesiologists want whole blood. The hematologists want factor VIII. How can we best resolve the conflict? We have to think about that.

2. Plasma can be transfused in the fresh frozen state (FFP) or as a byproduct of cryoprecipitation. In both cases the plasma is not available for fractionation and in the one case it is wasted from the point of view of hemophilia treatment. I want to emphasize here that the <u>transfusion of whole plasma</u> in the fresh frozen state is a waste of factor VIII; there is no patient who needs whole plasma and also factor VIII. Transfusing fresh frozen plasma is a total waste.

3. Fresh frozen plasma that is not transfused, can be used for <u>fractionation</u> for albumin and factor VIII. If the cryoprecipitate is separated from the plasma, the remaining plasma is good for albumin but it is not useful for factor VIII.

Let us consider the situation where 100 kg of albumin are needed annually for these million people. That is a relatively small amount compared with some countries but it is the norm in many other countries. It is easily produced from plasma derived from the whole blood resource. It is also possible from this source to meet a need of 200 kg albumin, but it is more difficult. If more than 200 kg is needed, an extra source of plasma must be found (plasmapheresis or over-collection of whole blood).

TABLE II. Factor VIII - Need and supply worldwide

World population	4,500,000,000
Hemophilia A cases	225,000
Factor VIII need per case	20,000 iu per year
Total factor VIII need	4,500,000,000 iu per year
Supply*	900,000,000 iu per year

*Supply = 20% of need.

Table II makes the point that the world supply of factor VIII is very much less than needed. The world resource is approximately equivalent to 4,000 units per patient per year. Recommended usage varies from country to country and is controversial. The lowest recommended usage is 10,000 units per patient and the highest is 250,000. So 4,000 is not enough; there is a serious lack of factor VIII. <u>Why is there this shortage? Why is there not enough factor VIII?</u>

Is it because in many countries, the <u>blood transfusion services are not fully developed</u>? Yes, this is a problem which needs attention.

Is the shortage of factor VIII because it is not possible to make sufficient amounts of cryo? The answer is no. This is not the reason.

It is possible to make enough cryoprecipitate to give every hemophilic patient 100,000 units per year, but this never happens in practice.

Is this shortage because the demand for cryoprecipitate is limited? Table III introduces us to another conflict situation, and shows why the answer to this question is 'yes'. Cryoprecipitate may concentrate about 400 units out of a liter of plasma, but the resulting product is inconvenient to use, particularly at home, is prone to allergic side-effects and has problems with control of dosage. The tendency is to prefer a purer product, and there are many good reasons for that. But the effect is that a limited resource is further reduced, because there is additional loss of factor VIII in the production of concentrates. There is a trade-off between the two priorities, the size of the supply and the quality of the supply. We must resolve this problem rationally, because it contributes to the shortage.

TABLE III. Factor VIII recovery *

Product	Recovery (units)
Fresh frozen plasma	1000
Cryoprecipitate	400
Concentrate	200

*Recovery from 1 liter fresh frozen plasma.

Is our problem that there is insufficient plasma? No. It is possible to increase the amount of plasma many times if the economics of fractionation will stand it. The plasma provision is the major cost in fractionation, much more expensive than the actual fractionation process.

TABLE IV. Transfusion of fresh frozen plasma (FFP)*

Year	FFP transfused	% increase
1974–75	192,840	–
1975–76	281,092	45.8
1976–77	381,822	35.8
1977–78	458,020	20.0
1978–79	576,823	25.9
1979–80	744,515	29.1

*Data from American Red Cross Blood Services.

Is the shortage because plasma is wasted? Table IV shows over a five-year period the growth of transfusion of fresh frozen plasma in the United States (nearly 300%). It now requires transfusion of about 20% of the whole blood resource to meet this demand. This is the most rapidly growing activity in blood transfusion. As I mentioned before, this is a waste. We need to control it.

If cryoprecipitate does not provide us with our answers, why not rely on concentrates? Why is this not the answer? Is there insufficient fractionation capacity to make more Factor VIII concentrate? The answer is no. The world's plasma fractionation is 7.1 million liters. The capacity of the fractionation facilities is about 13 million liters. The problem is not the lack of facilities. Existing <u>facilities are underutilized</u>.

TABLE V. Liters plasma produced for fractionation (in millions)

Source		Liters plasma (millions)			
		Fresh frozen	Other	Total	
USA	– commercial	3.75	–	3.75	} 5.0
	– not for profit	0.25	1.0	1.25	
Europe	– commercial	0.2	–	0.2	} 1.6
	– not for profit	0.6	0.8	1.4	
Rest	– commercial	0.2	–	0.2	} 0.5
	– not for profit	0.1	0.2	0.3	
	Total	5.1	2.0	7.1	

Is the shortage because <u>unsuitable plasma is being fractionated</u>? Yes, the factor VIII that we can produce from this 7.1 million liters is limited because only 5.1 million was in the fresh frozen state (Table V). Why was this extra 2 million liters fractionated? The answer is because this 'not fresh' plasma is inexpensive and is available to meet the albumin demand. Since albumin has such a significant role in the economics of fractionation, albumin demand sets the limit on the demand for plasma. This 7.1 million liters is not nearly sufficient for the world's factor VIII needs. We will not get beyond that level until there is a higher demand for albumin or the economics are such that factor VIII can support the costs of the total fractionation process. So all we can do with these numbers is try to increase the 5.1 towards the 7.1. We should not fractionate plasma if it is good only for albumin because the net effect is to depress the amount of factor VIII concentrate that can be produced and that is directly inimical to hemophilia treatment. The same is true of fractionation of placentas.

Table VI shows the relationship between albumin and factor VIII fractionation. The amount of albumin that can be produced from one liter of plasma is about 25 g, and the

TABLE VI. Relationship of albumin and factor VIII production

Albumin production (kg/million population/year)	Factor VIII production (units/person/year)	Equivalent Factor VIII availability (units/patient/year)
100	0.8	16,000
200	1.6	32,000
300	2.4	48,000
400	3.2	64,000
500	4.0	80,000
600	4.8	96,000

amount of factor VIII about 200 units. There is a linear relationship between the two, provided that all the plasma is fresh frozen. If there is plasma fractionated which is not fresh frozen, then the relationship is less favorable for factor VIII. If on the other hand the yield of factor VIII from the fractionation process is higher, perhaps 400 units per liter, then the relationship is much more favorable.

TABLE VII. Albumin usage by country (data from IFPMA)

Country	Albumin usage (kg/million population/year)
Germany (Fed. Rep.)	555
Switzerland	485
USA	296
Belgium	226
Sweden	117
Italy	115
UK	45

Table VII shows the enormous variation in usage of albumin in different countries; it is not difficult to see why most countries produce little factor VIII concentrate. Should albumin use be increased? It seems that the answer to this question must be 'no' because much of the existing use for albumin is of questionable validity.

I must conclude that improved management of the existing plasma resource is possible and desirable but that current technology and financial practices cannot satisfy for long the growing demand for factor VIII. We must be innovative.

As you all know, there is a long tradition of military spending on stock-piles of questionable value. Perhaps we can persuade the military to stockpile albumin! While admittedly useless, such a stockpile would have the merit of having no destructive capacity. If 3% of the United States defense budget was spent on making albumin, the world supply of factor VIII could increase by more than ten times. That is enough to treat all the world's hemophilic patients by the protocols used in the United States, approximately 40,000 units factor VIII per patient. This is a delightful phantasy!

We must find new ways of increasing the yield of factor VIII from fractionation. This is why the work using heparin as an anticoagulant is so significant. Perhaps there is also a future in chromatographic techniques for separating factor VIII or the use of monoclonal antibodies for solid phase separation; even centrifugation of plasma under weightless conditions in space has been suggested as a means of improving the efficiency of separation of the different protein fractions.

There is a technique that is being developed in the U.S. for separating cryoprecipitate from the donor and reinfusing the donor's own cryosupernatant plasma. That could free us of the albumin constraint. Factor VIII from non-human sources is being developed in the United Kingdom; that also could help. Possibly there is a future in the use of recombinant DNA-techniques for Factor VIII synthesis. A danger here is that it may be easier to use the same technology for making albumin and if that happens, the plasma fractionation industry is finished.

I have made a plea for technologic advances. That is what you are here for, to tell us about your research. So I will step down in anticipation of the many distinguished talks to follow.

INVITED SPEAKERS

Van Aken, W.G. *(moderator)*	– Central Laboratory of the Dutch Red Cross Amsterdam, The Netherlands
Von Bartheld, M.	– Red Cross Bloodbank Groningen-Drenthe Groningen, The Netherlands
Blumenstock, F.A.	– Union University Albany, USA
Breederveld, C.	– Wilhelmina Gasthuis Amsterdam, The Netherlands
Britten, A.F.H.	– American Red Cross Blood Services Albany, USA
Brozovic, M. *(moderator)*	– Central Middlesex Hospital London, UK
Ten Cate, J.W.	– Wilhelmina Gasthuis Amsterdam, The Netherlands
Cederbaum, A.	– The Memorial Hospital Worcester, USA
Cobert, B.L.	– New York, USA
Collins, J.A.	– Stanford University Stanford, USA
Das, P.C. *(moderator)*	– Red Cross Bloodbank Groningen-Drenthe Groningen, The Netherlands
Deinhardt, F.	– Max von Pettenkofer Institut München, FRG
Van Dijck, H. *(moderator)*	– President of the Dutch Society of Hemophilia Patients Leiderdorp, The Netherlands
Feldman, F.	– Armour Pharmaceutical Company Kankakee, USA
De Graaf, P.W.J.	– Dutch Society of Hemophilia Patients Voorburg, The Netherlands
Gueguen, M.	– Regional Blood Center Rennes, France
Gullbring, B.	– County Council Blood Transfusion Service Stockholm, Sweden
Haanen, C.A.M.	– St. Radboudziekenhuis Nijmegen, The Netherlands

Hemker, H.C.	- University of Limburg Maastricht, The Netherlands
Jones, P.	- Royal Victoria Infirmary Newcastle upon Tyne, UK
Kahn, R.A. (*moderator*)	- Regional Red Cross Bloodbank St. Louis, USA
Van Loghem, J.J. (*chairman*)	- Professor of Immunology Central Laboratory of the Dutch Red Cross Amsterdam, The Netherlands
Moss, G.	- Michael Reese Hospital Chicago, USA
Newton, D.E.F.	- University of Groningen Groningen, The Netherlands
Prothero, J.	- World Federation of Haemophilia London, UK
Rock, G.A.	- Red Cross Bloodtransfusion Service Ottawa, Canada
Silvergleid, A.	- Bloodbank of San Bernardino San Bernardino, USA
Sjamsoedin-Visser, E.J.M. (*moderator*)	- Medisch Centrum Berg en Bosch Bilthoven, The Netherlands
Stephan, W.	- Biotest Serum Institut Frankfurt, FRG
Suurmeijer, Th.P.B.M.	- University of Groningen Groningen, The Netherlands
Temperley, I.	- St. James's Hospital Dublin, Ireland
Vermijlen, C.	- Red Cross Bloodtransfusion Center Leuven, Belgium
Welbergen, H.	- Red Cross Bloodbank Groningen-Drenthe Groningen, The Netherlands

I. Blood coagulation and blood components

THE BIOCHEMISTRY OF BLOOD COAGULATION

H.C. Hemker

INTRODUCTION

Thrombin is the central enzyme in hemostasis and thrombosis. The study of its generation has been prompted by the many diseases in which hemostasis and thrombosis play a role. The bleeding disorders like hemophilia A are obvious but rare examples. Much more common is the other extreme: the excessive and unknown reaction of the hemostatic process known as thrombosis and its sequel embolism. Thrombosis on basis of atherosclerosis and thrombosis in the veins are very important pathological processes. Evidence is rapidly accumulating that not only (micro)thrombosis is an important complication of atherosclerosis but also plays a role, maybe even the main role, in the genesis of atherosclerosis. Thrombosis in one form or another may therefore be considered to be a key event in well over half of all deaths in the western society, including well-known diseases as coronary infarction, stroke, circulation disturbances in the legs, kidney disease etc. Thrombin generation therefore is a suitable subject of research in a biochemistry department of a medical faculty. On the other hand it shows so many novel features not recognized in enzymology until now, that it cannot fail to interest even the most basicly interested biochemist.

Since the middle of the last century, thrombin is known to clot blood, to cause a fibrinogen solution to turn into a jelly-like mass. This phenomenon is most impressing in vitro, but probably is of minor importance in hemostasis and thrombosis. Since the early sixties, it has been recognized that thrombocytes (blood platelets) play the major role in these processes. For some time this tended to obscure the role of thrombin. More recently, however, it became increasingly apparent that it is precisely the effect of thrombin on platelets that causes platelets to engage in thrombosis and hemostasis. Thrombin is not the only effector for these cells. Prostaglandins, ADP, serotonin etc. all play their role. Thrombin, however, is the agent that makes the platelet reactions irreversible and recent research in our laboratory has shown that it is involved much more early in the platelet reactions than has been supposed before. Anyhow, the view that clotting of blood is observed

in venous thrombi only and that therefore thrombin plays
a role in venous thrombosis only, although still widely
supported among practitioners and pathologists, is no
longer tenable.

WHAT IS THROMBIN?

Thrombin is a proteolytic enzyme of the serine protease
family. It is not unlike trypsin, in that it is specific
for bonds next to arginin. Its main or B-chain containing
the active serine shows extensive homologies with trypsin,
chymotrypsin and elastase as well as with the other pro-
teases of blood coagulation that we will discuss presently.
The B-chain contains aminoacids (in bovine material) and
is S-S linked to the A-chain, 58 residues in length. The
primary structure of both chains has been solved in the
laboratory of Magnusson.
    The function of the A-chain is as yet obscure. It can
be safely guessed that it will play a role in the striking
specificity of this enzyme. This specificity is already
illustrated by its action on fibrinogen. The large fibrinogen molecule (M.W. 360.000) contains scores of potential
vulnerable bonds next to its many arginins. Yet only two
of these are split by thrombin. This generates the fibrin
monomer that spontaneously polymerizes and thus causes
'clotting' per se. Thrombin has a multitude of other functions in hemostasis. It activates the fibrin stabilizing
factor (factor XIII). This factor in its activated form
links lysin residues to glutamic acid residues in adjacent
units of the polymer and thus covalently links the clot.
It also activates procoagulant factors (factors V and VIII)
and this is coupled in a positive feedback system to its
own generation. The way in which these factors act will be
discussed below.
    Thrombin also partakes in a negative feedback because
it splits its proenzyme (prothrombin = factor II) into a
product that is less readily activated than intact prothrombin. Thirdly, and perhaps most important, thrombin
acts on thrombocytes. It causes them to aggregate a basic
reaction of these cells in plugging a hole in a blood vessel as well as the first recognizable event in thrombosis
and probably in the generation of atherosclerosis. It also
causes them to make available the phospholipids that are
necessary for the clotting process: another form of positive feedback. Thrombin, of course, is as dangerous as it
is useful. When it is present in the blood stream even in
tiny amounts it causes a serious clinical picture known
as disseminated intravascular clotting, that often is the
final lethal complication in such diverse diseases as so-
lutio placentae, traumatic brain damage or leukemia. One
is not surprised to find a very efficient scavenger system
for thrombin in the plasma. The main component is antithrombin 3. It quickly combines with thrombin (and other
activated clotting factors) to form a stoichiometric pro-

duct with no enzymatic activity. An important recent event in blood coagulation research is the development of chromogenic substrates. These are tri- or tetrapeptides linked to a p-nitroanilide residue. They can be designed to be relatively specific for thrombin or other clotting esterases and thus make it feasible to estimate the enzymes by spectrophotometric assay. This circumvents much technical problems adherent to the study of the coagulation system by measuring clotting times.

WHAT IS PROTHROMBIN? HOW IS IT ACTIVATED? ROLE OF VITAMIN K

Prothrombin is the zymogen for thrombin. It is a single chain molecule of amino acid residues. The molecular weight is 72,000. It contains both the A- and the B-chain of thrombin but these only account for slightly more than half of the molecule.

In other words, there is an unusually large activation peptide. In order to generate the two chain trombin molecule it has to be split in two sites. The primary structure of prothrombin is known as well as the probable order of bond splitting during activation. In the activation peptide there is a site vulnerable to the action of thrombin. This splits the activation peptide in two parts, called fragment 1 and fragment 2. These regions have different and specific functions in the activation process. Fragment 2 can bind to factor V. Fragment 1 binds to phospholipid. Binding to factor V and phospholipid of the prothrombin molecule greatly enhances its liability of being activated as we will see later. Of particular interest is the way in which fragment 1, the N-terminal end of prothrombin, binds to phospholipid. For this function it is necessary that ten glutamic acid residues in this part of the molecule are converted into γ-carboxyglutamic acids. γ-carboxyglutamic acid (gla) residues are formed by carboxylation of glutamic acid residues in the polypeptide that but for these carboxylations is identical to prothrombin. This carboxylation is an unusual reaction in that it requires reduced vitamin K, O_2 and CO_2 but no biotin or ATP. Recently, the liver enzyme responsible for this reaction has been isolated in our laboratory. If by a lack of vitamin K or by the administration of vitamin K antagonists (the so-called oral anticoagulants, mostly coumarin derivatives) the carboxylation step cannot be carried out, no or at least not enough prothrombin is synthesized and the blood level drops. The precursor, i.e. the uncarboxylated prothrombin precursor either remains in the liver cell (as in the rat and chicken) or does not reach the blood stream (as in men and cows). This circulating descarboxy-prothrombin also known as Protein Induced by Vitamin K Absence, similar to factor II (PIVKA-II), may slowly generate thrombin and also in other ways disturb coagulation tests in anticoagulated patients. In fact, it was by these

effects that it was first recognized. It is one of the
factors that makes the control of oral anticoagulant treatment a difficult task and thus contributes to the occasional failure of this useful therapy. Apart from this, PIVKA-
II can be isolated from plasma and because it is completely
identical to prothrombin but for the capability to bind to
phospholipids, it is a perfect model to study the lipid
binding of this clotting factor. It may be mentioned already now that the other vitamin K dependent clotting factors (i.e. factors VII, IX and X) also show gla residues,
that also serve to bind them to phospholipid surfaces.
When no vitamin K is present (c.q. when its action is
blocked) analogs of these factors, called PIVKA-VII, PIVKA-
IX and PIVKA-X, occur in the blood stream.

The bonds that need to be split in prothrombin in order
to liberate thrombin are clipped by proteolytic enzymes.
This can be done by trypsin, by certain snake venoms or
by activated factor X. These reactions occur in free solution but are not very efficient. Under physiological circumstances a more sophisticated biochemical mechanism is
operative.

PROTHROMBINASE

The normal physiological activator of prothrombin consists
of factor X_a bound to a phospholipid surface next to a molecule of factor V_a. Factor X_a is the activated form of
factor X, one of the vitamin K dependent coagulation factors. This factor occurs in the blood in a two-chain form.
The heavy chain (MW 44,000) contains the active serine
and is S-S bound to the light chain (MW 17,000) that contains 12 gla residues in its N-terminal part. Upon activation, the mechanism of glycopeptides is removed from the
N-terminal part of the heavy chain. Unlike thrombin, this
activated enzyme in this case does possess a gla containing region, and it is via this region that it can bind to
phospholipid. Extensive comparisons carried out in our lab
between factor X and PIVKA-X, the decarboxy form of the
enzyme found in vitamin K deficiency, show that PIVKA-X
can be activated like factor X and then acquires properties indistinguishable from factor X_a when reactions are
studied that take place in free solution. When the reaction takes place at an interface, the properties are very
different indeed.

Factor V_a is a 100,000 MW two-chain protein that arises
from a 360,000 MW single-chain precursor in an as yet not
completely clear way. The activation under physiological
circumstances is carried out by thrombin.

It should be mentioned that no enzymatic activity of
factor V_a is known. Activation here does not mean a pro-
enzyme-enzyme conversion, as it does with all other coagulation factors except factor VIII. Early experiments
showed that factor X_a alone is capable of splitting prothrombin but that its catalytic action is enhanced up to

several thousand fold by the addition of phospholipids
and factor V_a that both are inactive as such.

Early kinetic experiments showed that prothrombinase
is formed by independent reversible adsorption of the
factors V_a and X_a on the phospholipid surface.

It thus appears that an interesting question in general
enzymology arises. Why is it that an enzyme (factor X_a)
is much more potent when it acts in concerted action with
an accessory factor, also called paraenzyme (factor V_a)
adsorbed at an interface? The question may be of much more
general importance than for the activation of prothrombin
alone. Not only does a similar situation occur in the activation of factor X, but also the same configuration is
encountered several times in the complement system. It
also can be recognized in oxidative phosphorylation and
it might indeed be a feature of many reactions occurring
at membrane-solution interfaces.

THE REACTIONS LEADING TO THE ACTIVATION OF FACTOR X

The factor X activated enzyme is the vitamin K dependent,
hence gla-containing, hence lipid binding factor IX_a. Precisely like factor X_a it needs for its full activity adsorption onto a phospholipid surface and a para-enzyme, in
this case factor VIII. Factor VIII remains a somewhat enig-
matic protein and I will not discuss it to any extent here.
It is sufficient to say that it probably is a polymer of
two different proteins, one of which is active in coagulation. Like factor V it is activated by thrombin.

Factor IX_a in its turn arises from factor IX in a reaction catalyzed by factor XI_a. The mechanism of formation
of factor XI_a has been unraveled in the last few years.
It is a direct consequence of contact of blood with negatively charged wettable surfaces.

In the presence of such a surface, factor XII adsorbs
from the plasma and in adsorbing undergoes a conformational change that makes it a suitable substrate for kallikrein. Kallikrein, however, does not act as such. In plasma it is bound to high molecular weight kininogen (HMWK).
Via HMWK that contains a domain of about 120 residues, 30%
of which are histidines, and that hence bears a strongly
positive charge, kallikrein binds to the negative surface,
next to factor XII and is capable of activating factor
XII. On the other hand, factor XII_a can activate prekallikrein when it adsorbs, also via HMWK.

This mutual activation leaves us with the question of
how the process starts. If both factor XII and prekallikrein were absolutely inactive pro-enzymes, the reaction
could not be triggered without the help of another enzyme.
At the moment we think that the proenzymes are not completely inactive, that some interaction is always possible
but that this is easily repressed by the antiprotease abundant in plasma.

By adsorption to a negative surface two phenomena occur

simultaneously:
  a. factor XII becomes a better substrate
  b. the concentration of the reactants near the surface
     is enhanced.
This the factors engage in a strongly non-linear interaction that breaks through the protective action of the an-
tiproteases.

Factor XII_a activates factor XI that like (pre)kalli-
krein is bound to the negatively charged surface by HMWK.
Factor XI_a then activates factor IX. The pathway here described is called the intrinsic pathway because no material
alien to the blood plays a role in it.

There is another pathway. A lipoprotein present in almost all cells and called tissue thromboplastin can interact with a vitamin K dependent plasma protein factor VII
to form a complex in all probability completely analogous
to the prothrombin and intrinsic factor X activating complexes that can activate factor X. Factor X_a in its turn
can activate factor VII and between these two proenzymes
a situation of reciprocal activation may exist not unlike
the situation between factor XII and factor XI described
above. Only here the reaction occurs at a phospholipid
solvable interface.

It becomes more and more clear that the factor VII dependent pathway is not completely independent of the intrinsic pathway. It has been known for a long time and
has been again found with modern methods that factor VII
acts upon factor IX. In fact under conditions that only a
limited amount of tissue thromboplastin is present, the
action of factor VII upon factor X is markedly enhanced
by the presence of the factors VIII and IX, but independent of the contact factors.

Factors VIII and IX thus seem to act as an accessory
factor X_a activator that can be triggered by factor VII
and tissue thromboplastin.

THE FUNCTION OF COMPLEX ENZYMES

The data in the literature only state that phospholipids
and factor V_a, each alone enhance the activity of factor
X_a as a prothrombin activator and that, when both are present together their action is markedly increased. We tried
to find out what the mechanism behind this phenomenon is.

To this end we purified factors X_a, V_a and II, and we
synthesized phospholipids of known composition. Then we
estimated the kinetic parameters of the conversion of factor II by the different possible activating enzymes, i.e.
factor X_a, factor X_a - phospholipid, factor X_a - factor V_a,
factor X_a - factor V_a - phospholipid. The rate of formation of thrombin at different prothrombin concentrations
was measured by subsampling from the incubation mixture
into a cuvette containing S 2238, a chromogenic substrate
for thrombin and assessing the amount of thrombin from
the rate of color production observed. In this way Line-

weaver-Burk plots of each of the enzymes could be obtained. It was seen that - but for a rare exception to be discussed later - straight Lineweaver-Burk plots were obtained.

We found that phospholipids decrease the K_m by about 1000-fold and that factor V increases V_{max} by about the same factor.

It is obvious that the overall rate enhancement attained by the combination of these effects can be enormous. The concentration of prothrombin in plasma is about 2 µM and it is seen that addition of phospholipid moves the K_m from above this value to well below it. Experiments on the factor X activating complex showed that completely comparable kinetics were observed here with factor X in the role of substrate and factors IX_a and VIII acting as enzyme and paraenzyme. The effects of the phospholipids and factor V are clearly different and the next task would be to seek a mechanistic explanation for the observed facts.

THE PHOSPHOLIPIDS

Already in 1967, we had found that excess phospholipid inhibits the formation of prothrombinase and we explained this phenomenon by assuming that the reaction of prothrombinase with prothrombin takes place in the two-dimensional compartment formed by the phospholipid-water interface. Addition of an excess of phospholipid increases this interface and dilutes the protein components in it. If this is the right explanation then the kinetic constants observed in bulk solution are only apparent constants and should be recalculated so as to represent the situation at the surface. For this we set out to determine the apparent K_m and V_{max} at a range of phospholipid concentrations.

It appeared that K_m shows a clear variation with the phospholipid concentration. From the literature the dissociation constant and the number of binding sites of prothrombin for the type of phospholipid we used could be obtained. With the aid of this constant the concentration of prothrombin at the surface could be calculated. It turned out that at every phospholipid concentration the variable apparent K_m calculated on basis of the bulk phase concentration corresponded to one fixed concentration of adsorbed prothrombin. The same phenomenon could be still more elegantly demonstrated with the factor X converting enzyme. Here we found a method to estimate the dissociation constant and the number of sites for factor X onto the phospholipid on the same day and in the same preparations as used for determination of the kinetic constants. This method is based on the fact that a proteolytic protein from the venom of Russells Viper (called in short RVV-X) activates factor X in free solution but does not act on the adsorbed enzyme. From the velocity of factor X formation in a mixture of phospholipid and factor X, the amount of free factor X thus be immediately assessed. When this is done in a series of concentrations a Scatchard plot can be constructed that yields both the dissociation constant and the number of binding sites for factor X on phospholipid.

Also in this case it became clear that the reaction shows its half maximal reaction velocity at a fixed number of substrate molecules adsorbed per amount of lipid. Apart from the substrate also the enzyme has to adsorb on the phospholipid. Under the conditions of our experiments with prothrombinase we saw that V_{max} increased slightly with the concentration of phospholipid. As V_{max} is proportioned to the enzyme concentration this was thought to reflect a more complete binding of the enzyme at higher phospholipid concentrations. The fact that this phenomenon is less pronounced than the effect on substrate concentration can be explained from the higher affinity of the enzyme (factor X_a) for the surface and from the fact that only small amounts of factor X_a are present i.e. the amount of lipid present is in excess over the amount of factor X_a and therefore the binding of factor X_a is favored.

These results all point in the direction that the reaction takes place between the adsorbed enzyme and the adsorbed substrate. The interface seems to form a 'two-dimensional reaction vessel' in which the molecules meet. Why should the reaction be favored by this arrangement. On first sight it is clear that the concentration at the surface is higher but a second thought learns that this as such will not increase the interaction velocity. For the molecules to interact they have to meet and it is not clear that adsorbed molecules are free to meet. Two arguments can be brought forward that favor the model proposed. The first is a theoretical one. From various types of experiments an estimate can be made of the lateral mobility of proteins adsorbed onto phospholipids. One can calculate the collision frequency and compare it to that in free solution. It turns out that the collision frequency of adsorbed protein may be easily some 100 to 1000 times higher than that in the free solution. The second argument in fact shows that an experimental change in diffusion coefficient does increase the reaction rate. We could show that the procoagulant activity of synthetic phospholipids sharply increases at the transition temperature of the phospholipids. As it can be assumed that the lateral diffusion coefficient increases sharply above the transition temperature, this can be accepted as evidence in favor of our model. Apart from increased collision frequency adsorption at an interface can act favorably by two other mechanisms. In free solution colliding molecules will make first contact at random places of their surfaces. When adsorbed they are oriented because one specific part of the molecules - the gla containing

N-terminal end – interacts with the phospholipids. Colliding adsorbed molecules therefore will make first contact at restricted places on their surface and the molecules may be so constructed that this causes more collisions to result in interaction.

Thirdly, the adsorption may cause conformational changes in the proteins and thus make them more reactive. This possibility is as difficult to refute as it is to prove and is only interesting when other explanations fail. In the contact activation mechanism it may be the only remaining possibility. It is as yet not absolutely necessary to postulate it in this case. We concluded that adsorption onto phospholipid increases the number of favorable collisions between the molecules, therefore acts as if increasing the concentration of substrate and thus causes a decrease of K_m.

THE PARAENZYMES

The activation of factor X involves the splitting of one peptide bond only. The k_{cat} of this reaction is increased by factor VIII, the accessory protein in this case. We therefore have to consider an influence of this protein on the reaction mechanism of the splitting.

Special attention should be paid to the possibility of the occurrence of noncovalent complexes. The increase of any forward rate constant in this mechanism will result in an increase of the observed k_{cat}. With small amide substrates acylation is the rate-limiting step. The rates that are observed with small substrates are explained by a k_{cat} of 10-100. Without factor VIII the k_{cat} of factor X activation is much lower (10^{-4}). With factor VIII k_{cat} is restored to about the level seen with small substrates (~2). This suggests that rather than accelerating the catalytic mechanism per se, factor VIII brings about conditions that make the enzyme as effective with large substrates as with small ones. This suggests that the mechanism of bond breaking as such is not involved, because this is not different in large and in small substrates. Rather would one expect an effect on interactions that are known to be different for these two types of substrates, i.e. the noncovalent interactions. We will see that in the case of prothrombin more arguments can be brought forward for this view.

The case of prothrombin is more complicated though. Here two peptide bonds have to be split in the substrate. The minimal possible reaction scheme therefore is:

It appears from an analysis of the reaction products obtained with different forms of prothrombinase that in the absence of factor V, P_2 + F is the main reaction product, whereas in its presence thrombin is formed directly.

So in the absence of factor V, P_2 dissociates readily from the enzyme but in its presence not. In order to discuss this phenomenon we will employ a simplified form of the reaction scheme:

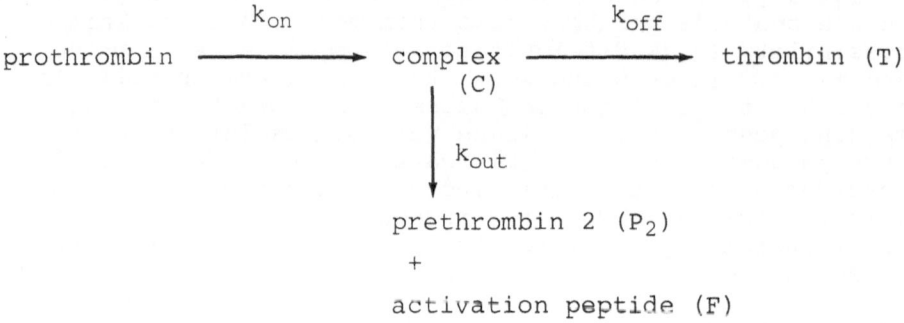

Factor V can prevent the production of P_2 in one of two ways. Either k_{out} is decreased or the steady state concentration of C is lowered by an increase of k_{off} relative to k_{on}. We cannot exclude that k_{out} is decreased by factor V. Actually binding of the activation peptide to factor V has been observed and it is also known that there is a relatively light noncovalent binding between F and P_2. It can be easily argued, however, that a decrease of k_{out} can not be the only mechanism involved. In the first place one would like to have a unifying explanation for the action of the paraenzymes in both complexes studied, but a decrease of k_{cat} can never explain the effect of factor VIII on factor X activation as only one bond splitting is involved there. In the second place k_{cat} of thrombin formation in the presence of factor V is about 50 s^{-1}. This means that both k_{on} and k_{out} should be at least 50 s^{-1}. The rate of P_2 formation in the absence of factor V was estimated by us to be 0.5 s^{-1} and the k_{cat} of thrombin formation was 0.05 s^{-1} under these circumstances. This is incompatible with forward rate constants of 50 s^{-1} or more. So one or both of the kinetic constants k_{on} and k_{off} have to be increased by factor V.

An interesting observation is that although the action of factor X_a on its natural substrate prothrombin is inhibited by the presence of a competing small substrate (S 2238), the action of factor X_a on the small substrate is not inhibited by the presence of prothrombin. Even when prothrombin is present at concentrations of about K_m so that one would expect that about 50% inhibitor would occur. In our opinion this can only be explained if prothrombin - factor X_a complexes occur that have the active center of factor X_a available for the splitting of a small

substrate. If this is true, then factor V would act by
diminishing the amount of that type of complexes. Unfortunately, technical difficulties prevent to investigate
the inhibition of S 2222 conversion by prothrombin in the
presence of factor V. Yet we may postulate that factor V
serves to diminish the level of prothrombin - factor X_a
complexes or thrombin - factor X_a complexes. That is,
factor V would act by guiding the large molecular weight ·
substrates to the active center of the enzymes.

THE ROLE OF THE PLATELET IN COAGULATION

Under physiological circumstances the phospholipids necessary for the coagulation reactions are provided by
the blood platelets. It has been shown that the plasma
membrane of the platelet is asymmetrical and that the
phospholipid composition of the outside has no significant procoagulant properties whereas those at the inside
have. Especially phosphatidyl serine (PS) is essential
in providing the negative charge that is a prerequisite
for binding of the K dependent clotting factors. This
phospholipid is almost entirely found at the inner surface of the membranes. It is wellknown that platelets that
are triggered for their hemostatic function show a release
reaction. As a part of this phenomenon factor V_a is transferred from storage vesicles inside the platelet to the
outside. We could show that if platelets are triggered
by thrombin and collagen, procoagulant phospholipids appear
at the outside of the plasma membrane. This phenomenon is
not accompanied by platelet breakdown as can be judged
from the fact that no platelet intracellular enzymes are
released. On the other hand the material stored in the
platelet granules (serotonin, factor V) is released. The
procoagulant phospholipids remain an integral part of the
platelet and, for more than 90% can be spun down with the
platelet. We hypothesize that parts of the plasma membrane
of the platelet turn inside out (flip-flop) so as to present their procoagulant inner surface when they are triggered. At the same time factor V_a becomes available from
the inside of the platelets. This explains the presence
of highly specific factor X_a binding sites at the surface
of activated platelets. The factor X_a at the surface of a
platelet is immune to activation by antithrombin 3. The
platelet reaction therefore provides a rich source of prothrombinase activity. Also because platelets active in
hemostasis stick to each other and to subendothelial structures, they create a sponge-like structure in the crevi-
ces of which flow will not wash away the thrombin formed.
Thrombin again will induce release and flip-flop in neigh-
boring platelets. The actions of blood platelets and the
blood coagulation factors thus mutually reinforce each
other.

CONCLUSION

From the biochemical point of view the blood coagulation mechanism offers the possibility of studying reactions and does cover patterns that are not easily found elsewhere.

Years of careful clinical observation have helped to sort out those illnesses that, as experiments of nature, can help in solving these questions. On the other hand, investigation of the basic phenomena underlying thrombin formation will in the end help in interfering with the processes of atherosclerosis, thrombosis, embolism, intravascular coagulation and bleeding tendencies, that together form largely more than half of the total death toll in our society at this moment.

REFERENCES

In view of the general nature of this overview further studies of the literature are best carried out on the hand of specialized review articles.

1. Hemker, H.C.: Capita Selecta: Vorming en functies van thrombine. Ned. Tijdschr. v. Geneesk., 126:198,1982.
2. Miletich, J.P., Majerus, P.W.: Properties of the factor Xa binding site on human platelets. J.biol.Chem. 253:6908, 1978.
3. Suttie, J.W., Jackson, C.M.: Prothrombin structure activation and biosynthesis. Physiol. Rev. 57:1. 1977.
4. Zwaal, R.F.A.: Biochim.biophys.Acta 515:163, 1978.
5. Zwaal, R.F.A., Hemker, H.C.: Blood cell membranes and haemostasis. Haemostasis, 11:12,1982.

BLOOD COAGULATION: LABORATORY PRACTICE

M. Brozović

Assessment of blood coagulation and general hemostasis is
undertaken by the clinical laboratory for three major reasons: to diagnose and treat acute hemostatic failure, to
diagnose, investigate and if necessary treat a patient with
bleeding tendency, and finally, to monitor the effects of
blood component therapy. The tests used and the interpretations made depend on the clinical context. Therefore each
of the three clinical situations will be discussed separately.

ACUTE HEMOSTATIC FAILURE

Acute hemostatic failure is a common emergency in surgical,
medical and obstetric practice. There is usually no time
for complicated tests: all investigations must be simple,
quick and reliable; their significance should be familiar
to both laboratory and clinical emergency staff. The tests
commonly used are: one stage prothrombin time (PT), activated partial thromboplastin time (PTT), thrombin time (TT)
or fibrinogen determination and platelet count. Using these
four variables, the common causes of acute hemostatic failure are easily distinguished (Table I).

TABLE I. Common diagnostic patterns in acute hemostatic failure

Test \ Diagnosis	DIC	Stored blood transfusion	Liver disease	Vitamin K deficiency	Undiagnosed Thrombo-cytopenia	Undiagnosed hemo-philia
PT	↑↑	↑	↑↑	↑↑	N	N
PTT	↑↑	↑↑	↑↑	↑	N	↑↑
TT	↑↑	N	↑	N	N	N
Platelet count	↓↓	↓	↓	N	↓↓	N

Laboratory and medical staff easily recognize the patterns
shown on this table (4).
    There are, however, many pitfalls with these relatively

simple tests. The problems may arise with samples, techniques or interpretation of results obtained.

Samples. It is often difficult to obtain a satisfactory venous sample from a peripherally collapsed patient: hemolyzed or partly clotted samples are common. Samples are sometimes collected from indwelling catheters. Such samples are not suitable for investigation of hemostasis, as all artificial surfaces adsorb plasma proteins (5). Fibrinogen, factors VIII, XII and XI are adsorbed, thrombin is generated via the intrinsic pathway with gradual formation of a fibrin monolayer and platelet aggregates. We have studied the effect of collection through a catheter on the assays of factors VIII and V. Activation of the intrinsic pathway is present within 10 minutes of insertion. Even with repeated flushing, blood obtained through catheters may contain traces of activated factors and is unsuitable for coagulation tests and platelet counting.

Another commom problem is the contamination with heparin, either added to keep the catheters patent, or remaining in the needle if the same site was used to collect a sample for blood gas estimation. Reptilase or Arvin are useful reagents in distinguishing long times due to heparin from those due to true hemostatic failure.

Problems related to laboratory techniques are well recognized and have been extensively reviewed. Good quality, stable and standardized reagents, adequate normal and abnormal controls, familiar procedures, and experienced operators are all equally important. Quality control schemes are run by many national and international authorities. Participation in such schemes ensures that individual laboratories maintain their standards of performance.

The emergency tests are also open to interpretation errors. Common sources of such errors are: (i) The tests used are global and only reflect severe defects. For example, the majority of PTT reagents only detect factor VIII levels of below 20 iu/dl (3). Thus it is possible for a mild hemophiliac with a factor VIII: C level of 25 iu/ml to experience severe post-operative bleeding due to lack of factor VIII and have normal PTT. (ii) In early stages of DIC or of acute liver failure, the presence of activated clotting factors may give rise to false normal clotting times. A few hours later all clotting times may be grossly prolonged. (iii) The combination of heparin in plasma and low platelet count may mean DIC in a heparinized patient, or heparin-induced thrombocytopenia. Many such examples can be quoted. The errors of interpretation can be minimized with close cooperation between the laboratory and the clinical staff.

Emergency tests can also be used to monitor the therapy of acute hemostatic failure as illustrated on Fig. 1 in a case of stab injury to the liver with severe hemostatic disturbances. In general DIC is monitored with serial fibrinogen estimations, effects of massive transfusion with PTT, and acute vitamin K_1 deficiency with PT. If sufficient plasma is available all emergency tests should be repeated as

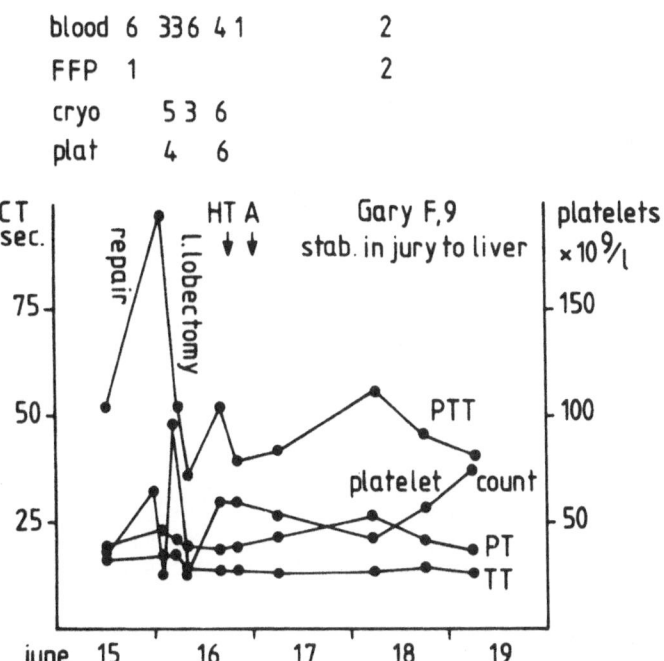

Fig. 1. Management of acute hemostatic failure with emergency tests.
A nine year old boy was admitted deeply shocked and bleeding from a
small abdominal wound having fallen over a sharp fence. He was resuscitated with blood and fresh frozen plasma and taken to theater where
a large tear in the left lobe of the liver was repaired. Postoperatively he began to ooze from all catheter and injection sites and bled
profusely from the wound. The hemostatic abnormalities were corrected
with blood, cryoprecipitate and platelet concentrates, and generalized
bleeding stopped, but the wound continued to drain large amounts of
blood. He underwent second laparotomy 12 hours later; left lobectomy
was carried out. He developed right hematothorax and required more
blood, cryoprecipitate and platelets. His general condition gradually
improved and he was discharged home one month later.

often as possible, as combination defects, such as DIC followed by problems of massive transfusion or vice versa, are
common.

DIAGNOSTS AND MANAGEMENT OF ABNORMAL BLEEDING

In situations when more time, more blood and a relatively
well patient are available, more complex tests can be used.
The usual practice is to take a detailed and careful clinical and family history, and then carry out a small number
of screening tests. These tests may vary from laboratory
to laboratory but generally include platelet count, bleeding

time, PT, PTT, TT, fibrinogen determination and a clot solubility test. When the results of the screening tests and
the analysis of the history are available, it is usually
clear what type of second line tests are required. The general outline of second line tests is shown on Table II.

TABLE II. Second line tests in the investigation of bleeding tendency

Screening abnormality	Second line test	Likely diagnosis if low or abnormal
Isolated long PTT	(1) FVIIIc, RAg	Classical hemophilia
	(2) FIXc	FIX deficiency
	(3) FXI	FXI deficiency
	(4) Assays of other contact factors	FXII deficiency, Fletcher, Fitzgerald factor defect
Isolated long PT	(1) FVII	FVII deficiency
Long PT and PTT	(1) Stypven time, FX	FX deficiency
	(2) FV	FV deficiency
	(3) Prothrombin assay and immunological tests	Hypo- or dysprothrom-binemia
Long PT, KPTT and TT; low or absent fibrinogen	(1) Clot weight	Afibrinogenemia or dysfibrinogenemia
	(2) Polymerization studies	
	(3) Immunological studies	
	(4) FpA and Fp release	
Increased clot solubility	(1) Biochemical assay of FXIII	FXIII deficiency
	(2) Immunological assay	
Long bleeding time long PTT	(1) FVIIIc, RAg, RiCoF	Von Willebrand's syndrome
	(2) Crossed IEF of VIII RAg	
	(3) Platelet aggregation	
Long bleeding time	(1) Platelet morphology	
	(2) Platelet aggregation studies	
	(3) VIIIc, RAg, RiCoF	
	(4) Membrane glycoproteins	Glanzmann's
	(5) Prostaglandin pathway	
	(6) ATP, ADP content	Storage pool disease
	(7) Release reaction	
	(8) Electron microscopy	

All second line tests require careful collection of
specimens, meticulous techniques, stable and standardized
reagents, reliable normal and abnormal controls, and accurate end point assessment. Coagulation factor assays, whether biological or immunological, require in addition reliable standards, preferably freeze dried and calibrated

by more than one laboratory. Furthermore, plasma concentration of coagulation factors varies with age, sex, oral
contraceptive usage, and the presence of stress or acute
phase reaction. All these variables must be taken into account when assessing the hemostatic function and in particular when studying possible heterozygotes. For reliable
interpretation of immunological tests, high quality, well
purified antisera are essential.

The most widely used of the <u>platelet function test</u>, platelet aggregation, varies widely from laboratory to laboratory. The results are easily affected by the pH of blood,
length of storage of blood prior to testing, aggregometer
temperature, type, and even size and shape of the stir-bar
(3). In addition, detailed questioning about drugs is often

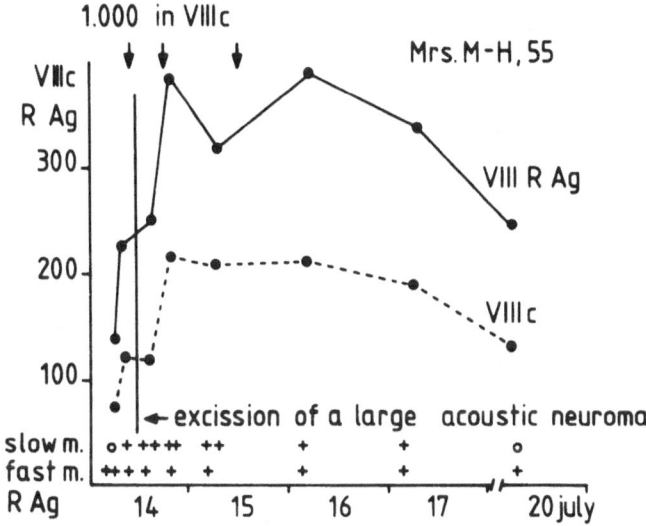

Fig. 2. Management of a patient with a severe congenital platelet
function defect undergoing neurosurgery.
A 37 year old woman, a known case of Hermansky-Pudlak syndrome with
severe bleeding tendency was admitted for excision of a large acous-
tic neuroma. Preoperative tests disclosed that in addition to the abnormal aggregation to ADP and collagen, her platelets also failed
to aggregate to 1.2 mg Ristocetin per ml and that the defect was
corrected on addition of factor VIII. The operation was covered with
platelets and factor VIII and lasted for 6 hours. Towards the end of
the procedure surgeons reported difficulties with hemostasis and additional platelets and factor VIII were given. Hemostasis remained
satisfactory and laboratory tests showed complete correction of all
defects. She recovered uneventfully.

omitted. Many unexplained abnormalities of platelet behavior are due to drugs such as antihistamines, tranquilizers
and β-blockers. The effects of these drugs on platelets vary
from individual to individual, and are not widely recognized by the medical and laboratory staff.

Finally, if the pattern of abnormality obtained on secondary testing does not fit into a recognizable pattern
even after excluding the possibility of technical or cleric-
al error, one of the more unusual combined defects may be
present (2).

TESTS FOR MONITORING BLOOD COMPONENT THERAPY IN HEMOSTATIC
DEFECTS

In the majority of cases the therapy is monitored using

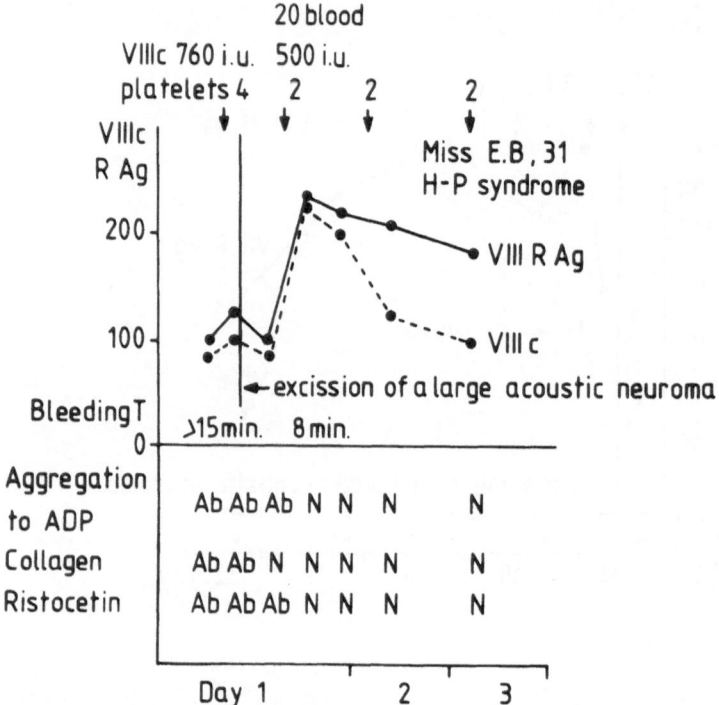

Fig. 3. Management of a patient with Von Willebrand's disease undergoing neurosurgery.
This 55 year old woman was a known case of Von Willebrand syndrome
with FVIIIc and FVIII RAg levels varying on different occasions between 10-20 iu/dl; platelet aggregation to Ristocetin was absent and
the crossed IEF disclosed an abnormal fast moving factor VIII RAg
only. In 1981 she was admitted for excision of a large rapidly growing
cystic glioma. On this occasion her factor VIIIc and RAg were normal,
although VIII RAg remained abnormal in IEF mobility. The operation
was covered with factor VIII concentrate. A malignant glioma was partially excised and there were no problems with hemostasis. She made
an uneventfully post-operative recovery, but deteriorated after dis-
charge and died 3 months later.

specific coagulation assays, i.e. factor VIII: C assay to
monitor the replacement with factor VIII: C in a hemophiliac,
factor IX: C assay to monitor the administration of factor
IX concentrate (6). In a small proportion of cases more
complex testing is required. This is usually the case with
variants of Von Willebrand's syndrome or severe congenital
platelet defects, as illustrated in Fig. 2 and 3.

Monitoring may also be necessary to recognize and prevent the side effects of blood component therapy. A list
of common hemostatic side effects of therapy with blood
components and their usual clinical and laboratory manifestations is shown on Table III.

TABLE III. Hemostatic side effects of therapy with blood components

Replacement with	Side effect	Clinical or laboratory signs
Clotting factors	Inhibitors	Poor recovery in vivo. Resistance to therapy. Positive in vitro inhibitor tests. Rarely positive immunopre-cipitation tests.
Factor VIII materials of low and interme-diate purity	Excessively high fibrinogen	Paradoxical prolongation of PTT. Increased plasma viscosity.
Factor IX concentrates	Thrombogenicity	Thrombotic events. Low grade DIC. Laboratory signs of DIC, in particular reduced platelet count.
Platelet concentrates	Isoimmunization	Resistance to therapy. Allergic or febrile reactions. Demonstration of antiplatelet antibodies.

SUMMARY

A good laboratory should be able to provide simple and
quick tests for the immediate diagnosis and management of
acute hemostatic failure. There must be a clear cut policy
on the use and interpretation of such tests. These tests
must be available in all hospitals with acute admissions.

When investigating a patient with abnormal bleeding tendency, two types of tests are required: the screening tests
and the more elaborate second line tests. In the majority
of patients screening tests, factor VIII: C and VIII RAg
assays and platelet aggregation studies can establish the
diagnosis. The remaining patients require further, often

complex, investigations. The screening procedures, factor VIII assays and platelet aggregation tests should be available in most if not all hospitals. Further tests can only be carried out successfully in specialized centers, where both the laboratory and the medical expertise are available.

The treatment of hemostatic defects with blood components must be monitored with appropriate assays. The incidence of side effects is sufficiently high to warrant a policy of systematic simple screening for inhibitors and continuous watching of responses in all patients treated with factor concentrates.

REFERENCES

1. Austen, D.E.G., Rhymes, I.L.: A Laboratory Manual of Blood Coagulation. Blackwell Scientific Publications Oxford, 1975.
2. Bloom, A.L.: Inherited disorders of blood coagulation. Haemostasis and Thrombosis, edited by A.L. Bloom and D.P. Thomas, Churchill Livingstone, Edinburgh, 1981, p. 321.
3. Bowie, E.J.W., Owen, C.A.: The significance of abnormal preoperative hemostatic tests. Progress in Hemostasis and Thrombosis, volume 5, edited by T.H. Spaet, Grune & Stratton, New York, 1980, p. 179.
4. Brozović, M.: Acquired disorders of haemostasis. Haemostasis and Thrombosis, edited by A.L. Bloom and D.P. Thomas, Churchill Livingstone, Edinburgh, 1981, p. 411.
5. Forbes, C.D.: Thrombosis and artificial surfaces, ibid, p. 761.
6. Rizza, C.R.: Management of patients with inherited blood coagulation defects, ibid, p. 371.

THE MAGIC OF FRESH WHOLE BLOOD

R.A. Kahn

With the development of plastic blood collection bags that permit several containers to be integrally connected and sterilized as a unit, separating whole blood into its components became possible. The availability of blood components fostered their utilization and the concept of 'component therapy', or transfusion of the specific fraction of the blood which the patient lacks, has become an increasingly important part in today's practice of blood transfusion.

Table I shows the trend in component production within the American Red Cross Blood Services. In 1976 only 45% of the blood collected was centrifuged into packed red blood cells (PRBC). In each successive year, however, the proportion has increased, and in 1980 nearly three-quarters of the blood collected was destined for component production.

TABLE I. American National Red Cross whole blood and component production (units in thousands)

	1976	1977	1978	1979	1980
Whole blood	2568	2365	2011	1624	1454
Red blood cells	2123(45%)	2581(52%)	3044(60%)	3591(69%)	3981(73%)
Platelets	903	1101	1256	1419	1564
FFP	812	1106	1321	1518	1719
Cryo	293	254	244	241	254

* Data derived from the Operations Report of the American National Red Cross. Fiscal year 1980/1981.

What does component therapy mean to patients? First, and foremost, it means that more patients can be treated with the blood collected from one donor. Improving the efficiency with which this valuable resource is used is essential if the transfusion needs of all patients are to be adequately met.

Second, the transfusion of components rather than whole blood insures that patients receive precisely what is needed, and at its optimal dosage and functional capability. To fully appreciate the value of components it is worthwhile at this point to briefly discuss the course of events from the time a unit of blood is collected to the time it can be released for transfusion.

In the United States the majority of blood is collected at sites away from the processing center. Usually only a few hours elapse from collection to the time when the unit reaches the Center, so that component production can be initiated in a relatively short period of time. Regardless of whether the blood is destined to be made into components, processing the unit takes a long time. The donor's name must be checked against a deferral list to insure that there is no record of previous involvement in a case of viral hepatitis; it must be ABO and Rh typed; the plasma tested for unusual antibodies; and a test for syphilis performed. Most time consuming is the test for hepatitis B surface antigen - an assay that takes at least five hours. After all tests are completed the data must be collated and the unit properly labelled. It should be obvious that all of this activity takes an inordinate amount of time; at our Center, blood is available for issue approximately 15-20 hours after collection.

During the processing time, if the unit is kept as whole blood, many of the components are adversely affected. Within 10 hours of collection the concentration of many of the clotting factors in plasma, particularly Factor VIII, have declined significantly (7,13). Platelet function also is impaired, since the chilling of blood to maintain red cell viability has an adverse effect on platelets if the unit should be rewarmed (8). Granulocyte function is also compromised; investigations have shown that harvesting leukocytes from whole blood that has been stored for only a short time adversely affects their function (9, 12). Thus, keeping the unit as whole blood is detrimental to all components with the exception of red cells. The remedy for this problem is to harvest each component in a timely fashion and in a manner that will maintain their functional capability. To this end, platelet concentrates are prepared within four hours of collection by centrifugation of whole blood at room temperature (5,14). Concentrates prepared in this manner can be stored for up to three days at ambient temperature (14,2,11) with far less deterioration than would be seen if these cells were kept as part of whole blood.

Plasma, also harvested by differential centrifugation, is frozen solid within six hours of collection and can be kept in this state (-20°C or colder) for up to 12 months, preserving all of the coagulation factors as well as the albumin fraction. Fresh frozen plasma can also be fractionated to make a concentrated, lyophilized, Factor VIII preparation or be used for the production of cryoprecipitate. Alternatively, newer methods are now available to directly prepare purified Factor VIII from fresh frozen plasma without going through complex fractionation techniques (1,15).

In summary, preparing components from whole blood insures that each will be as functional as possible, given the time constraint of processing. If, however, processing could be shortened to only a couple of hours, would fresh whole blood then be the product of choice?

The answer to that question is that the use of components is still, in nearly all situations, better therapy. Let us examine the indications for each blood component in relation to whether it could be properly transfused as part of fresh whole blood or by itself.

RED CELL TRANSFUSION

It must be kept in mind that the only reason for transfusing red cells is to increase the oxygen carrying capacity of the blood. If necessary, a restoration of blood volume can simultaneously be accompanied by the transfusion of red cells. In assessing the need for replacement of red cells, several clinical factors are involved and should be considered. These are (1) the extent of red cell loss; (2) the rate of loss, acute or chronic; (3) the oxygen requirements of the patient; (4) the response of the circulation, especially the cardiac output; (5) the state of tissue perfusion; and (6) the desired rate of restoration, for example, preparation for surgery or recovery of acutely lost volume.

Few patients really need a whole blood transfusion. Those that do are primarily patients who have acute massive blood loss in which there is no time to prepare or obtain the component needed. More importantly, whole blood is indicated for patients who need both increased oxygen carrying capacity and restoration of blood volume. Even if 'fresh' whole blood were available there is no difference between this product and PRBC as far as red cell viability and function is concerned (10), but as shown in table II there are many undesirable features of whole blood. For example, it contains higher concentrations of unneeded electrolytes, citrate, as well as potential allergens. Also, the potential for volume overload in the elderly or debilitated patient is greater using whole blood than PRBC; on a pure volume basis, PRBC will raise the hematocrit to a higher level than will a unit of whole blood. PRBC are the product of choice for the patient with severe anemia who does not require restoration of blood volume. However, the addition of crystalloid (normal saline) can be used to increase the volume transfused as well as improve the transfusion flow rate. Because most of the plasma is removed, PRBC will lessen the incidence of allergic and febrile transfusion reactions. The fact that all red cell products must have 70% survival, 24 hours after transfusion, insures that regardless of the age of the product, a good response will be achieved.

TABLE II. Composition of whole blood and packed red cells (PRBC)

Composition	Whole blood	PRBC
Volume	521 ml	250 ml
Red cell mass	200 ml	200 ml
Hemoglobin	30 g	30 g
Plasma volume	225 ml	75 ml
Albumin	12.5 g	2 g
Citrate	67 ml	22 ml
Plasma sodium	45 mEq	15 mEq
Plasma potassium	15 mEq	4 mEq
Protein antigens and antibodies	Maximal	Minimal

PLATELETS

Platelet therapy is related to the level of thrombocytopenia and the underlying disease process. There is little risk of spontaneous hemorrhage in individuals with platelet counts above 30,000/μl, in the absence of trauma or surgery. For most surgical procedures a count of at least 100,000/μl is usually necessary. Since one unit of platelets (as a concentrate or in 'fresh' whole blood) will raise the patients platelet count by only 7-10,000/μl (6), thrombocytopenic patients require multiple unit transfusions. Administration of 5 or 10 units of whole blood would obviously be an inefficient way to provide platelets; 10 units of platelet concentrate are contained in a volume of 500 milliliters, 10 units of whole blood is nearly 5000 milliliters.

GRANULOCYTE TRANSFUSION

Granulocytes are indicated for patients who have a circulating granulocyte count below 500/μl, who have evidence of infection, and who have not responded to antibiotic therapy. Granulocytes have been of proven benefit only in the treatment of Gram-negative infections (3,4).

Although the most effective dose of transfused granulocytes has not been established, clinical improvements in infected patients have been demonstrated when the number of granulocytes transfused per day was greater than 8×10^9 (3,4). Transfusion of whole blood, or even the extraction of granulocytes from whole blood to achieve this dosage, has been proven very inefficient and cumbersome (whole blood contains approximately 2.5×10^9 granulocytes). Thus, only by a leukapheresis technique, in which donor blood is processed for large quantities of granulocytes, can a sufficient number of these cells be obtained.

FRESH FROZEN PLASMA

This product contains all of the coagulation factors and the albumin fraction of plasma. It is used mainly in the replacement of fluid volume in emergency situations and to replace deficient coagulation factors not available in purified form. Its use as a volume expander has been replaced by other substances such as dextran, hydroxyethyl starch and albumin. The major advantage of these fluids is that they do not carry the risk of hepatitis. In addition, albumin can be obtained bottled in a 25% concentration; far greater than its concentration in plasma (i.e. 3-5%).

FFP is rich in clotting factors V, VIII and XI. In patients with undefined hereditary deficiencies of clotting factors, FFP may be useful to control bleeding until a definite diagnosis is made. Since FFP is the only available source of Factor V, this product is indicated in the treatment of this rare disorder. On the other hand, there is little indication for FFP in the treatment of hemophilia A or B, since much more concentrated preparations of Factor VIII or prothrombin complex are available.

It must be remembered that FFP carries a far higher risk of transfusion reactions than most other volume expanders or fluid replacements, since it contains all the antigens and antibodies of plasma. It also contains approximately 25 mEq of citric acid which can result in hypocalcemia if many units are transfused.

FRESH WHOLE BLOOD

The preceding discussion has focused on the virtues of blood components and moreover, the fallacy of using 'fresh' whole blood (were it available) instead of components. There are, however, some indications for the use of fresh blood. In patients with acute massive blood loss when there is no time to prepare or obtain components, when both oxygen and increased volume are needed, and when the labile clotting factors may be helpful - fresh whole blood is warranted.

Also, neonatal blood exchange is a clear indication for the use of fresh whole blood as the most efficient replacement medium. Whereas an adult may be able to accomodate the by-products that are produced when blood is stored, neonates cannot. The immature neonatal liver and kidney can be overwhelmed by transfusing the metabolites that accumulate in units that are less than fresh. Rapid infusion of high concentrations of potassium, ammonia, and acid may produce severe physiologic decompensation. Transfusing components in neonatal exchange would be inefficient because the small volume of blood to be given would result in considerable waste, thereby defeating the economy of component production.

Both of the conditions outlined above, occur infrequently, and thus the use of fresh blood is for all practical purposes unwarranted. This product can do no more, nor does it contain any more, than the properly prepared blood component. *There is no magic in fresh whole blood.*

REFERENCES

1. Das, P.C., Smit Sibinga, C.Th.: Thaw siphon technique for Factor VIII cryoprecipitate. Lancet 2:273, 1978.
2. Filip, D.H., Aster, R.H.: Relative hemostatic effectiveness of human platelets stored at 4° and 22°C. J. Lab. Clin. Med. 91:618, 1978.
3. Granulocyte transfusions - an established or still an experimental therapeutic procedure. An International Forum. Vox. Sang. 38:40, 1980.
4. Higby, D.J., Burnett, D.: Granulocyte transfusions: current status Blood 55:2, 1980.
5. Kahn, R.A., Cossette, I., Friedman, L.I.: Optimum centrifugation conditions for the preparation of platelet and plasma products. Transfusion 16:162, 1976.
6. Kahn, R.A., Meryman, H.T.: Storage of platelet concentrates. Transfusion 16:13, 1976.
7. Kasper, C.K., Myhre, B.A., McDonald, J.D., Nakasako, Y., Feinstein, D.I.: Determinants of factor VIII recovery in cryoprecipitate. Transfusion 15:312, 1975.
8. Kattlove, H.E., Alexander, B., White, F.: The effect of cold on platelets. II. Platelet function after short-term storage at cold temperatures. Blood 40:688, 1972.
9. Lane, T.A., Windle, B.: Granulocyte concentrate function during preservation: effect of temperature. Blood 54:216, 1979.
10. Mollison, P.L.: Blood Transfusion in Clinical Medicine. 6th Edition. Blackwell, London, 1979, p. 66.
11. Murphy, S., Sayar, S.N., Gardner, F.H.: Storage of platelet concentrates at 22°C. Blood 35:549, 1970.
12. Price, T.H., Dale, D.C.: Neutrophil transfusion: effect of storage and of collection method on neutrophil blood kinetics. Blood 51: 789, 1978.
13. Slichter, S.J., Counts, R.B., Henderson, R., Harker, L.A.: Preparation of cryoprecipitated factor VIII concentrates. Transfusion 16:616, 1976.
14. Slichter, S.J., Harker, L.A.: Preparation and storage of platelet concentrates. I. Factors influencing the harvest of viable platelets from whole blood. Brit. J. Haemat. 34:395, 1976.
15. Smit Sibinga, C.Th., Welbergen, H., Das, P.C., Griffin, B.: High-yield method of production of freeze-dried purified factor VIII by blood banks. Lancet 2:449, 1981.

BLOOD COMPONENTS: WHY AND WHAT FOR?

W.G. Van Aken

INTRODUCTION

Blood is a complex mixture of cellular elements, plasma
proteins, electrolytes and water, each with a different
and important function. Disturbances in any of these functions may, at least in theory, be corrected by the transfusion of whole blood. Clinical experience has shown however that the relevant component in the blood donation is
often present at a concentration too low to be effective.
Increasing the volume of transfused blood, in an attempt
to overcome this problem, is frequently accompanied by the
danger of circulatory overload and other side effects. The
development of techniques and equipment for the isolation,
concentration and preservation of specific blood components
has opened the possibility to individualize blood transfusion practice so that only the blood component which is
lacking, can be administered.

The advantages of blood component therapy over the
transfusion of whole blood are numerous:

1. The components can be concentrated to the extent
that with a restricted transfusion volume, the blood level meets the therapeutic purpose.

2. The risk of immunologic transfusion reactions decreases when plasma components instead of whole blood are used.

3. The preservation of labile proteins e.g. coagulation
factors, can be improved by freeze-drying.

4. The danger for transmitting infectious diseases, notably posttransfusion hepatitis, is lower at least in immunoglobulin and albumin preparations.

5. Aggregates of platelets and leukocytes which are
formed during the storage of blood and which may give rise
to respiratory problems, can be removed prior to transfusion.

6. Since most patients usually require replacement of
only one specific component, remaining parts of the donor
blood can be used to treat other patients thus affording
the maximum use of donated blood.

7. Logistic problems of blood banks and blood transfusion centers are less frequent since the introduction of
blood component therapy.

8. Safety control of blood products is often easier to

perform on components rather than on whole blood.

The safe and effective application of blood and blood components requires first of all knowledge of the pathophysiology of the condition being treated. In addition information about the storage stability and in vivo survival of blood components, the function of these components and an understanding of the hydrodynamic aspects of the circulation are required.

In general, the clinical conditions in which transfusion of blood or its components is required, can be grouped in one of the following types:

a. the need to restore and maintain circulating blood volume e.g. in patients with hemorrhagic and traumatic shock; transfusion of cellular and plasma components can be started without delay and if necessary 'bridge' the period required to collect fresh whole blood

b. the need to supply some specific cellular or protein component which is deficient in the patient; it goes without saying that this is the area 'par excellence' for blood component therapy

c. special situations such as exchange transfusion to remove toxic materials from the blood, and extracorporeal circuits used for open heart surgery; again blood components can be used in most of these circumstances.

In this brief survey a selected number of blood components, used in the management of bleeding disorders, will be discussed in terms of indications, safety and quality control.

PLATELET TRANSFUSION

Normal platelets are required for adequate hemostasis. Platelet transfusions are given to prevent or stop bleeding in the presence of thrombocytopenia or thrombocytopathy. Usually no bleeding problem will be anticipated until the circulating level falls below 30,000 per mm^3 provided that platelet function is not disturbed and humoral blood coagulation remains intact.

Platelet transfusion is indicated in all patients with overt bleeding due to thrombocytopenia (platelet count less than 50,000 per mm^3). There is one exception to this rule; in patients with diffuse intravascular coagulation, transfusion of platelet concentrates apart from being ineffective, may even potentiate the in vivo thrombin and fibrin formation. Once heparin therapy is instituted to stop further fibrin deposition in these patients, it may be advisable to administer platelet concentrates in cases of severe thrombocytopenia.

When thrombocytopenia is caused by impaired bone marrow production (e.g. aplasia and leukemia) or antibody mediated destruction, the concomitant institution of corticosteroid therapy may help to restore hemostasis and decrease the requirement for platelet transfusion.

It should also be stressed that in patients with thrombocytopenia caused by posttransfusion purpura and in case of neonatal thrombocytopenia, only compatible platelets should be transfused.

Conditions in which bleeding is caused by platelet function defects (bleeding time more than 15 minutes) are also candidate for platelet transfusion. However, in those patients in which functional platelet defects are secondary to uremia, paraproteinemia or drug treatment, the effect of platelet transfusion is at best only transient. Treatment of the underlying disease, if possible, or discontinuation of drug therapy, will largely determine the longterm result of treatment. Similarly, platelet transfusion is of limited value in conditions with increased peripheral destruction of platelets and a normal or increased bone marrow production, such as hypersplenism.

In patients undergoing surgery, platelet transfusion appears indicated when platelet count has dropped to less than 50,000 per mm^3 (in the absence of functional platelet defects) or when thrombocytopathy (bleeding time more than 15 minutes) is present. Disturbed hemostasis during surgical procedures or in severely traumatized patients may be caused by thrombocytopenia. In such circumstances it rather often occurs that massive transfusion has been given before thrombocytopenia is detected. Platelet transfusion may help to restore hemostasis but it should be kept in mind that concomitant coagulation abnormalities may be present which require additional treatment.

Although there is some evidence that prophylactic platelet transfusion reduces the incidence of bleeding and morbidity in patients with severe thrombocytopenia due to impaired bone marrow production (6), the real value of this approach has not been fully elucidated (see contribution by Silvergleid). As a consequence a number of protocols for prophylactic platelet transfusion are currently used. In our hospital patients with platelet counts of less than 10,000 per mm^3 (due to impaired platelet production) are considered candidates for such prophylactic platelet transfusions.

The major complications of platelet transfusion are alloimmunization to donor platelet antigens, transmission of infectious diseases (e.g. cytomegaly), graft vs host reaction and septicemia due to bacterial contamination. Alloimmunization to platelet antigens with the development of clinical resistance is likely to be more frequent and may have serious consequences when platelet transfusions are frequently used. In this respect the quality of platelet suspensions is critically related to the degree of leukocyte contamination. The platelet concentrates used in our hospital contain less than 1 leukocyte per 10,000 platelets, which is about one tenth of the standard used in the USA.

When refractoriness arises it may be possible to select serologically matched donors, based upon HLA-typing. Notably family related blood donors, in which cytapheresis allows the collection of sufficient platelets may be used in this situation. When insufficient platelet recovery after transfusion occurs this may be caused by platelet specific antibodies which can be detected by the platelet suspension immunofluorescence technique (3).

The availability of platelet concentrates has led to a sharp and still continuing increase in the number of platelet transfusions. Although many clinicians would agree that this has facilitated the treatment of certain hemorrhagic complications, it should also be emphasized that there are still many questions to be answered before the efficacy and indications of platelet therapy can be defined.

CRYOPRECIPITATE

The treatment and prevention of bleeding episodes in patients with hemophilia A presented many problems until Pool et al. in 1964 succeeded in developing a technique for the preparation of a factor VIII-concentrate called cryoprecipitate (5). Besides factor VIII, a number of other coagulation factors (notably fibrinogen and factor XIII) and a platelet adhesion factor are present.

The preparation of cryoprecipitate is rather simple, does not require extensive equipment and results in yields of about 400 IU factors VIII per liter plasma depending on the quality of the starting plasma, the anticoagulant and freeze and thawing conditions (16,17).

Cryoprecipitate can be used for the prevention and treatment of almost all bleeding complications in patients with hemophilia A. The only exceptions are patients with an inherited or acquired inhibitor to factor VIII and patients with allergic reactions to the administration of cryoprecipitate. In these cases factor VIII concentrate is indicated.

Despite its attractions cryoprecipitate has also some disadvantages which become notably apparent during home treatment. It must be stored at low temperature, it is rather inconvenient to reconstitute and administer by the patient himself, accurate dosage is impossible because yields are extremely variable and occasionally allergic reactions occur. However, the inconvenience of storage at low temperature can be overcome by freeze-drying.

Cryoprecipitate is also indicated in the treatment of hemorrhage by several other causes. Von Willebrand's disease is an inherited abnormality of the hemostatic process associating a defect in the platelet plug formation and a factor VIII deficiency. In patients with moderate severe disease, administration of cryoprecipitate and DDAVP (des-amino-D-arginine-vasopressine) will increase factor VIII-activity in the circulation. In severe forms of Von Willebrand's disease very high doses of cryoprecipitate may be required to correct the bleeding time (13). However, such correction has not been observed after infusion of factor VIII concentrate.

Factor XIII deficiency, platelet storage pool deficiency and uremia are also candidates for cryoprecipitate (4, 7).

FACTOR VIII CONCENTRATE

Most of the available factor VIII concentrates are produced from (fresh) frozen plasma using cryo-alcohol, polyethylene glycol, amino acid precipitation and combinations of these procedures (12). It should be stressed that the yield of factor VIII in such concentrates is considerably lower than that in cryoprecipitate. In so-called intermediate purity concentrates the factor VIII yield is about 200-300 IU per liter, whereas in high purity preparations the yield drops to less than 150 IU per liter fresh frozen plasma.

Factor VIII concentrates have certain distinct practical advantages when compared to cryoprecipitate. They are usual ly more potent per unit volume than cryoprecipitate and can be dispensed and administered in standard doses with a syringe. Therefore, they are selected with some preference for home treatment and also for the management of bleeding in patients with inhibitors to factor VIII. The latter situation occurs in about 5 to 10% of hemophiliacs after treatment. When it is possible to obtain circulating levels of factor VIII in patients with factor VIII inhibitors, treatment with factor VIII concentrates is the treatment of choice. The major features which determine this response to treatment are the titer of the factor VIII antibody and the immune responsiveness of the patient. With low titer inhibitor in poor immunological responders reliable treatment with increased doses of factor VIII concentrate is feasible (2). However, in brisk immunological responders, factor VIII treatment may result in an anamnestic response; here activated prothrombin complex concentrate appears to be effective in the control of bleeding (11).

The usage of factor VIII concentrates goes not without disadvantages. Besides the low recovery of factor VIII during the preparation of factor VIII concentrate which has a bearing on costs, it should also be mentioned that such concentrates are derived from a larger pool of donated plasma. As a consequence, the risk of post-transfusion hepatitis (both hepatitis B and non-A non-B) is increased. This risk is even considerably larger when plasma from paid donors is used. Blood from paid donors is associated with a four to eight fold higher incidence of both hepatitis B and non-A non-B hepatitis in recipients than blood from volunteers (1).

Similarly plasma products prepared from paid donors or from plasma of unknown origin, possibly collected in countries where viral hepatitis is highly endemic, are asso-

ciated with a high incidence of posttransfusional hepatitis. In Sweden the usage of a commercial factor VIII concentrate caused non A non B hepatitis in 40% of patients
receiving replacement therapy for the first time (10).

PROTHROMBIN COMPLEX CONCENTRATES

Prothrombin complex concentrates containing factors II,
IX, X and VII are obtained by fractionation of pooled
plasma. A distinction has been made between 'regular' (un-
activated) prothrombin complex concentrate, a product in-
tended primarily for use in patients with hemophilia B,
and 'activated' prothrombin complex concentrate, a product
that is processed to contain a higher proportion of activated clotting factors for use in patients with factor
VIII inhibitors.
    'Regular' prothrombin complex concentrate is indicated
in the treatment of patients with factor IX deficiency to
arrest serious bleeding and to prevent operative and post-
operative bleeding. It is also suitable for use in similar
circumstances for congenital deficiencies of factors II,
VII and X. Hemorrhage due to multiple clotting factors deficiency induced by overdosage of coumarin-type drugs can
also be treated with such concentrates. However, the correction of the coagulation defect after prothrombin complex concentrate is only temporarily and administration
of vitamin K is required to permanently normalize factors
II, VII, IX and X.
    Activated clotting factors may be present in some pre-
parations of this concentrate. These are not removed efficiently in patients with liver disease and in neonates.
Because of the risk of thrombin and diffuse intravascular
coagulation, the quality of prothrombin complex is critically related to the potential benefit in such patients.
In addition the risk of hepatitis B virus transmission is
present despite the fact that all plasma used in its preparation has been tested and found negative for hepatitis
B surface antigen.
    Both 'regular' and 'activated' prothrombin complex con-
centrate have been used in the treatment of bleeding in patients with factor VIII inhibitors. The manner in which
they promote hemostasis has not yet been elucidated. Factor Xa, thrombin, factor VIIa and platelet activity have
all been held responsible (8). Recent controlled studies
suggest that regular prothrombin complex concentrates may
be effective in roughly half of the bleeding episodes
treated (9) and the 'activated' concentrates may be more
effective (11).

PRESENT AND FUTURE DEVELOPMENTS

Plasma components that have been purified and currently
are tested for their clinical efficacy include antithrombin III, plasminogen, α_1-antitrypsin and fibronectin. In

addition progress is made to ascertain that side effects can be reduced. The assays of small quantities of endotoxin, vasoactive substances, degradation products, activated coagulation factors and the use of animal models should be included in quality control programs.

Post-transfusion hepatitis remains a considerable hazard notably for multitransfused patients. Attempts to reduce the incidence of such infections can be grouped in three categories. First, the addition of hepatitis B immunoglobulin to a clotting factor concentrate has been shown, at least in experimental studies performed in chimpanzees, to remove the hepatitis B virus infectivity (15). Recent data from our laboratory demonstrate that even at a much lower dosage of specific immunoglobulin than used in the former study, this protective effect is still present (Brummelhuis, personal communication). Secondly, the availability of hepatitis B vaccins permits the immunization of patients and donors against hepatitis B (14).

Lastly, the risk of non A non B hepatitis can be reduced once specific serological tests for non A non B hepatitis are available.

It is also to be expected that the advent of recombinant DNA-technology in the next few years will open new areas for the production of plasma components.

REFERENCES

1. Aach, R.D., Lander, J.J., Sherman, L.A., Miller, W.V., Katess, R.A., Gitmide, G.L., Hollinger, F.B., Werch, J., Szmuness, W., Stevens, C.E., Kellner, A., Weiner, J.M., Mosley, J.W.: Transfusion transmitted viruses: interim analyses of hepatitis among transfused and non-transfused patients. In: Viral Hepatitis, editors A. Vyas et al. Franklin Institute Press, Philadelphia, 1978, p. 383.
2. Bloom, A.L.: Current status and trends in treatment of hemophilic patients with inhibitors. Hemophilia and Hemostasis, editors D. Menaché et al. Alan R. Liss, New York 1981, p. 123.
3. Borne, A.E.G.Kr. Von Dem, Verheugt, F.W.A., Oosterhof, R., Riesz, E. Von, Brutel de la Rivière, A., Engelfriet, C.P.: A simple immunofluorescence test for the detection of platelet antibodies. Brit. J. Haematol. 39:195, 1973.
4. Gerritsen, S.W., Akkerman, J.W.N., Sixma, J.J.: Correction of the bleeding time in patients with storage pool deficiency by infusion of cryoprecipitate. Brit. J. Haematol. 40:153, 1978.
5. Hershgold, E.J., Pool, J.G., Rappenhagen, A.R.: The potent antihemophilic globulin concentrate derived from a cold insoluble fraction of human plasma: characterization and further data on preparation and clinical trial. J. Lab. Clin. Med. 67:23, 1966.
6. Highby, D.J., Cohen, E., Holland, J.F.: The prophylactic treatment of thrombocytopenic leukemic patients with platelets. Transfusion 14:404, 1974.
7. Janson, P.A., Jubelirer, S.J., Weinstein, M.J., Deykin, D.: Treatment of the bleeding tendency in uremia with cryoprecipitate. N.

Engl. J. Med. 303:1318, 1980.

8. Kasper, C.K.: Management of inhibitors to factor VIII. In: Progress in Hematology, editor E.B. Brown. Grune and Stratton, New York, 1981, p. 143.

9. Lusher, J.M., Shapiro, S.S., Pallascak, J.E., Rao, A.V., Levine, P.H., Blatt, Pl. M.: Hemophilia Study Group. Efficacy of prothrombin-complex concentrates in hemophiliacs with antibodies to factor VIII. New Engl. J. Med. 303:421, 1980.

10. Norkrans, G., Widell, A., Teger-Nilsson, C., Kjellman, H., Frösner, G., Iwarson, S.: Acute hepatitis Non-A, Non-B following administration of factor VIII concentrates. Vox Sang. 41:129, 1981.

11. Sjamsjoedin, L.J.M., Heynen, L., Mauser-Bunschoten, E.P., Van Geylswijk, L., Van Houwelingen, H., Van Asten, P., Sixma, J.J.: The effect of activated prothrombin-complex concentrate (FEIBA) on joint and muscle bleeding in patients with hemophilia A and antibodies to factor VIII. New Engl. J. Med. 305:717, 1981.

12. Smith, J.K., Bidwell, E.: Therapeutic materials used in the treatment of coagulation defects. Clin. Haematol. 8:183, 1979.

13. Sultan, Y.: Rationale for the treatment of Von Willebrand disease. Hemophilia and Hemostasis, editors D. Menaché et al. Alan R. Liss, New York, 1981, p. 149.

14. Szmuness, W., Stevens, C.E., Harley, E.J.: Hepatitis B vaccine: demonstration of efficacy in a controlled clinical trial in a high-risk population in the United States. New Engl. J. Med. 303:833, 1980.

15. Tabor, E., Aronson, D.J., Gerety, R.J.: Removal of hepatitis B virus infectivity from factor IX complex by hepatitis-B immune globulin. Lancet 2:68, 1980.

16. Vermeer, C., Soute, V.A.M., Ates, G., Brummelhuis, H.G.J.: Contributions to the optimal use of human blood. VII. Increase of the yield of factor VIII in four-donor cryoprecipitate by an improved processing of blood and plasma. Vox Sang. 30:1, 1976.

17. Vermeer, C., Soute, V.A.M., Ates, G., Hellings, J.A., Brummelhuis, H.G.J.: Contributions to the optimal use of human blood. VIII. Stability of blood coagulation factor VIII during collection and storage of whole blood and plasma. Vox Sang., 31(suppl. 1):55, 1976.

Discussion

Moderator: J.J. van Loghem

P.J.W. De Graaf, Voorburg:

I would like to thank Dr. Britten for his friendly words on
the fact that we succeeded in 'clotting' together as a national society for 10 years now. I would like to thank the
World Federation of Hemophilia for its vital role in the
starting phase and it is still very important for us from
a moral and from a practical point of view.
My question is: In view of the fact that all the different
factors mentioned in your lecture are present in every
country, may be different in magnitude and nature, do you
believe that a national approach should prevail from a logistic point of view, or do you think that some formal international agreement on logistic factors should be part of
the national approach.

A.F.H. Britten, Albany, USA:

I think that there is some confusion about the term 'national selfsufficiency' which is widely used. I feel, and this
is just my opinion, that the important aspect of national
selfsufficiency is that the source material for whatever
product one is considering, should be generated within each
nation or in larger countries, within each region of appropriate size. If we take factor VIII as the prototype for this
discussion, it is the ability to generate the appropriate
amount of fresh frozen plasma.
It is much less important where this plasma is processed.
If you consider a small country like Iceland, it is ridiculous to require selfsufficiency in fractionation in Iceland. On the other hand, if you take a large country like
the Soviet Union, it is ridiculous to consider that as one
entity.

C.A.M. Haanen, Nijmegen:

Dr. Hemker explained very beautifully the loop which exists
in the activation of the intrinsic or the final pathway by
activation of factor VII through tissue thromboplastin. I
still do not understand why people with factor XII or XI, or
plasma kallikrein insufficiency do not bleed and people with
factor IX and VIII deficiency do.

H.C. Hemker, Maastricht:

The most simple way to explain this is, that the essential
operation in our opinion at the moment is the extrinsic
pathway. Factors VIII and IX constitute a reinforcement
loop, something that helps the extrinsic pathway. That is
necessary in those cases where only a small amount of factor VII is activated. The question remains: what is small
amount? Probably everything that is released during trauma
in vivo is considered a small amount in vitro, in a testtube. So to summarize: the extrinsic pathway is the pathway
that is operative, but it does need the reinforcement
brought about by VIII and IX.

R.A. Kahn, St. Louis, USA:

There is another partial answer to that question in a report in 'Blood'[*], in which classical hemophiliacs who were
not taking any drugs and who were not receiving infusion
within the previous 48 hours, had bleeding time measurements
performed.
In fact in almost all of them the bleeding time was indeed
significantly longer than an equivalent controlled population. The last study as I recall was in 1969[**] indicating
that the bleeding time in classical hemophiliacs was normal
related to a control population. With the newer template
procedures to perform the bleeding time test as well as a
little more control on the hemophiliac population itself,
there is clear evidence from this study that indeed bleeding
time is longer in the hemophiliac.

J.G. Jolly, Chandigarh, India:

Dr. Britten has rightly surveyed the factor VIII situation.
I had the opportunity to visit Moscow recently. The USSR
has adopted as a matter of principle the yield of cryoprecipitate rather than factor VIII concentrate.
I would like to have the opinion of dr. Britten as to what
should be the strategy in smaller countries where factor
VIII concentrate production is not a possibility today, but
cryoprecipitate can be prepared by most of the bloodbanks.

A.F.H. Britten, Albany, USA:

This is a question that can be applied to almost every country. The technology involved in the preparation of cryoprecipitate as you know, is much more easily accessible than
the technology of plasma fractionation.
As I mentioned in my talk, the existing facilities for factor VIII fractionation are substantially greater than the

[*] Eyster, M.E. et al., Blood 1981, 58, 719.
[**] Kaneshiro, M.M. et al., New Engl. J. Med. 1969, 281, 1039.

amount of fractionation that can be done, because of the albumin demand. So I would not recommend creating new fractionation facilities without a very earnest and deep study of the situation in question. It is not a difficult thing to translate a bloodtransfusion service into a cryoprecipitate service, so that is by far the quickest way of solving the hemophilia problem on a local basis.

E.H. De Nooij, Utrecht:

In my opinion very often red cell concentrate is transfused with practically all the leucocytes and thrombocytes. Dr. Kahn, I missed from your table about the composition of red cells, what on the average is the number of leucocytes and thrombocytes in your packed cells. That is very important because of all transfusion reactions quite a number is caused by the leucocytes and thrombocytes in the packed cells. Besides, a number of pulmonary problems which occur in intensive care patients after surgery, can be avoided as well by removing the leucocytes and the thrombocytes from the packed cells. Technically that seems to be very difficult. What are your experiences?

R.A. Kahn, St. Louis, USA:

You are absolutely right in a number of points. Indeed, when we prepare packed red blood cells, quite often, if we just harvest the plasma alone, the white cells and platelets are still in the red blood cell concentrate. Fortunately, most blood transfused is given to relatively healthy individuals. The frequency in transfusion reactions is very low. You are right again, in the sense that leucocytes and platelets can pose a problem to debilitated patients, but fortunately the frequency of these kinds of reactions are low as well. What do you do in circumstances like that? You can order of course for the patient who does have a transfusion reaction, products called leucocyte-poor red blood cells, usually obtained through inverted centrifugation or filtration. This seems to clear up the problem considerably. There does not seem to be any new method, to my knowledge, on the horizon to overcome this problem in the situations that it does occur despite transfusion of leucocyte poor red blood cells.

F. Feldman, Kankakee, USA:

I like to comment on one of the tables shown by dr. Van Aken. The table on intralaboratory variation in the factor VIII assay. The variation you showed is incredible and in fact raises questions as to the validity and potential of measuring patient in vivo recovery and half lifes. I would like to say that at Armour, we have been working for the last 2 years to attempt to minimize variation such as you have shown. Currently we can say that we are within 5% differences with laboratories such as Oxford, NIBS and the Bureau of Biologics laboratory in Bethesda. I would further like to say that I completely agree with your statement as how one arrives at that state.

Without assaying a tremendous number of replicate samples, taking special care to insure parallelism between unknown and standards, and calibration of samples and standards in reagents between the laboratories involved it will never be possible to attain better results than what you have shown. Could you comment on the variation that you have shown and the problems that it raises in terms of inter-preting results in the patient in vivo.

W.G. Van Aken, Amsterdam:

In fact I wanted to make very clear that the variation can be very large, if one is not aware of the problems related to this assay.

During the follow-up of this study, when the participating centers tried to come together and finalize the protocol in which a number of these variables were more or less put into place, the range of variation became tremendously small. The interindividual variation is now about 15%.

But still, one should keep control every year because it proves that gradually variables move in again and increase the variation rate.

We have indirect evidence now that the assay we are using correlates very well with in vivo recovery, but we need more experiments in order to make that statement very firm.

C. Orthner, Bethesda, USA:

I wonder if dr. Hemker would comment on recent studies that indicate that factor V-a is the platelet receptor for factor X-a and how this fits into your model?

H.C. Hemker, Maastricht:

I simplified my presentation a little bit. In fact what platelets do are two things. They move out factor V-a with the release reaction and they flip-flop membrane. You can differentiate between these two things by looking at the platelet procoagulant activity in presence of a large amount of factor V-a. It then becomes quite clear that there is still a time-dependent flip-flop process, that also can be demonstrated with direct chemical methods.

What has been called the platelet factor X-a receptor, in our opinion should be replaced in more mechanistic terms. Simultaneously there is a platelet flip-flop and a release of factor V, factor V binds to the available phospholipid and both together create a site to which factor X-a can bind.

B. Gullbring, Stockholm:

I would like to comment on what dr. Britten told us: 'we want to make components but some surgeons still want whole blood'.
One of the difficulties of red cell concentrates is the rather high hematocrit and the viscosity. In our country, at the present time we use quite a lot of blood of which we remove the buffy coat and add a salt-adenine-glucose-manitol (SAG) solution. So we have a red cell storage time of 35 days.
In Sweden 'SAG' solution is used in 20% of bloodtransfusion. In the 'SAG' solution the hematocrit is 55%, which makes it more acceptable for clinicians to use, particularly in surgery. In the solution there is about 1% of protein left after the preparation.
I would like to ask dr. Kahn: Do the clinicians agree to use red cell concentrates, or is part of it out-dated?

R.A. Kahn, St. Louis, USA:

The proportion that outdates is the same for whole blood as it is for red cells. One comment on your 'SAG'-solution. I think that is the answer to salvaging more plasma and keeping the viscosity of the unit low. Probably this saline-adenine-glucose additive will soon be used throughout the United States as well, as soon the companies can get it licenced and marketed.

II. Platelet function and platelet therapy

PLATELET FUNCTION TESTS

J.W. Ten Cate

The following platelet function tests are discussed:
bleeding time, platelet retention tests, platelet aggregation, and radio-immunoassays for platelet release products, such as β thromboglobulin (βTG), and platelet factor 4 (PF4).

As soon as a lesion is produced, platelets adhere almost immediately at the exposed subendothelial collagen
tissue. Adhesion is coincided with an explosive extrusion
of platelet granular contents, as for example serotonin,
ADP and calcium. ADP is a strong challenger of platelet
aggregation as is TXA_2 an intermediate product of prostaglandin metabolism which is produced during adhesion and
release. These compounds induce shape change of platelets,
rendering sticky platelets, followed by aggregation at
the site of the vessel wall lesion. The formed platelet
mass, or hemostatic plug, results in arrest of bleeding.
Figure 1 shows a transection of a normal platelet. The
next figure (Fig. 2) shows the platelets having undergone
the release reaction and have taken part in the formation
of a platelet aggregate.

One of the main tests to evaluate this process is the
bleeding time test, as long as it is well performed. The
bleeding time measures the time it takes for the arrest
of bleeding upon infliction of a standard wound at the
volar site of the under arm. A sphygmomanometer cuff
around the upper arm is inflated to a constant pressure
of + 40 mm mercury. Two techniques are reliable, the
original of Ivy with a standard puncture wound of 3 mm
deep, producing normal values of 4 min and the Mielke (10)
technique with standardized incision of 9 mm long and 1
mm deep. The bleeding time is prolonged (Table I) in congenital and acquired platelet disorders, Von Willebrand's
disease and what should also be kept in mind at low hematocrit. Congenital platelet disorders like Glanzmann's disease and Bernard-Soulier Syndrome are extremely rare, storage pool disease is less rare, however, still an infre-
quent finding in specialized laboratories. In this disease
is lacking the contents of the platelet granules, like
ADP and serotonin.

Of much more relevance are the acquired platelet defects, like in chronic uremia, liver cirrhosis, in Gram-

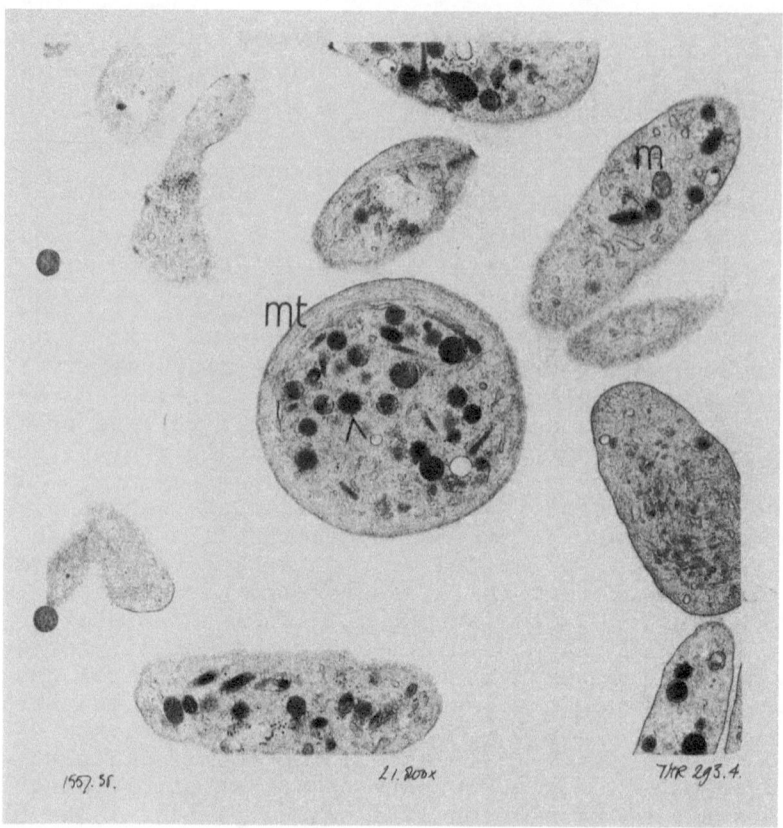

Fig. 1. Transmission electron microscopy of human blood platelets.
Magnification 21,800. Reduced for reproduction 69%.
mt = microtubular system. M = mitochondria. ∧ = platelet granules.

negative septicemia, and in hematological disorders such
as leukemia, paraproteinemia, and myeloproliferative disorders. The most frequently encountered acquired platelet
defect is induced by drugs, such as aspirin. Under all
these circumstances the bleeding time may be more or less
prolonged and bleeding may occur. It is of interest to
note that the prolonged bleeding time can be corrected by
the infusion of cryoprecipitate, red cells and platelets
(Table II).

Platelets adhere and aggregate at the site of the glass
surface in a similar fashion as at collagen tissue. Several
platelet tests involving the measurement of retention of
platelets in glass bead filters have been designed, two
test systems those of Hellem (7) using native blood and
the one of Bowie (2) using heparinized blood are still in
use. After passage of blood through these filters less
platelets are retained in Von Willebrand's disease, Factor

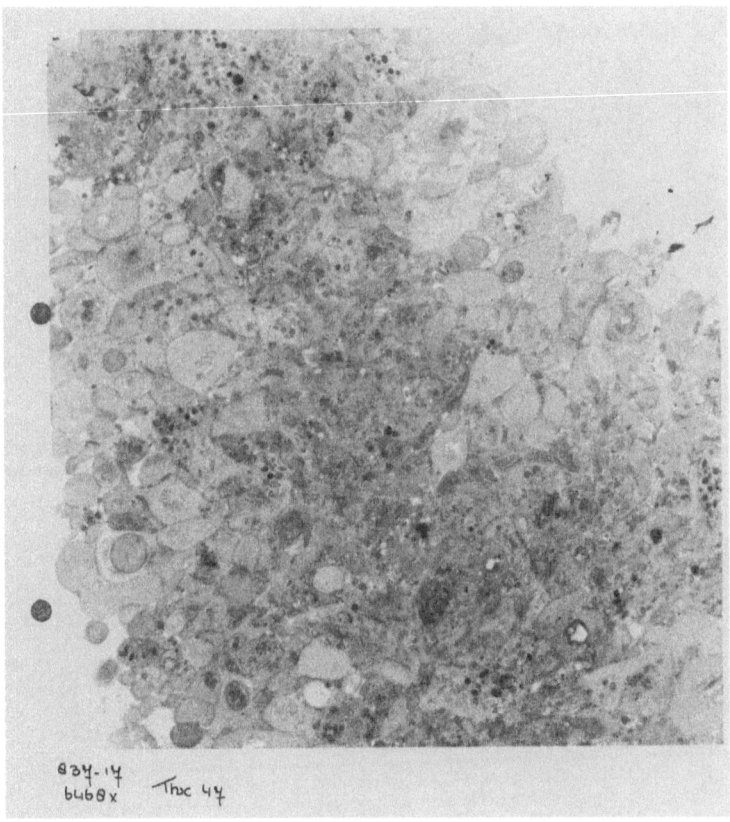

Fig. 2. Transmission electron microscopy of a platelet aggregate.

TABLE I. Prolonged bleeding time in:

- congenital platelet disorders
- acquired platelet disorders
- Von Willebrand's disease
- Low hematocrit

TABLE II. Correction of prolonged bleeding time

IN:	BY:
Aspirin induced platelet defect	cryoprecipitate
Hermansky-Pudlak Syndrome	cryoprecipitate
Uremic platelet defect	cryoprecipitate
Von Willebrand's disease	cryoprecipitate
Low hematocrit	packed cells
All other platelet disorders	platelet suspensions

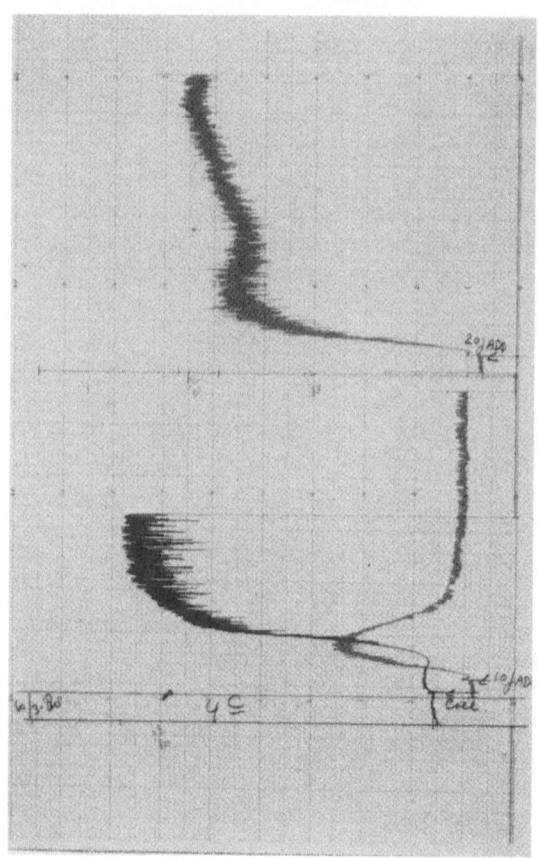

Fig. 3. ADP and collagen-induced aggregation.

XII deficiency, severe platelet disorders and low hematocrit. This test is therefore of similar clinical relevance
as the bleeding time test, although isolated retention abnormalities, with a normal bleeding time and a mild bleeding tendency may occur.

The next platelet test to discuss is the platelet aggregation test developed by Born in 1962 (1). When citrated blood is slowly centrifuged, the supernatant plasma is
enriched in platelets: platelet-rich plasma of PRP. This
plasma is continuously stirred in a spectrophotometer cuvette at 37°C. Addition of aggregating agents such as ADP
results in visible aggregate formation and a decrease of
the optical density. Depending upon the concentration added, three different patterns may be observed (Fig. 3).
Low concentrations induce a small and reversible response.
Increasing the dosage results in immediate aggregation followed by a second wave of aggregation which is induced by
the substances released during the first wave of aggregation. This process is irreversible and is associated with
degranulation of the platelets. Decreased aggregation res-

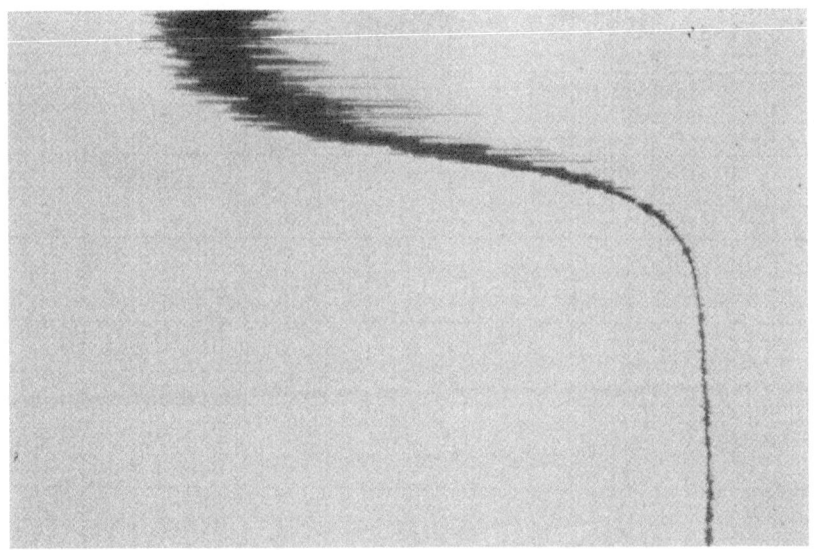

Fig. 4. Spontaneous platelet aggregation.

ponse towards ADP and collagen occurs in many acquired
platelet disorders. Reversible responses are occurring in
storage pool disease and in the 'aspirin-like' platelet
defect, because during the aggregation induced by any
agent no release occurs and therefore the second wave of
aggregation is lacking.

Another peculiar phenomenon is the so-called spontaneous platelet aggregation (Fig. 4). This aggregation is
induced just upon stirring. It was first described in a
patient with thrombocythemia having attacks of painful
fingers and toes (13). Aspirin abolished not only spontaneous aggregation but also the painful attacks. Interruption of aspirin treatment resulted in the recurrence of
the attacks and of spontaneous aggregation. Treatment of
these patients with aspirin has shown to offer protection
against recurrent thrombo-embolic disorders. Thereafter
SPA has shown to occur in cerebrovascular disorders (5,6,
8,14) (40%), carcinoma (12) (40%), diabetes (11) (40%) and
also in healthy normals, however to a much lower extent
(5%). This phenomenon has, however, only clinical relevance
in thrombocythemia and in the 'Hammerstein Syndrome'.
This syndrome occurred in a lady with severe arterial lesions (5) (Fig. 5 and 6). Note the severe stenotic lesions
in the carotid and brachial arteries. She had transient
ischemic attacks and microinfarctions in the nail bed
(Fig. 7) and spontaneous aggregation. Aspirin treatment
abolished the TIA, infarctions and SPA. Withdrawal of ASA
resulted in prompt recurrence of these phenomena. She is
now 6 years under treatment without further symptoms of
her severe arterial disease.

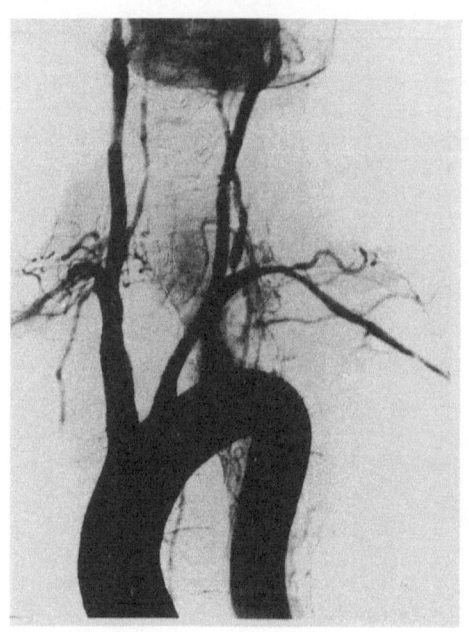 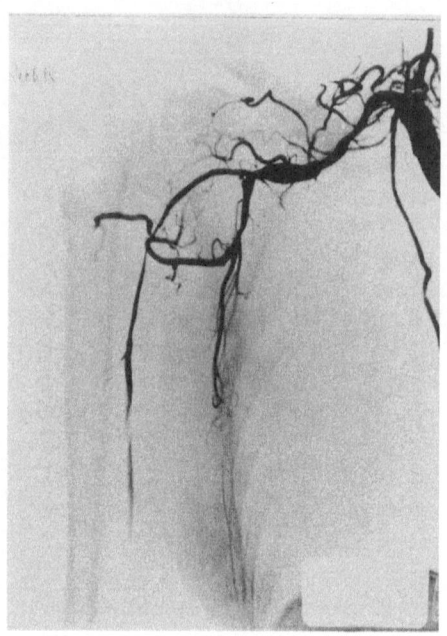

Fig. 5. Angiography of the aortic arch. <u>Note</u>: the multiple stenotic lesions of the carotid and subclavian arteries.

Fig. 6. <u>Note</u>: the severe and multiple stenotic lesions of subclavian and brachial artery.

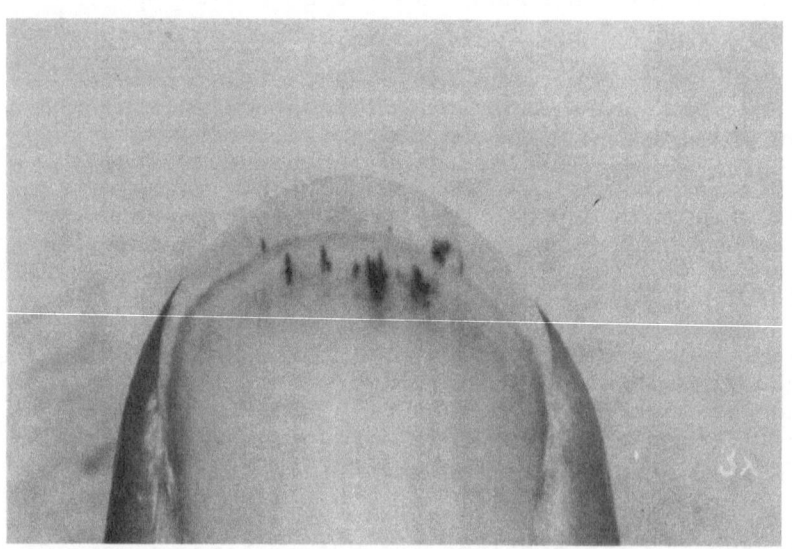

Fig. 7. Microinfarctions in the nailbed of the thumb.

The last tests to discuss are the radio-immunoassays for βTG and PF-4. Both proteins are released during platelet adhesion and aggregation. Increased plasma levels of βTG are encountered in arterial and venous thrombosis. There is still much controversy regarding the clinical value of these tests, however, I am convinced that they may find application in studies on the effects of anti-aggregating drugs, such as aspirin. For example in this family (Table III), two members had complications of arterial thrombosis at a relatively early age. All three had increased levels of plasma βTG. The 26 year old girl suffered from the Wallenberg syndrome after a cerebrovascular accident. She had a normal angiography. The βTG was 140 μg/ml. Treatment with low dose aspirin resulted in complete correction of the high βTG levels (Table IV). A higher dose of aspirin was as ineffective as placebo (blind cross-over study).

TABLE III. Family S, 5 members investigated

3 had increased βTG levels with respectively:
1 cerebrovascular incident (age 26)
1 myocardial infarction (age 39)
1 asymptomatic

TABLE IV. M.S. Wallenberg Syndrome

Treatment (1 week)	
No	: 140 μg/ml
Placebo	: 135 μg/ml
500 mg ASA	: 120 μg/ml
80 mg ASA	: 17 μg/ml

My conclusion is that at this aspirin dose the continuous in vivo platelet-platelet and possible platelet-vessel wall interaction is effectively blocked. More studies of this kind will reveal the future potency of these test systems.

REFERENCES

1. Born, G.V.R.: Quantitative investigation into the aggregation of blood platelets. J. Phys. 62:67, 1962.
2. Bowie, E.J.W., Owen Jr, C.A., Thompson, J.H., Didisheim, P.: Platelet adhesiveness in Von Willebrand's disease. Am. J. Clin. Path. 52:69, 1969.
3. Ten Cate, J.W.: Platelet function tests. Clinics in Haematology 1:283, 1972.
4. Ten Cate, J.W., De Vries, S.E., Sixma, J.J., Van Berkel, W.: Reproducibility and normal values of various platelet function tests.

Folia Med. Neerl. 15:10, 1972.

5. Ten Cate, J.W., Vos, J., Prenger, D., Jenkins, C.S.P.: Spontaneous platelet aggregation in cerebrovascular diseases. Thromb.
   Haem. 39:223, 1978.

6. Ten Cate, J.W., Jenkins, C.S.P.: The investigation of platelet
   functions. In: Blood Coagulation and Haemostasis, Ed. J. Thompson,
   1979.

7. Hellem, A.J.: The adhesiveness of human blood platelets in vitro.
   Scan. J. Clin. Lab. Invest., 12:suppl. 51, 1960.

8. Hoogendijk, E.M.G.: Platelets in cerebrovascular disease: a study
   on platelet functions and on inhibition of platelet functions.
   Thesis, University of Amsterdam, 1980.

9. Ludlam, C.A., Bolton, A.E., Moore, S., Cash, J.D.: New rapid method for diagnosis of deep vein thrombosis. Lancet ii:259, 1975.

10. Mielke Jr, Kaneshiro, M.M., Naher, I.A., Weiner, J.M., Rapaport,
    S.I.: The standard normal Ivy bleeding time and its prolongation
    by aspirin. Blood 34:204, 1969.

11. Porter, N.R., Preston, F.E.: Platelet abnormalities in diabetic
    peripheral neuropathy. Lancet ii:1274, 1975.

12. Peuscher, F.W.: The significance of fibrinopeptide A in patients
    with cancer and venous thrombo-embolism. Thesis, University of
    Amsterdam, 1980.

13. Vreeken, J., Van Aken, W.G.: Spontaneous platelet aggregation of
    blood platelets as a cause of idiopathic thrombosis and recurrent
    painful toes and fingers. Lancet ii:1394, 1971.

14. Wu, K.K., Hoak, J.C.: Spontaneous platelet aggregation in arterial
    insufficiency: Mechanisms and implications. Thromb. Haem. 35:702,
    1976.

BETA-THROMBOGLOBULIN: A STORY OF VALUE?

B.L. Cobert, C.Th. Smit Sibinga and P.C. Das

INTRODUCTION

Beta-thromboglobulin (BTG), since its isolation and characterization in 1975, has stirred much interest because of
its intimate association with the platelet release reaction
and because of the increasingly recognized role platelets
play in various disease states.

THE PLATELET RELEASE REACTION

Platelets contain three different types of storage granules: dense bodies, alpha granules and lysozymol enzyme
granules. Platelets may be stimulated to adhere to various
substances or to themselves by four groups of inducers.
The first includes low molecular weight compounds such as
epinephrine, vasopressin and ADP. The second includes larger substances such as collagen, immune complexes and viruses among others; the third group includes compounds
such as trypsin, thrombin and plasmin. The fourth includes
physical factors such as ultrasound.
   Of the three granules involved, the one that concerns
us here is the alpha granule which contains fibrinogen,
platelet factor 4, potassium, BTG and several other factors
(19,22).

BETA THROMBOGLOBULIN

Beta-thromboglobulin, BTG, is a protein composed of four
subunits each with 8 amino acids and a total molecular
weight of about 35,000 (5,30). It is related to platelet
factor 4. The two proteins have similar amino acid structures and antigenic components. Excision of the terminal
four amino acids in the NH_2 terminal of platelet factor 4
produces a new NH_2 terminal which is identical to the NH_2
terminal of BTG. It has been suggested that BTG is derived
from platelet factor 4 by proteolytic action (23,34).

BTG IN NORMALS

Several groups have studied BTG levels in normals. Normal
values have been found in plasma to range from 3 to 185

ng/ml, though most values fall between 10 and 65 ng/ml (24)
The mean values found are consistently around 20 to 35 ng/
ml (10,24,47). Values are slightly higher in women and older people but usually not significantly so (24,46). However, not all studies have been controlled for these variables. Healthy pregnant women in the 3rd trimester have
been found to have normal BTG levels.

BTG is found in urine at levels of one two-hundredth
of those in plasma. The half-life in plasma is about 100
minutes at 37°C (10). Excretion appears to be predominantly renal (8). BTG is found almost exclusively in platelets.
Concentrations found in other organs (Table I) are from 30
to 30,000 times less (24). BTG appears in synovial and amniotic fluid in the same concentrations as in plasma. Since
these fluids normally contain no platelets, the plasma concentration is probably in a steady state with these body
fluids. Hence elevations in plasma BTG are felt to reflect
only on the BTG released by platelets (10).

TABLE I. BTG content in various human tissues

Organ	Patient 1	Patient 2
	(ng BTG/g wet weight)	
Psoas muscle	74	4.0
Left ventricle	37	9.0
Liver	1,430	40.0
Spleen	33,900	92.0
Kidney	2,500	5.6
Lung	680	30.4
Ileum	3,600	4.2

Platelets 1,240,000
(Ludlam, C: Brit. J. Haematol, 41:271, 1979)

Interestingly, no specific biologic action for BTG has
yet been found. It may function as a packing substance or
filler in the alpha granule (5).

A radioimmunoassay has been developed and commercially
marketed for BTG. It is relatively easy to perform but
does require clean venous blood drawing through a large
bore needle into a plastic syringe containing EDTA, theophylline and prostaglandin E_1. Attention must also be given to rates of centrifugation and proper temperature control (2,40).

BTG IN PERIPHERAL ARTERIAL DISEASE AND CEREBROVASCULAR
DISEASE

Plasma BTG has been found to be significantly elevated in
patients with peripheral artery disease though overlap between the patients and controls was large. The magnitude

of elevation of the BTG was directly correlated with severity of the disease (46,48).

In cerebrovascular disease, one report indicated that in acute cerebrovascular disease and transient ischemic attacks plasma BTG was elevated (27). In patients with remote cerebrovascular disease of at least three to six months, the BTG levels were the same as controls (8).

BTG, HEART DISEASE AND CARDIAC VALVE PROSTHESES

BTG has been shown to be elevated in patients with acute myocardial infarction although overlap with controls is high (11,27,35). In another study of patients at least three months after myocardial infarction, BTG was noted to be about twice normal. Unfortunately the patients are not described nor are their treatment or concomitant diseases (31).

Patients who have received cardiac prostheses had increased BTG levels regardless of whether or not these patients had porcine, disc or double valve replacement or whether they received warfarin therapy (9,25).

BTG, DIABETES MELLITUS AND HYPERLIPIDEMIA

BTG has been found to be elevated in diabetes. Because of problems with controls and assay techniques the results must be interpreted cautiously but data suggest that diabetics with retinopathy have greater BTG levels than those without this complication. Patients adequately treated with diet, insulin or hypoglycemic agents do not have lower or normal BTG values. Hemoglobin AIC levels do not correlate with BTG levels either (28).

In the hyperlipidemias BTG has been found to be elevated particularly in type IIa hyperlipoproteinemia (45). This raises the possibility that the platelet release reaction may play a role in hyperlipidemias.

BTG AND VENOUS DISEASE

Acute deep vein thrombosis seems to be associated with elevated BTG levels (29). Treatment (35) and/or remote or chronic venous disease are not associated with elevated levels (8,35).

BTG AND RENAL DISEASE

Plasma BTG is elevated in glomerulonephritis (37). Plasma BTG rises as the glomerular filtration rate falls (12,15). In one interesting study of renal failure patients with elevated BTG before dialysis, the BTG level was shown to rise after hemodialysis with the Travenol cuprophane dialyser but not after dialysis with the Cordis-Dow regenerated cellulose machine. Hence the choice of the dialysis filter seems to influence platelet interactions (1). Peritoneal dialysis does not elevate BTG levels (32).

BTG AND OTHER DISEASES

Elevated BTG levels have been found in a variety of other
diseases including pre-eclampsia (41), myeloproliferative
disorders and secondary thrombocytosis (7), sickle cell
disease (29) and disseminated intravascular coagulation
(16,27).

In one report, a diverse group of patients with malignant disease had elevated BTG levels which decreased
(though never totally back to normal) after chemotherapy.
This BTG fall occurred after the first chemotherapy session when the platelet count remained normal and again
decreased after the second chemotherapy treatment in which
the platelet count fell (6). BTG has been found to be elevated in Raynaud's phenomenon. Levels fell after plasma
exchange and remained low for several months after cessation of therapy. Low BTG levels were associated with improvement of symptoms (36,42,48).

From these studies several points are raised. First,
methodological problems involved in blood drawing can be
important especially involving inclusion of prostaglandin
E_1, EDTA and theophylline for anticoagulation. Second, the
controls are critical. Sex, age, presence of coronary artery disease, hyperlipidemias and other yet unknown factors may play a significant role in BTG evaluations. Any
study should attempt to account for and control these factors. Third, although there is evidence that BTG is a useful marker of the platelet activation and release reaction,
it is not clear whether platelet involvement in any of
these disease states is a cause or an effect. That is,
platelets may play an active role in the etiology and pathogenesis of the disease or may be the result of an on-
going disease process. Nevertheless, we felt that it might
be useful to use the BTG levels as an in-vitro indication
of the platelet reaction in stored platelets.

USE OF BTG IN QUALITY CONTROL OF PLATELETS

In work done at the Red Cross Blood Bank Groningen-Drenthe
several studies were undertaken to evaluate platelet concentrates.

Platelet rich concentrates are prepared in the usual
manner (3,14) and are used for transfusion in the University Hospital and other hospitals in this region of the
Netherlands. These platelet concentrates are prepared
from the platelets of 4 to 6 donors. The platelets are
stored at room temperature and are discarded at 48 to 72
hours if not used.

As part of routine evaluation of quality control of
these preparations, several studies were done. Samples
were drawn in a sterile manner in plastic syringes from
random platelet concentrates at four hours, one, two,

and five days after donation.

Platelet counts as done on the Coulter Counter revealed acceptable levels through 48 hours though standard deviation was high (Table II), pH was measured and also found to remain within acceptable limits (Table III). Clot retraction in-vitro as induced by thrombin may reflect the in-vitro ability of platelets to draw injured blood cell walls together to decrease bleeding. We measure clot retraction at three and again at 24 hours. Results show good retraction at three and 24 hours with a small but steady drop-off as platelets age (Table IV and V).

TABLE II. Platelet counts

Age	n	Mean count	S.D.	
4 hours	15	1,082,330	641,580	
1 day	17	1,256,000	431,000	NS
2 days	15	1,059,000	275,000	NS
5 days	3	713,000	213,000	$P < 0.05$

TABLE III. pH of platelet concentrates

Age	n	Mean pH	S.D.	
4 hours	9	7.33	0.12	
1 day	17	6.94	0.22	NS
2 days	15	6.42	0.54	$P < 0.05$

TABLE IV. Thrombin induced clot retraction at 3 hours

Age	n	% retraction	S.D.%
4 hours	15	73.5	9.7
1 day	17	76.2	7.6
2 days	18	58.7	28.6
5 days	6	10.4	17.7

TABLE V. Clot retraction at 24 hours

Age	n	% retraction	S.D.%
4 hours	12	82.6	3.4
1 day	13	80.5	4.4
2 days	18	63.8	28.7
5 days	6	10.4	17.7

[14]C radiolabeled serotonin uptake by platelets was studied. Normal platelets take up over 90% of the serotonin

TABLE VI

Age	n	% uptake	S.D.%
4 hours	18	99.1	0.3
1 day	13	98.8	0.4
2 days	14	98.0	2.3
5 days	6	95.7	3.5

(26). Our studies showed normal uptake in the 95 to 99%
range (Table VI).

Hence we felt that these platelet concentrates were
acceptable for clinical use as judged by these in-vitro
techniques.

Finally we studied BTG using the RIA Kit manufactured
commercially by the Radiochemical Centre in Amersham, U.K.
(2). First we looked at six randomly selected sacs of
platelet concentrates. Three had been prepared 15 hours
earlier and three had been prepared 72 hours earlier. In
both cases BTG levels were about 10 times our normal values (Table VII). Since we noted elevated BTG levels in
platelets that were only 15 hours old, we next attempted
to determine how early the BTG levels rise.

TABLE VII. Platelet concentrates

Age	n	BTG mean	S.D.	
15 hours	3	313.3	32.0	
72 hours	3	320.0	10.8	NS

In 8 randomly selected blood donors, an extra tube (as
provided by the manufacturer of the BTG kit) of blood was
taken for BTG determination. The plastic sacs of blood
were handled routinely and were collected for processing.
At one hour after donation 5 cc of blood were taken ste-
rily from each sac and placed in the manufacturer's tubes
for BTG determinations. Plastic syringes and 16 gauge
needles were used to withdraw the blood. Platelet poor
plasma was prepared and BTG levels were then determined
in duplicate and the mean value used. All determinations
were within the 7.5% coefficient of variation as noted
by the manufacturer for reproducibility of results (Table
VIII).

TABLE VIII. Single donor whole blood

Age	n	BTG mean	S.D.	
fresh	8	24.1	5.0	
1 hour	8	213.4	94.3	$P < 0.05$

Plasma from fresh whole blood had normal levels of BTG as expected. Yet after only one hour of routine handling, the BTG levels were already about 9 times higher. Presumably further BTG is released later on to attain the somewhat higher level noted at 15 and 72 hours.

We thus concluded that significant amounts of BTG are released within an hour of collection of donor blood and that BTG assay as in in-vitro quality control test of platelet is not useful.

In summary, beta thromboglobulin is a platelet specific protein liberated into the blood during the release action and whose measurement may be of some use in diseases in which platelets are felt to play a significant role.

ACKNOWLEDGEMENT

Appreciation is expressed to Ms. Maria Mausser for aid in preparation of the manuscript.

REFERENCES

1. Adler, A., Ludin, A., Friedman, A., Berlyne: Effect of hemodialysis on plasma beta thromboglobulin levels. Trans. Am. Soc. Artif. Intern. Organs XXV:347, 1979.
2. Anonymous: Beta Thromboglobulin Radio-Immunoassay. Manufacturer's Instructions, Amersham, 1977.
3. Anonymous: Blood Component Therapy - A Physician's Handbook. The American Association of Blood Banks, Washington D.C., 1975.
4. Anonymous: Editorial - Platelets, Beta-thromboglobulin and diabetes mellitus. Lancet i:250, 1978.
5. Begg, G., Pepper, D., Chesterman, C., Morgan, F.: Complete covalent structure of human thromboglobulin. Biochemistry 17:1739, 1978.
6. Bidet, J., Ferriere, J., Besse, G., Chollet, P., Gaillard, G., Plagne, R.: Evaluation of β-thromboglobulin levels in cancer patients: effects of antitumor chemotherapy. Thromb. Res. 19:429, 1980.
7. Boughton, B., Allington, M., King, A.: Platelet and plasma β-thromboglobulin in myeloproliferative syndromes and secondary thrombocytosis. Brit. J. Haematol. 40:125, 1978.
8. Cella, G., Zahavi, J., De Haas, H., Kakkar, V.: Thromboglobulin, platelet production time and platelet function in vascular disease. Brit. J. Haematol. 43:127, 1979.
9. Cella, G., Schivazappa, L., Casonato, A., Molaro, L., Girolami, A., Westwick, J., Lane, D., Kakkar, V.: In vivo platelet release reaction in patients with heart valve prosthesis. Haemostasis 9:263, 1980.
10. Dawes, J., Smith, R., Pepper, D.: The release, distribution and clearance of human β-thromboglobulin and platelet factor 4. Thrombos. Res. 12:851, 1978.
11. Denham, M., Fisher, M., James, G., Hassen, M.: Letter. Lancet i:1154, 1977.
12. Depperman, D., Andrassy, K., Seelig, H., Ritz, E., Post, D.: Beta-

thromboglobulin is elevaled in renal failure without thrombosis.
Thromb. Res. 17:63, 1980.

13. Fabris, F., Casonato, A., Randi, M., Girolami, A.: Plasma and
    platelet beta-thromboglobulin levels in patients with May-Hegglin
    anomaly. Haemostasis 9:126, 1980.

14. Gardner, F.: Preservation and clinical use of platelets. In: He-
    matology, editor: W.Williams. McGraw-Hill, New York, 1977.

15. Green, D., Santhanam, S., Krumlovsky, F., Del Greco, F.: Elevated
    β-thromboglobulin in patients with chronic renal failure: effect
    of hemodialysis. J. Lab. Clin. Med. 95:679, 1980.

16. Han, P., Turpie, A., Genton, E.: Plasma β-thromboglobulin: Dif-
    ferentiation between intravascular and extravascular platelet
    destruction. Blood 54:1192, 1979.

17. Holmsen, H.: Collagen-induced release of adenosine diphosphate
    from platelets incubated with radioactive phosphate in vitro.
    Scand. J. Clin. Lab. Invest. 17:239, 1965.

18. Holmsen, H., Day, H., Stormorken, H.: The blood platelet release
    reaction. Scand. J. Hematol. Suppl.8:1, 1969.

19. Holmsen, H.: Biochemistry of the platelet release reaction. In:
    Biochemistry and Pharmacology of Platelets. Ciba Foundation Sym-
    posium, 35, Amsterdam, Elsevier. North Holland Biomedical Press,
    1975, p. 175.

20. Holmsen, H., Day, H.: The selectivity of the thrombin induced
    platelet release reaction. J. Lab. Clin. Med. 75:840, 1970.

21. Jones, N., Zahavi, J., De Haas, H., Clark, S., Leyton, J., Kakkar,
    V.: Platelet function in arterial vascular disease. Thromb. Hae-
    mostas. 42:147, 1979.

22. Kaplan, K., Broekman, J., Chernoff, A., Lesznick, G., Drillings,
    M.: Platelet ɑ granule proteins: studies on release and subcel-
    lular localization. Blood 53:604, 1979.

23. Kaplan, K., Nossel, H., Drillings, M., Lesznick, G.: Radioimmuno-
    assay of platelet factor 4 and β-thromboglobulin: development and
    application to studies of platelet release in relation to fibri-
    nopeptide A generation. Brit. J. Haematol. 39:129, 1978.

24. Ludlam, C.: Evidence for the platelet specificity of β-thrombo-
    globulin and studies on its plasma concentrations in healthy in-
    dividuals. Brit. J. Haematol. 41:271, 1979.

25. Ludlam, C., Allen, N., Blandford, R., Dowdle, R., Bentley, N.,
    Bloom, A.: β-Thromboglobulin and platelet survival in patients
    with rheumatic disease and prosthetic heart valves and their
    treatment with sulfinpyrazone. Thromb. Haemostas. 42:329, 1979.

26. Massini, P., Luscher, E.: The induction of the release reaction
    in human blood platelets by close cell contact. Thrombosis et
    Diatheses Haemorrhagica 25:13, 1971.

27. Matsuda, T., Seki, T., Ogawara, M., Miura, R., Yokouchi, M., Mu-
    rakami, M.: Comparison between plasma levels and β-thromboglobu-
    lin and platelet factor 4 in various diseases. Thromb. Haemostas.
    42:288, 1979.

28. Matthews, J., O'Connor, J., Hearnshaw, J., Wood, J.: Beta-throm-
    boglobulin and glycosylated haemoglobin in diabetes mellitus.
    Scand. J. Haematol. 23:421, 1979.

29. Mehta, P.: Significance of plasma β-thromboglobulin values in pa-
    tients with sickle cell disease. J. Pediatrics 97:941, 1980.

30. Moore, S., Pepper, D., Cash, J.: The isolation and characteriza-

tion of platelet specific β-globulin (β-thromboglobulin) and the detection of anti-urokinase and anti-plasmin released from thrombin-aggregated washed human platelets. Biochim. Biophys. Acta 379:360, 1975.

31. Muhlauser, I., Schernthaner, G., Silberbauer, K., Sinzinger, H., Kaliman, J.: Platelet proteins (β-TG and PF 4) in atherosclerosis and related diseases. Artery 8:73, 1980.

32. Niewiarowski, S., Guzzo, J., Rav, A., Berman, I., James, P.: Increased levels of low affinity platelet factor 4 in plasma and urine of patients with chronic renal failure. Thromb. Haemostas. 42:416, 1979.

33. Niewiarowski, S., Senyi, A., Gillies, P.: Plasmin-induced platelet aggregation and platelet release reaction. Effects on haemostasis. J. Clin. Invest. 52:1647, 1973.

34. Niewiarowski, S., Walz, D., James, P., Rucinski, B., Kueppers, F.: Identification and separation of secreted platelet proteins by isoelectric focusing. Evidence that low-affinity platelet factor 4 is coverted to β-thromboglobulin by limited proteolysis. Blood 55:453, 1980.

35. O'Brien, J., Etherington, M., Shuttleworth, R.: Letter - β-thromboglobulin and heparin-neutralising activity test in clinical conditions. Lancet i:1153, 1977.

36. O'Reilly, M., Zahavi, J., Dubiel, M., Cotton, L., Kakkar, V.: Plasmapheresis and platelet function and Raynaud's phenomenon. Thromb. Haemostas. 42:338, 1979.

37. Parbtani, A., Frampton, G., Cameron, J.: Measurement of platelet release substances in glomerulonephritis: A comparison of beta-thromboglobulin (β-TG), platelet factor 4 (PF4) and serotonin assays. Thromb. Res. 19:177, 1980.

38. Pfuller, S., Luscher, E.: Studies on the mechanism of the human platelet reaction induced by immunological stimuli. II. The effects of Zymosan. J. Immunol. 112:1211, 1974.

39. Prowse, C., Vigano, S., Borsey, D., Dawes, J.: The release of beta-thromboglobulin from platelets during the clotting of whole blood. Thromb. Res. 17:433, 1980.

40. Rasi, V.: β-Thromboglobulin in plasma: false high values caused by platelet enrichment of the top layer of plasma during centrifugation. Thrombos. Res. 15:543, 1979.

41. Redman, C., Allington, M., Bolten, F., Stirrat, G.: Letter - Plasma β-thromboglobulin in pre-eclampsia. Lancet ii:248, 1979.

42. Talpos, G., Horrocks, M., White, J., Cotton, L.: Plasmapheresis in Raynaud's disease. Lancet i:416, 1978.

43. Williams, A., Chater, B., Allen, K., Sherwood, M., Sanderson, J.: Release of β-thromboglobulin from human platelets by therapeutic intensities of ultrasound. Brit. J. Haematol. 40:133, 1978.

44. Williams, A., Chater, B., Sanderson, J., Taberner, D., May, S., Allen, K., Sherwood, M.: Letter - β-thromboglobulin release from human platelets after in-vivo ultrasound irradiation. Lancet ii: 931, 1977.

45. Zahavi, J., Betterridge, D., Jones, N., Galton, D., Leyton, J., Kakkar, V.: β-Thromboglobulin, platelet factor 4 and malondialdehyde formation in hyperlipidemic patients. Thromb. Haemostas. 42:424, 1979.

46. Zahavi, J., Cella, G., Dubiel, M., Kakkar, V.: The variability

of plasma β-thromboglobulin in healthy individuals. Thromb. Haemostas. 40:565, 1979.

47. Zahavi, J., Jones, N., Leyton, J., Dubiel, M., Kakkar, V.: Enhanced in-vivo platelet 'release reaction' in old healthy individuals. Thromb. Res. 17:329, 1980.

48. Zahavi, J., Kakkar, V.: β-Thromboglobulin - a specific marker of in-vivo platelet release reaction. Thromb. Haemostas. 44:23, 1980.

PLATELET THERAPY

A.J. Silvergleid

INTRODUCTION

In the twenty or so years since platelets first became
available in a highly concentrated form for transfusion
to thrombocytopenic patients, platelet therapy has established itself as an integral and vital component in the
management of such patients. Dramatic changes in medical
practice, and the full-fledged development of medical on-
cology as a separate discipline, owe much to the expanding
blood component technology which has provided them with
highly concentrated preparations of viable and hemostatically competent platelets. Surgery, trauma, chemotherapy and
radiotherapy have, as well, all been altered by the ready
availability of platelet concentrates. Whereas in the 1960s,
over 75% of deaths in acute leukemia were the result of hemorrhage directly attributable to thrombocytopenia (37),
this figure has been radically lowered to no more than 10%
to 20%, at this time. Chemotherapy and radiotherapy continue to push to the limits of bone marrow tolerance, and
surgery is undertaken in thrombocytopenic patients former-
ly considered inoperable.
   Two recent symposia (42,82) very beautifully defined
the 'state of the art' as regards platelet transfusions
(in 1978) and are highly recommended for the breadth and
depth of their coverage. This review attempts, on a smaller
scale, to provide an overview of platelet transfusion therapy with a heavy emphasis on the clinical aspects of platelet transfusions. The variables affecting platelet recovery, the importance of a pretransfusion and posttransfusion estimate of compatibility, the complications of
platelet transfusions, and the various special preparations
available will be discussed, albeit cursorily, after major
emphasis has been placed on the specific indications for
(and contraindications to) platelet transfusion therapy.

INDICATIONS FOR PLATELET TRANSFUSION

Platelet transfusions are indicated for the prevention and/
or treatment of hemorrhage which is associated with either
thrombocytopenia or a functional (qualitative) platelet defect (Table I). Actually, the etiology of the thrombocyto-

TABLE I. Indications for platelet transfusions

1. Prophylaxis or treatment of hemorrhage

   A. Thrombocytopenia from impaired production
      aplastic anemia, primary hematologic malignancy
      marrow infiltration, marrow suppression (chemotherapy, ra-
         diotherapy)

   B. Qualitative (intrinsic) platelet dysfunction
      thrombasthenia, storage pool disease, Bernard Soulier syndrom
      Hermansky Pudlak, Aspirin, impaired release reaction

2. Surgery

   A. Patients in category I A or B

   B. Special situations:
      Cardiopulmonary bypass
      Aspirin

3. Massive transfusions (dilutional thrombocytopenia)

4. Other: Factor V inhibitor

penia is as important as the fact of it, for, in general, platelet transfusions are valuable when thrombocytopenia is the result of diminished platelet production, while they are of questionable value when thrombocytopenia is a reflection of excessive platelet destruction, or seques-tration.

In assessing the need for platelet transfusions the two most valuable laboratory diagnostic tests are the platelet count and the template bleeding time (50,67). These highly standardized and reproducible procedures, when used appro-priately, can provide an accurate assessment as to the re-lative risk of bleeding on the basis either of thrombocy-topenia or platelet dysfunction. In addition, they provide a convenient and sensitive means for monitoring the effi-cacy of platelet transfusion therapy, the effectiveness of which is gauged by either restoration of hemostasis (re-flected in normalization of the bleeding time), or eleva-tion of the platelet count. The tests must be used wisely, however, in order to provide as much information as possi-ble with minimal risk to the patient. The platelet count, which is noninvasive, and which correlates in almost a li-near fashion with the template bleeding time when the pla-telet count is less than $100,000/mm^3$ (50) should be the first test obtained in the clinical evaluation of the pa-tient with either a proven, or suspected, hemostatic de-fect. When hemostasis appears inadequate in the face of a normal platelet count, or out of proportion to the degree of thrombocytopenia, the template bleeding time should be performed, as this is the most sensitive clinical indica-tor of platelet function (51). A bleeding time should al-

most never be performed in a severely thrombocytopenic patient, since, generally, it will add little new information (thrombocytopenic patients, except for those recover-
ing from splenectomy in ITP or chemotherapy-induced marrow
suppression (92), should have a prolonged template bleeding time), tends to produce disfiguring scars, and may
serve as a source of infection in a patient who is neutro-
penic as well as thrombocytopenic. The exception to this
generalization is in the thrombocytopenic patient who is
being considered for surgery, and in whom the efficacy of
preoperative platelet transfusions are to be judged by
their ability to normalize (or shorten) the bleeding time.

The platelet count below which the template bleeding
time progressively prolongs, and the risk of clinical
bleeding progressively increases, is $100,000/mm^3$ (50).
Most major and minor surgery can still be safely performed with platelet counts maintained above 30,000-60,000/
mm^3 (96), and the risk of spontaneous, serious bleeding
becomes great only at platelet counts below $20,000/mm^3$
(37). These figures are, of course, only generalizations,
and clinical bleeding may be as much a function of the nature of the thrombocytopenia, as the degree. In the circumstance where the platelet count is dropping rapidly,
spontaneous bleeding might be evident with counts as high
as $50,000-70,000/mm^3$; while in situations associated with
a rapidly rising platelet count, adequate hemostasis might
be achieved with counts as low as $10,000-20,000/mm^3$ (50,
92).

PREPARATION OF THE HEMOSTATICALLY INCOMPETENT PATIENT FOR
SURGERY

The preoperative evaluation and management of hemostatically compromised patients was extensively reviewed by
Simpson in 1978 (96), and his chapter is highly recommended for its thorough and critical review of the available
literature, some of which will be summarized here. Patients
who are anticipating surgery and who are either thrombocytopenic (on the basis of diminished platelet production)
or who have an intrinsic platelet functional defect (inherited or acquired) are candidates for preoperative prophylactic platelet transfusions. It is imperative that the
ability to achieve adequate hemostasis via platelet transfusions (as indicated by either a rise in platelet count
to levels between $30,000-60,000/mm^3$ or by a shortening of
the template bleeding time to less than twice the upper
limit of normal, i.e. ⪕ 15 minutes) be well demonstrated
prior to subjecting such patients to surgery. For most
adults, this can be accomplished with approximately six
to eight units of random platelet concentrates, though
the exact number may vary somewhat depending upon the size
of the patient. If adequate hemostasis cannot be achieved
with platelet transfusion, the implications are that the
patient: (1) is allosensitized, and may respond to fresh,

histocompatible platelets; (2) has an extrinsic qualitative platelet disorder (i.e. uremia (80), dysproteinemia
(59)), and attention will have to be directed towards alle-
viating the underlying condition; or (3) has a hemostatic
abnormality, or long bleeding time, on the basis of a non-
platelet disorder (i.e. Von Willebrand disease (12)) which
is not correctable by platelet transfusions (118). If adequate hemostasis is achieved at surgery there is no particular need for prophylactic platelet transfusions postoperatively; they should be reserved for patients with
clinical bleeding and either a platelet count below 50,000-
60,000/mm^3 or a prolonged template bleeding time.

There are two groups of patients with somewhat unique
platelet requirements in relation to surgery which deserve
special mention:

Cardiopulmonary bypass surgery

Patients who are subjected to extracorporeal circulation
may experience excessive bleeding postoperatively in spite
of low normal (100,000-150,000/mm^3) platelet counts and
normal coagulation parameters. The etiology of this postbypass hemorrhagic diathesis is unknown, and in fact, its
existence may well be arguable. Simpson, after carefully
reviewing the available evidence, concluded that 'routine
or prophylactic administration of platelet transfusion to
postbypass patients cannot be justified on the basis of
any current data', and that 'the same indications should
be applied to the use of platelet transfusion in bypass
patients as in any other surgical situation' (96). This
approach appears to be quite reasonable, and is to be recommended. Nevertheless, there are a number of studies
which appear to indicate that there is a platelet functional disorder following cardiopulmonary bypass (11,13,
48,65,66,71) such that a thorough evaluation of hemostasis (platelet count, template bleeding time) is warranted,
and, if indicated (by a prolonged template bleeding time),
platelet transfusions given in spite of a normal, or low
normal, platelet count.

Aspirin-related bleeding

Occasionally, a patient with no prior history of a bleeding
disorder, will undergo surgery and experience severe and
persistent bleeding in spite of a normal platelet count.
A careful review of the patient's medication history will
often reveal that the patient has regularly consumed aspirin (acetylsalicylic acid). Although the hemostatic in-
competence might have been detected with a preoperative
template bleeding time, this is not routinely obtained for
patients with a negative bleeding history and a normal preoperative platelet count. Such patients clearly have an
acquired platelet functional disorder secondary to aspirin
(117,119) which will not normalize for several days, without intervention. Since hemostasis can be normalized if as

few as 20% of circulating platelets have not been exposed
to aspirin (102), this aspirin-induced hemorhagic diathesis is eminently reversible by the transfusion of six to
ten units of random platelets, and such an approach is to
be recommended in this setting.

Intrinsic platelet functional disorders

Inherited qualitative platelet disorders, such as Glanzmann's thrombasthenia, storage pool disease, Bernard-Soulier syndrome, Hermansky-Pudlak syndrome, and a variety of
release reaction abnormalities (38), may be associated
with spontaneous bleeding, if the abnormality is particularly severe. For the most part, however, patients with
these disorders rarely require platelet transfusions unless they are traumatized, or require surgery. Surgical
management of these patients is no different from that of
any other patient with impaired hemostasis, except that
their life-long platelet requirement may lead to their
being allosensitized, and thus they may require histocompatible platelet support. The crucial aspect of·their management is to shorten the bleeding time into a hemostatic
range prior to surgery, transfusing as many platelets as
this may require.

Thrombocytopenia resulting from impaired production

Among the multiple etiologies of decreased platelet production, those which are most commonly encountered in clinical practice are: aplastic anemia, primary hematologic
malignancies (i.e. acute leukemia), marrow infiltration
secondary to a primary tumor (i.e. lymphoma, carcinoma),
and marrow hypoplasia as a temporary or permanent concomitant of chemotherapy and/or radiotherapy (8). Patients
with these disorders are the major 'consumers' of platelets in most hospitals. These patients require, and will
respond to, platelet transfusion support during surgery,
or should they experience a bleeding episode related to
their thrombocytopenia. Special consideration must be given to determining the appropriate dose of platelets, since
these patients frequently have fever, sepsis, or splenomegaly, and will require a larger dose (sometimes as high as
12 to 16 units), in order to achieve circulating platelet
levels which are hemostatic. In addition, these are the
patients who become allosensitized and for whom histocompatible platelet support is often necessary.
The major consideration in the management of these chronically thrombocytopenic patients, however, is the necessity for the use of prophylactic platelet transfusions. Based originally on the landmark study of Gaydos et al.(37),
in which the risk of serious or fatal hemorrhage in such
patients was shown to be directly related to the degree of
thrombocytopenia, and supported by two prospectively randomized trials demonstrating that prophylactic platelet
transfusions reduce the incidence of bleeding and morbidi-

ty (54,73), it has become 'standard' practice at most major medical centers to provide prophylactic platelet support to patients either chronically thrombocytopenic (e.g.
with aplastic anemia) or temporarily thrombocytopenic (during acute leukemia induction therapy, or as a result of
chemotherapy and/or radiotherapy) with an aim towards keeping the platelet count above 15,000-20,000/mm^3. On the
basis of another study, this one by Roy et al. (81), it
has been accepted that for purposes of prophylaxis moderate doses of platelets (e.g. four to six units per transfusion) are adequate, and adoption of this practice has
resulted in a substantial reduction in platelet usage
with no noticeable increase in morbidity (1).

Considering the hazards of platelet transfusions and,
particularly in the chronically thrombocytopenic patient,
the extra hazard associated with the development of refractoriness, there is still some debate as to the wisdom
of the universal application of prophylactic platelet
transfusions. It is significant, in this regard, that
Higby (54) noted in his study that hemorrhagic events
were often related to complications such as fever or infection, and a subsequent study by Soloman et al. (98)
demonstrated no difference in morbidity in patients receiving prophylactic platelet support versus those receiving therapeutic platelet transfusions for bleeding (or
a rapidly falling platelet count). It may well be that we
will shortly be in a position to refine our indications
for prophylactic platelet transfusions so as to protect
only those patients who are most at risk. At present,
however, given the limitations of our clinical acumen,
and the lack of any truly dependable prognostic indicator,
it would seem that patients chronically (or temporarily)
thrombocytopenic on the basis of impaired production should
receive prophylactic platelet support to try to keep their
platelet count above 15,000-20,000/mm^3.

One interesting point, occasionally overlooked, is that
granulocyte concentrates are extremely rich in platelets
($5-7 \times 10^{11}$), and patients who are receiving daily granulocyte concentrates as part of the management of a septic
episode are thus unusually well supplied with platelets
and will not require separate transfusion of this component.

Massive transfusion

Massive blood replacement, as occurs in the setting of
trauma, severe gastrointestinal hemorrhage, or ruptured
aortic aneurysm is frequently associated with a characteristic hemorrhagic diathesis of which both thrombocytopenia and a platelet functional defect are components (58,
63,68,100). Because it has been difficult to define the
precise cause of the bleeding disorder accompanying large
volume blood replacement, and, therefore, the optimal approach to its management, various recommendations for re-

placement therapy have included platelet concentrates, fresh frozen plasma (106), and even 'fresh warm blood' (89,106). Recently, Counts et al (23) prospectively studied the coagulation profile and hemostatic competence (platelet count, template bleeding time) of 27 patients requiring massive transfusion with whole blood and determined that: (1) the transfusion of large volumes of whole blood of random age to trauma patients does not cause clinically significant clotting factor deficiencies; (2) clinically significant thrombocytopenia (platelet counts < 100,000/mm^3) is likely to develop only after the transfusion of 15 to 20 units of platelet-depleted whole blood (1.5 to 2.0 times the patient's blood volume); and (3) the most useful parameter for estimating the need for platelet transfusion was the platelet count. The bleeding time, which has been shown to be prolonged in all patients by the time they receive five units of blood (68), is of no value in anticipating the onset of microvascular bleeding. A fibrinogen level is useful as a sensitive indicator of the presence of disseminated intravascular coagulation, for in the absence of that complication fibrinogen levels are usually normal even in patients with large volume replacement. From Counts' study, one can conclude that massively transfused patients may safely be managed with whole blood (regardless of age) and, if thrombocytopenia develops, platelet transfusions to elevate the platelet count above 100,000/mm^3. Fresh frozen plasma does not appear to be indicated.

In this regard, another recent study (94) in which the coagulation factor activity in platelet concentrates was evaluated, is worth mentioning. Simon and Henderson have documented that hemostatic levels of all coagulation factors (including V and VIII) are transfused with stored platelet concentrates. Considering the fact that when eight to ten units of platelets are transfused this is accompanied by 400 ml to 500 ml of essentially fresh plasma, it can be readily appreciated that platelet concentrates are not only a rich source of platelets, but are as well a rich source of coagulation factors. In fact, in the patient with both thrombocytopenia and coagulation factor deficiency, it may well be that the most appropriate therapy is platelet concentrates alone, reserving fresh frozen plasma for those situations for which platelets are not required, or for which Factor V is the critically required ingredient.

POSSIBLE INDICATIONS

In addition to the well-defined indications for platelet transfusion, discussed above, and the somewhat questionable indications (or contraindications), to be discussed, there is a small group of clinical situations for which platelet transfusions may be indicated, though at the present time there is neither sufficient, nor compelling, data to sub-

stantiate such an indication. One of these situations is
in the presence of a coagulopathy caused by an acquired
inhibitor to Factor V. Chediak et al. (18) recently reported on the successful management of a patient with such
an inhibitor via the transfusion of multiple units of platelets, and postulated that the platelet membrane provided receptor sites for the inhibitor such that it was
cleared from the plasma, allowing the coagulopathy to resolve temporarily. This intriguing application of the use
of platelet concentrates for this fortunately exceedingly
rare clinical condition awaits further substantiation.

Another possible application of platelet transfusions,
unrelated to thrombocytopenia, might be in the pretrans-
plant patient in whom, as it seems clear, exposure to
blood products seems to predispose to better graft survival (78). If it can be shown that exposure to transplantation (HLA) antigens is the critical feature, then platelet concentrates, which represent an excellent readily
available source of highly concentrated transplantation
antigens, might be the component of choice for these patients.

QUESTIONABLE INDICATIONS AND CONTRAINDICATIONS

As noted above, platelet transfusions are most valuable
in the treatment of the hemorrhagic diathesis resulting
either from thrombocytopenia, which is caused by diminished platelet production, or from an intrinsic platelet functional defect, and the use of platelets in these
disorders has already been considered. Platelet transfusions are of significantly less value in the management
of thrombocytopenia which is caused by excessive platelet
destruction (or sequestration), or the hemorrhagic diathesis resulting from an extrinsic platelet functional defect. In the first category are such entities as idiopa-
thic thrombocytopenic purpura (ITP), immune-mediated drug
purpura, posttransfusion purpura and neonatal isoimmune
thrombocytopenic purpura (unless P1^{A1}-negative platelets
are available for these latter two), hypersplenism, thrombotic thrombocytopenic purpura (TTP), and disseminated intravascular coagulation (DIC). All of these disorders are
characterized by rapid removal or sequestration of circulating platelets and moderate to marked thrombocytopenia.
In spite of the thrombocytopenia, routine or prophylactic
platelet transfusions are not indicated (or are contrain-
dicated) for the following reasons:
1. Because of the rapid platelet utilization, most of the
   circulating platelets are younger, and, therefore, are
   considered to be hemostatically more effective (92).
   That this is true is somewhat substantiated by the decreased clinical bleeding seen in these disorders (with
   the exception of DIC and TTP), and the relative dis-
   cordance between the profound thrombocytopenia and the
   only moderately prolonged template bleeding time (50,

92). Platelet transfusions will thus be unnnecessary unless the thrombocytopenia is accompanied by active bleeding.

2. Transfused platelets will be rapidly cleared (as are the autologous platelets) and their effectiveness is minimized.

3. In certain of these disorders (isoimmune neonatal purpura, DIC, TTP) platelet transfusions may prolong or exacerbate the pathologic process.

4. Repeated platelet transfusions will allosensitize the patient (leading to refractoriness), such that adequate (histocompatible) platelet support during a hemorrhagic crisis may be nearly impossible to guarantee.

In summary, the general approach to the management of these disorders is to avoid platelet transfusions unless the patient has a serious or uncontrollable bleed, at which time, there is really no other option than to transfuse high doses of platelets in hopes of achieving hemostasis. Bleeding patients with immune thrombocytopenia have occasionally been seen to respond to a slow, constant infusion of platelets, and highly allosensitized patients, as these patients often are, may temporarily suppress their alloantibody titer sufficiently to allow for a hemostatic response to a second bolus of platelets, if they are first primed with an extremely large dose (i.e. 20 units) which will serve to bind all free antibody (75).

The second category alluded to above, the extrinsic qualitative platelet functional disorders, includes uremia (80), and the dysproteinemias (59). In these disorders, platelets which are intrinsically normal are rendered hemostatically incompetent either by virtue of a circulating toxin (in uremia) or by an immunoglobulin coating (in the dysproteinemias). Platelet transfusions are useless in these settings, and appropriate management includes dialysis (76) or plasmapheresis (59).

DOSE RESPONSE

Platelet dose

The number of platelets in a platelet concentrate, or 'unit', prepared as a byproduct of whole blood collection, is required (by the FDA) to be greater than 5.5×10^{10} in at least 75% of concentrates prepared in any facility (35). In practice, most centers routinely prepare concentrates which contain roughly $7\text{-}8 \times 10^{10}$ platelets (85,123), harvesting 70% to 80% of the 1×10^{11} platelets from a unit of freshly drawn blood. When determining dose-response curves, therefore, most people assume that 7×10^{10} platelets constitute a 'unit'.

Platelet concentrates harvested via platelet apheresis range in quantity from 2.5×10^{11} to 6.5×10^{11} (2,41,57, 77,105), with the quantity being influenced by the donor's prepheresis platelet count, the type of equipment used, and either the number of cycles performed (Haemonetics), or the duration of the procedure (IBM, Fenwal). In most experienced centers the number of platelets routinely harvested by plateletapheresis ($4-6 \times 10^{11}$) represents the equivalent of six to eight units prepared from individual whole blood donations.

Anticipated rise in platelet count

For the individual who has none of the complications known to have a detrimental effect on platelet recovery after transfusion (e.g. fever, sepsis, splenomegaly, allosensitization, medication), it is relatively easy to calculate the rise in platelet count to be anticipated after transfusion with platelet concentrates. A precise calculation would involve dividing the total number of platelets transfused by the blood volume (estimated by multiplying the body weight in grams by 0.07 ml/g) and then multiplying the result by 2/3 (to allow for the fact that 1/3 of the transfused platelets will immediately be sequestered in the spleen) (9).

$$\text{Anticipated Platelet Increment} = \frac{\text{Total number of platelets transfused}}{\text{Blood volume (body weight, g} \times 0.07 \text{ ml/g)}} \times 2/3$$

In practical terms, the standard 70 kg (weight), 1.75 m^2 (body surface area), 5,000 ml (blood volume) patient should expect to experience a 5,000 to 10,000/mm^3 increment in platelet count for each 'unit' transfused; presuming, again that there are no adverse variables which would diminish platelet recovery. It is important that recovery be checked with a count taken approximately one hour after completion of the transfusion so as most accurately to assess the response to the transfusion (25). Counts done after any considerable time lapse (e.g. 12 hours, 24 hours) reflect platelet survival rather than platelet recovery (e.g. responsiveness) and may be strongly influenced by factors other than those which affect immediate recovery (Table II)

TABLE II. Variables affecting platelet recovery after transfusion

---

Compatibility
  ABO, Rh
  HLA, platelet specific antigens
Fever/infection
Spleen size
Medications
Storage duration
Rapid utilization
Filters

VARIABLES AFFECTING RECOVERY

ABO compatibility

Although there have been a substantial number of studies specifically addressing the role of ABO compatibility in clinical platelet transfusions there is neither unanimity, nor agreement, as to the interpretation of the results of these studies. Several early studies purported to demonstrate the presence of ABO blood group antigens on platelet membranes (45,61) and the effect of the presence of these antigens was shown to be decreased recovery of transfused, ABO incompatible platelets both by Aster (4), and also by Pfisterer et al. (79). In contrast, Freireich (36), Shulman (90), Cohen (19), Lohrmann (64), Tosato (109), and Van Eys (114) have all published data suggesting that ABO compatibility has little, if any, effect on platelet recovery. Most recently, Duquesnoy et al. (28) reported studies in alloimmunized, thrombocytopenic patients which indicated that ABO incompatibility between donor and recipient accounted for approximately a 23% decrease in the mean 24-hour platelet recovery in patients receiving platelets from donors who were either HLA-compatible or selectively mismatched for cross-reactive HLA antigens.

This author's own interpretation of the above data, and of clinical data collected at Stanford University Hospital, would lead to the following suggested guidelines:

1. In the setting of a single transfusion exposure to platelets (e.g. hemostasis in an acute situation), ABO compatibility (of the platelet concentrates) may safely be ignored. However, minor side incompatibility (e.g. group 0 platelet concentrates given to a patient who is either group A, B or AB) should probably be avoided, because of the problems that may result from hemolysis, or the development of a positive direct antiglobulin test in a patient who may require further transfusions. Although this will represent more of a problem for children than for adults, it may be avoided, or circumvented, in either group simply by pooling and packing the platelet concentrates prior to administration.
2. Plateletpheresis donors, either random or HLA-matched, should probably be ABO compatible (major and minor side) considering the large plasma volume, the heavy red blood cell contamination (especially with the Haemonetics Model 30), and the approximate 20% loss of platelets when concentrates are spun so as to remove incompatible red blood cells.
3. Plateletpheresis-harvested concentrates for alloimmunized, thrombocytopenic patients should almost certainly be ABO compatible to maximize platelet recovery and minimize the potential for a transfusion reaction, although in the event that the only available donors are HLA compatible but ABO incompatible (on the major side), pheresis of such donors is reasonable and to be recommended.

Rhesus

Rh antigens have not been demonstrated on platelets (3, 46,60), and survival studies (79,90) have shown no dif- ference in survival of Rh-positive and Rh-negative pla- telets given to Rh-negative patients, including $Rh_0(D)$- sensitized patients with potent anti-D antibodies (133). Thus, the major concern with respect to the role of the Rh system in platelet transfusion is the risk of sensi- tizing an Rh-negative patient to the D antigen via trans- fusion of Rh-positive platelet concentrates (which are in- variably contaminated with red blood cells). Goldfinger and McGinniss (40) reported an $Rh_0(D)$-sensitization rate of 7.8% in a population of immunosuppressed Rh-negative patients who had been transfused with Rh-positive plate- let concentrates, a low figure which contrasts sharply with the 70% to 80% sensitization rate reported for nor- mal volunteers given a similar antigenic stimulus (44, 101,116). Since at that time (1969 through 1971) platelet concentrates were generally reserved for critically ill patients with a limited life expectancy, the consequences of Rh sensitization were considerably less, even consi- dering the decreased risk of such sensitization.

At the present time, however, with platelet concentra- tes used routinely for patients considerably less immuno- suppressed than in Goldfinger's study, the risks for, and the consequences of, Rh-sensitization are significant, and if at all possible, Rh-negative females with child-bearing potential should receive platelet concentrates prepared from Rh-negative donors. Apparently the FDA recognizes the validity of this position, since they are proposing to amend the labeling requirements for platelet concen- trates to include the donor's Rh type (34). In the event that one cannot possibly avoid giving Rh-positive plate- let concentrates to an Rh-negative female of child-bearing potential, this author recommends calculating an appropr- riate dose of, and administering, Rh-immune globulin to the patient in an effort to prevent Rh sensitization.

HLA

HLA antigens are unquestionably expressed on platelets (21,104), although the expression may be variable (10, 32,62) and appears to be limited to the HLA-A and HLA-B antigens: HLA-C, -D, and DR antigens have not been demon- strated on platelets (31,115). Refractoriness to random donor platelet transfusions, which can be anticipated in roughly 60% to 70% of patients who receive repeated trans- fusions of platelets from random donors over a prolonged period (56), results primarily from alloimmunization to the antigens of the HLA system. Refractoriness is mani- fested by the failure to achieve a rise in circulating platelet count one hour after infusion of adequate numbers of platelets, and is often accompanied by the development of lymphocytotoxic antibodies. That alloimmunized patients

frequently respond successfully to platelet transfusions
from donors matched for HLA-A and -B antigens (64,107,
122,123), and that the response is directly proportional
to the number of HLA antigens shared between donor and
recipient, is the best evidence for the predominant role
of the HLA system in the development of the refractory
state which characterizes the alloimmunized patient.

Considering the highly polymorphic nature of the HLA
system (more that 60 antigens have been identified), it
is virtually impossible to guarantee sufficient numbers
of HLA-typed donors so as to be in a position to provide
HLA-matched platelets for all alloimmunized, thrombocytopenic patients. Fortunately, serologic crossreactivity
has been demonstrated among antigens in the HLA system
(70,103), and Duquesnoy et al. (30) have shown that platelet transfusions from donors mismatched for crossreactive antigens are as effective as perfectly matched platelets in providing hemostasis. As a result of these observations, the donor pool necessary to sustain a matched-
platelet program can be reduced dramatically to manageable
numbers (108).

Although the HLA system appears to be the most important system with respect to the development of refractoriness, the relationship between refractoriness and sensitization to HLA antigens is not absolute, for there are
numerous instances in which poor transfusion results are
obtained in the presence of a perfect HLA match and, conversely, there are instances in which excellent transfusion results are obtained in the presence of a major HLA
mismatch. In the former circumstance, it is postulated
that platelet antigens other than HLA (e.g. platelet-specific antigens, ABO antigens) are influencing the poor
recovery, while in the latter circumstances it is hypo-
thesized that the good results are a function of:
1. A restricted pattern of alloimmunization, in which antibodies are produced against only a very few antigen
   specificities in spite of a broad transfusion exposure.
   In particular, patients who are HLA-A2 negative seem
   to become so highly immunized against HLA-A2 that they
   will have substantially better recoveries of HLA-A2-
   negative donors (in spite of refractoriness to random platelets) than will patients who are HLA-A2-posi-
   tive and who, therefore, have not 'restricted' their
   immune response to HLA-A2 (29).
2. The variable expression of HLA antigens on the platelet
   surface, particularly HLA-B12 (62).

Two other components within, or closely related to, the
HLA system have been evaluated for their effects on the development of refractoriness. HLA-C antigens, so far as can
be determined, do not appear to be as immunogenic as HLA-A
or HLA-B antigens, or are not so strongly expressed on
platelets, since matching for HLA-C, in addition to HLA-A
and -B, does not appear to be necessary (31). The Bw4/Bw6

antigen system, a simple diallelic system in which each
antigen appears to be closely associated with a distinct
group of HLA-B locus antigens, appears to explain certain
instances of refractoriness, when the presence of anti-
Bw4 or anti-Bw6 correlated with poor recoveries of platelets containing the associated HLA-B antigens (32).

A final note with respect to HLA is that there is reasonably convincing evidence that lymphocytes and monocytes
are more immunogenic than platelets and that the refractoriness to 'platelet' transfusions may partially reflect
an immune response predominantly aimed at the HLA antigens
on leukocytes. The evidence for this is based on a study
by Brand et al. (16), in which they demonstrated a markedly decreased rate of alloimmunization to random donor platelets which had been subjected to a slow centrifugation
in order to effect removal of contaminating leukocytes.
In addition, Herzig et al. (53) were able to improve significantly the transfusion response to HLA-matched platelet concentrates by performing a similar maneuver (to remove the leukocytes). Such an approach would appear to be
justified for selected patients in whom it is impossible
to produce an adequate response even to HLA-matched platelets.

Platelet-specific antigens

Although several platelet-specific antigens have been well
defined, including $Pl^{A1}(2)$, $Pl^{E1}(2)$, and $Ko^{A,B}(91,113)$,
there is almost no information regarding the role of platelet-specific antigen incompatibility in transfusion support of highly alloimmunized patients. Antibody to Pl^{A1} is
capable of inducing rapid clearance of Pl^{A1}-positive platelets, and is the etiologic factor in posttransfusion purpura (7). Nevertheless, there have as yet been no reported
cases in which chronically thrombocytopenic patients have
developed refractoriness to Pl^{A1}-positive platelets. In
spite of the lack of supportive evidence for a role for
platelet-specific antigens, their importance has been inferred because of the more than occasional failure of HLA-
A and HLA-B matched platelets to produce a good response
in a refractory patient, and because in vitro 'compatibility'
tests other than lymphocytotoxicity (presumably based on
determining compatibility for platelet-specific antigens)
are sometimes of predictive value.

OTHER VARIABLES

Other variables which may adversely affect platelet recovery and function after transfusion (Table II) include fever (36,43), splenomegaly (5,49,52), certain medications
(including Acetaminophen (Tylenol) (33), Methacillin (87),
possibly Carbenicillin (83)), length of storage of the concentrates (122), rapid utilization, or consumption e.g.
in hemorrhage (6) or disseminated intravascular coagulation

(DIC) (14,95), or the use of ultrapore filters (72).

PRETRANSFUSION ESTIMATION OF COMPATIBILITY

Pretransfusion testing is not necessary prior to administering platelet concentrates to a patient who is not alloimmunized. Attention should be directed towards the ABO
group and Rh type (for reasons enumerated above), but no
additional testing is either required or recommended.
There are, however, two settings in which compatibility
testing may be necessary. The first of these pertains to
the apheresis-harvested platelet concentrate which is heavily contaminated with red blood cells. In this situation,
a major crossmatch is recommended. Since some of the newer,
continuous-flow pheresis apparatuses (particularly the IBM
2997, when a double channel is used) are capable of harvesting platelets with virtually no red blood cell contamination, the necessity for performing a crossmatch may be
eliminated even for pheresis concentrates. Our general approach is to recommend a crossmatch if there are sufficient
red blood cells in a small segment of the tubing to make a
crossmatch possible.
   The second situation which may require some pretransfusion estimate of compatibility is in the highly alloimmunized patient who is refractory to random donor platelets.
Although on most occasions these patients will respond to
HLA-matched platelets (64,69,107,122,123), approximately
25% of the time they will have no response to platelets
from donors with whom they are perfectly matched at the
HLA-A and HLA-B loci, while approximately 1/3 of the time
they will have excellent responses to platelets from donors with them they have a major HLA incompatibility (108,
109). Selection of donors via HLA typing alone is, thus,
far from infallible, although it has proven clinically
very useful and moderately dependable. Because of the somewhat less than totally predictable results obtained with
the use of HLA-matched platelets for the support of highly
allo-immunized patients, investigators have sought to develop and evaluate in vitro assays which could reliably
predict the response to transfusions. Among the assays described have been lymphocytotoxicity (39), mixed lymphocyte
culture (120), platelet aggregometry (121), platelet fluorescence (15), ^{14}C-adenine and ^{3}H-serotonin release (97),
a radioimmunoassay to detect platelet-bound IgG (79), gra-
nulocytotoxicity, microleukoagglutination, and platelet
migration inhibition (110). There are problems with all of
these assays, including: their lack of 100% correlation
with the response to transfusion, their expense, the necessity for fresh platelets for testing (requiring a potential
donor to make two trips to the blood center), and the time
required for the assay. Nevertheless, the assays have proven valuable when used in the appropriate clinical situation.
   The following outline summarizes the in vitro correlates

of refractoriness and the appropriate flow of responses
to adjust to this difficult situation:

1. Lymphocytotoxic antibodies develop quite early in patients (including immunosuppressed patients) regularly
   transfused with platelets (86), and the development of
   these antibodies correlates quite well with the development of refractoriness to random platelets.
2. For refractory patients, providing HLA-matched platelets
   will result in a good response better than 60% of the
   time. Unfortunately, approximately 25% of the HLA-matched transfusions will be unsuccessful.
3. Patients apparently unresponsive to HLA-matched platelets should receive fresh ABO compatible, leukocyte-
   free, HLA-matched single donor concentrates as the first
   approach.
4. It is presumed that the failure to respond to HLA-matched, lymphocytotoxicity-negative platelet transfusions
   is a function of incompatibility for either platelet-
   specific antigens or some as yet unidentified marker
   system, and that this incompatibility may be predicted,
   or detected, by an in vitro crossmatch.
5. For truly refractory patients, therefore, HLA matching
   and lymphocytotoxicity should probably be combined with
   a platelet crossmatch (one of the assays mentioned above)
   in hopes of detecting compatible donors and predicting
   a successful response to transfusion.

POSTTRANSFUSION ESTIMATION OF COMPATIBILITY

This section is included in order to emphasize the importance of a one-hour posttransfusion platelet count (increment) as an index of platelet compatibility. Hemostatic
effectiveness of transfused platelets may be evaluated by
their ability to shorten a bleeding time which is prolonged
as a result either of thrombocytopenia, or aspirin ingestion. Viability of transfused platelets can be assessed
either directly, by [51]Chromium-labeling platelets prior to
infusion so that survival may be measured, or indirectly,
by following serially obtained platelet counts. For practical reasons, however, invasive tests (bleeding time) and
costly, radioisotopic procedures ([51]Chromium survival) are
rarely used in thrombocytopenic patients except as inves-
tigative tools, and most clinicians (justifiably) assume
that a sustained rise in platelet count after transfusion
will be associated with hemostatic effectiveness. Therefore, posttransfusion platelet counts represent the most
widely used measure of the effect and effectiveness of platelet transfusion. Of paramount importance in this regard
is the elapsed time between the transfusion and the assessment of the platelet increment. As mentioned earlier, and
stressed here, platelet compatibility (or recovery) is
most accurately assessed with a platelet count done approximately one hour after transfusion (25), because this will
generally eliminate from consideration conditions which

affect survival rather than recovery. It is imperative
that all platelet transfusions to chronically thrombocytopenic patients be followed with a one-hour platelet
count as the most reliable clinical index of responsive-
ness/refractoriness. Random donors should not be abandoned,
nor a patient declared refractory, unless a persistent
failure to achieve a measurable one-hour posttransfusion
platelet increment after transfusion with adequate numbers
of 'fresh' ($\leqslant$ 24 hours old) platelets can be documented.

COMPLICATIONS OF PLATELET TRANSFUSION

Criteria for the use of platelet transfusions must be well
defined, and (then) adhered to rigidly for, much as with
any other blood product, there are certain well-defined
risks attendant upon the transfusion of platelet concentrates (Table III). While most of these complications
would be anticipated in the wake of transfusion with almost any blood product, a few of them are uniquely associated with platelet transfusions, as a consequence either
of the peculiar storage conditions, or the type of patients
for whom the product is most often required. It must be
kept in mind that, in spite of this impressive list of
complications, platelet transfusions are by and large relatively free from serious risk.

TABLE III. Complications from platelet transfusions

Infection
  Hepatitis, bacterial
Non-hemolytic transfusion reactions
  urticarial, leukoagglutinin
Granulocytopenia
Graft vs. host
Hemolysis/positive DAT
Allosensitization

SPECIAL PREPARATIONS

For most clinical situations in which platelet transfusions
are indicated, there is no need to perform any special ma-
nipulations on the platelet concentrates. There are, however, certain settings in which specialized handling, or
preparations, of the platelets is either recommended or
obligatory. In this section, the types of special platelet
preparations will be reviewed (Table IV), as will the indications for their preparation and use.

TABLE IV. Special platelet preparations

Pooled/packed
Washed
Monocyte-poor
Irradiated
Frozen
Single donor

Pooled/packed

Individual platelet concentrates may be pooled, spun (5,000 RPM for five minutes), and resuspended in 30 ml to 50 ml of plasma prior to transfusion. This is indicated for patients (particularly children) who need platelets but are unable to tolerate a fluid load. It is also indicated in situations in which there is a potentially significant ABO incompatibility. Lastly, this technic may enable allosensitized (to plasma proteins) patients to avoid urticarial transfusion reactions. As with any blood product the container of which has been entered, pooled/packed platelets should be transfused as soon as possible after preparation.

Washed

A platelet-washing technic has been described (93) which enables highly allosensitized patients to be transfused with concentrated, hemostatically effective platelets in a plasma protein-free medium. This specialized product is only indicated for patients with severe transfusion reactions to even the minimal amount of plasma protein present in pooled/packed platelet concentrates.

Monocyte-poor

Platelet concentrates may be pooled and made monocyte-poor by subjecting the pooled concentrate to a short, soft spin (700 RPM for three minutes, modified from Herzig) (53). This same technic may also be applied to pheresis-harvested single donor platelet concentrates. Monocyte-poor platelet concentrates are indicated primarily for those patients who are experiencing transfusion reactions (of the leukoagglutinin type) or refractoriness as a result of allosensitization to leukocyte (predominantly HLA) antigens. It is also possible (though untested) that monocyte removal might provide an alternative to irradiation as a means of preventing GVHD in immunocompromized patients.

Irradiated

All blood products, including platelet concentrates, may be irradiated to destroy T-lymphocytes, apparently without deleterious effects on cell survival or function (17,55,88). Although clear-cut indications for irradiated platelet con-

centrates are not yet well defined, it is possible that
all severely immunocompromized patients may one day be
transfused strictly with blood products which have been
irradiated so as to prevent GVHD. As yet, there is neither
agreement that this is necessary nor any consensus as to
the appropriate dose.

Frozen

Although technics for platelet cryopreservation are still
evolving, current methodology provides us with viable and
hemostatically effective platelets after frozen storage for
periods of up to three years (20,24,26,27,47,74,84,99,111,
123,124). Allosensitized (refractory) patients who enter
a remission of their primary disease may provide autologous
platelets for freezing and use during subsequent thrombocytopenic episodes (relapses), thereby circumventing the
difficulties imposed by their refractoriness. In addition
to autologous platelets, it is possible that HLA typed (and
matched) homologous platelets will be frozen to provide an
immediate supply of compatible platelets for patients who
become refractory to random donor platelets. A well-stocked
platelet freezer should also provide an excellent inventory
and supply buffer, particularly on long weekends and holi-
day periods. Platelet cryopreservation, therefore, represents a critically important technical advance, the full
benefits of which we have only begun to appreciate.

Single donor

Single donor platelet concentrates, harvested by apheresis,
represent an extremely valuable resource, particularly for
the allosensitized patient refractory to random donor platelets (64,85,109,123). Additionally, it has been argued
(without any substantial data) that single donor platelets
should have an even wider application; i.e. that they are
appropriately used from the very onset of platelet support
for chronically thrombocytopenic patients. The presumed advantages of such an approach are derived from the fact that
the patient is exposed to fewer donors, and, therefore, is:
(1) less likely to develop hepatitis; and (2) more likely
to develop a restricted pattern of alloimmunization (i.e.
to fewer HLA antigens), enabling the clinician to switch donors with a reasonable assurance that the patient is not
broadly refractory. Although this application of single donor platelets already has many adherents, and it is super-
ficially very attractive, a carefully controlled clinical
study on the efficacy of such an approach has yet to be
published, and, considering the expense differential between single donor and random concentrates, it would seem
that there is an urgent need for such a study. The final
(current) application of single donor platelets is as a
source of supply and inventory control, enabling large
numbers of platelets to be prepared from a limited number
of donors, and with a limited staff. How important this ap-

plication will ultimately prove to be is as yet unclear.

SUMMARY

This review has concentrated mainly on clinical aspects of platelet therapy, and I have therefore intentionally avoided discussing many important aspects of platelet physiology and function, including platelet collection and storage variables, techniques and applications of plateletpheresis, and platelet cryopreservation methodology. Comprehensive discussions of these subjects may be found in the references cited in the introduction (42,82). It is my hope that the clinician and/or transfusionist who is interested in a rationale for the appropriate use of platelet therapy will have found such a rationale in the preceding discussion.

REFERENCES

1. Aisner, J.: Clinical use of platelet transfusions for patients with cancer. In: Platelet Physiology and Transfusion. Washington, D.C., American Association of Blood Banks, 1978, p.39.
2. Aisner, J., Schiffer, C.A., Wolff, J.H. et al.: A standardized technique for efficient platelet and leukocyte collection using the Model 30 Blood Processor. Transfusion 16:437, 1976.
3. Ashurst, D.E., Bedford, D., Coombs, R.R.A.: Examination of human platelets for the ABO, MN, Rh, Tj^a, Lutheran and Lewis system of antigens by means of mixed erythrocyte-platelet agglutination. Vox. Sang. 1:235, 1956.
4. Aster, R.H.: Effect of anticoagulant and ABO incompatibility on recovery of transfused human platelets. Blood 26:732, 1965,
5. Aster, R.H.: J. Clin. Invest. 45:645, 1966.
6. Aster, R.H.: The Platelet. Baltimore, Williams and Wilkins, 1971, p. 153.
7. Aster, R.H.: Hematology. New York, McGraw-Hill, 1977, p. 1341.
8. Aster, R.H.: Hematology, ed. 2. New York, McGraw-Hill Book Co. Inc., 1977, p. 1317.
9. Aster, R.H., Jandl, J.H.: Platelet sequestration in man. I. Methods. J. Clin. Invest. 43:843, 1964.
10. Aster, R.H., Szatkowski, N., Liebert, M. et al.: Expression of HLA-B12, HLA-B8, w4, and w6 on platelets. Transplant. Proc. 9:1965, 1977.
11. Bachman, F., McKenna, R., Cole, E.R. et al.: The hemostatic mechanism after open-heart surgery. J. Thorac. Cardiovasc. Surg. 70:76, 1975.
12. Barbui, T., Baudo, F., Ciavarella, N. et al.: Spectrum of Von Willebrand's disease: a study of 100 cases. Br. J. Haematol. 35:101, 1977.
13. Bick, R.L., Schmalhorst, W.R., Arbegast, N.R.: Alterations of hemostasis associated with cardiopulmonary bypass. Thromb. Res. 8:285, 1976.
14. Bowie, E.J., Owen, C.A. Jr.: Hemostatic failure in clinical medicine. Semin. Hematol. 14:341, 1977.
15. Brand, A., Van Leeuwen, A., Eernisse, J.G. et al.: Platelet trans-

fusion therapy. Optimal donor selection with a combination of lymphocytotoxicity and platelet fluorescence tests. Blood 51:781, 1978.

16. Brand, A., Van Leeuwen, A., Eernisse, J.G. et al.: Platelet immunology with special regard to platelet transfusion therapy. Excerpta Medica Int. Congress Series No. 415:639, 1978.

17. Button, L.N., De Wolf, W., Newburger, P. et al.: The effect of irradiation upon blood components. In: Proceedings of the 17th International Congress of Hematology, in press.

18. Chediak, J., Maxey, B., Desser, R.: Successful management of bleeding in a patient with a Factor V inhibitor by platelet transfusions, abstracted. Blood 54:273a, 1979.

19. Cohen, E., Feliciano, H., Glidewell, O.: Platelet increments following transfusion of ABO group specific and nonspecific platelets. Transfusion, 8:310, 1968.

20. Cohen, P., Gardner, F.H.: Platelet preservation. II. Preservation of canine platelet concentrates by freezing in solutions of glycerol plasma. J. Clin. Invest. 41:10, 1962.

21. Colombani, J.: Blood platelets in HL-A serology. Transplant. Proc. 3:1078, 1971.

22. Coombs, R.R.A., Bedford, D.: The A and B antigens on human platelets demonstrated by means of mixed erythrocyte platelet agglutination. Vox. Sang. 5:11, 1955.

23. Counts, R.B., Haisch, C., Simon, T.L. et al.: Hemostasis in massively transfused trauma patients. Ann. Surg. 190:91, 1979.

24. Daly, P.A., Schiffer, C.A., Aisner, J. et al.: Successful transfusion of platelets cryopreserved for more than 3 years. Blood, 54:1023, 1979.

25. Daly, P.A., Schiffer, C.A., Aisner, J. et al.: Platelet transfusion therapy: One-hour posttransfusion increments are valuable in predicting the need for HLA-matched preparations. JAMA 243:435, 1980.

26. Dayian, G., Pert, J.H.: A simplified method for freezing human blood platelets in glycerol-glucose using a statistically controlled cooling rate device. Transfusion 19:255, 1979.

27. Dayian, G., Rowe, A.W.: Cryopreservation of human platelets for transfusion: A glycerol-glucose, moderate rate cooling procedure. Cryobiology 13:1, 1976.

28. Duquesnoy, R.J., Anderson, A.J., Tomasulo, P.A. et al.: ABO compatibility and platelet transfusion of alloimmunized thrombocytopenic patients. Blood 54:595, 1979.

29. Duquesnoy, R.J., Filip, D.J., Aster, R.H.: Influence of HLA-A2 on the effectiveness of platelet transfusions in alloimmunized thrombocytopenic patients. Blood 50:407, 1977.

30. Duquesnoy, R.J., Filip, D.J., Rodey, G.E. et al.: Successful transfusion of platelets 'mismatched' for HLA antigens to alloimmunized thrombocytopenic patients. Am. J. Hematol. 2:219, 1977.

31. Duquesnoy, R.J., Filip, D.J., Tomasulo, P.A. et al.: Role of HLA-C matching in histocompatible platelet transfusion therapy of alloimmunized thrombocytopenic patients. Transplant. Proc. 9:1827, 1977.

32. Duquesnoy, R.J., Testin, J., Aster, R.H.: Variable expression of w4 and w6 on platelets. Possible relevance to platelet transfusion therapy of alloimmunized thrombocytopenic patients. Transplant.

Proc. 9:1829, 1977.

33. Eisner, E.V., Shahidi, N.T.: Immune thrombocytopenia due to a drug metabolite. N. Engl. J. Med. 187:376, 1972.

34. Federal Register, Proposed Rules. Washington, D.C., Jan. 15, 1980 Vol. 45, No. 10, p. 2852.

35. Food and Drug Administration: Code of Federal Regulations, Platelet concentrates (human), Sect. 640.24, Processing, p. 119.

36. Freireich, E.J., Kliman, A., Gaydos, L.A. et al.: Response to repeated platelet transfusion from the same donor. Ann. Intern. Med. 59:277, 1963.

37. Gaydos, L.A., Freireich, E.J., Mantel, N.: The quantitative relation between platelet count and hemorrhage in patients with acute leukemia. N. Engl. J. Med. 266:905, 1962.

38. Gloster, E.S., Strauss, R.A.: Clinical Hematology for Blood Bankers. Inherited and acquired platelet disorders, p. 183-213, 1979.

39. Gmur, J., Von Felten, A., Frick, P.: Platelet support in polysensitized patients: Role of HLA specificities and crossmatch testing for donor selection. Blood 51:903, 1978.

40. Goldfinger, D., McGinniss, M.H.: Rh-incompatible platelet transfusions - risks and consequences of sensitizing immunosuppressed patients. N. Engl. J.Med. 284:942, 1971.

41. Graw, R.G. Jr., Herzig, G.P., Eisel, R.J. et al.: Leukocyte and platelet collection from normal donors with the continuous flow blood cell separator. Transfusion 11:94, 1971.

42. Greenwalt, T.J., Jamieson, G.A. (eds.): The Blood Platelet in Transfusion Therapy. New York, Alan R. Liss Inc., 1978.

43. Grumet, F.C., Yankee, R.A.: Long-term platelet support of patients with aplastic anemia. Ann. Intern. Med. 73:1, 1970.

44. Gunson, H.H., Stratton, F., Cooper, D.G. et al.: Primary immunization of Rh-negative volunteers. Br. Med. J. 1:593, 1970.

45. Gurevitch, J., Nelken, D.: ABO groups in blood platelets. J. Lab. Clin. Med. 44:562, 1954.

46. Gurevitch, J., Nelken, D.: Studies on platelet antigens III. Rh-Hr antigens in platelets. Vox. Sang. 2:342, 1957.

47. Handin, R.I., Valeri, C.R.: Improved viability of previously frozen platelets. Blood 40:509, 1972.

48. Harbury, C.B., Galvan, C.: Surgically acquired platelet storage pool deficiency, abstracted. Proceedings of the 18th Annual Meeting of the American Society of Hematology, 1975, p. 195.

49. Harker, L.A.: The role of the spleen in thrombokinetics. J. Lab. Clin. Med. 77:247, 1971.

50. Harker, L.A., Slichter, S.J.: The bleeding time as a screening test for evaluation of platelet function. N. Engl. J. Med. 287:155, 1972.

51. Hathaway, W.E.: Bleeding disorders due to platelet dysfunction. Am. J. Dis. Child. 121:127, 1971.

52. Hester, J.P., McCredie, K.B., Freireich, E.J.: Platelet replacement therapy: A clinical assessment. The Blood Platelet in Transfusion Therapy. New York, Alan R. Liss Inc. 1978, p. 281.

53. Herzig, R.H., Herzig, G.P., Bull, M.I. et al.: Correction of poor platelet transfusion responses with leukocyte-poor HLA-matched platelet concentrates. Blood 46:743, 1975.

54. Higby, D.J., Cohen, E., Holland, J.F. et al.: The prophylactic treatment of thrombocytopenic leukemic patients with platelets: A

double blind study. Transfusion 14:440, 1974.

55. Holley, T.R., Van Epps, D.E., Harvey, R.I. et al.: Effect of high doses of radiation on human neutrophil chemotaxis, phagocytosis, and morphology. Am. J. Pathol. 75:61, 1974.

56. Howard, J.E., Perkins, H.A.: The natural history of alloimmunization to platelets. Transfusion, 18:496, 1978.

57. Koepke, J.A., Wu, K.K., Hoak, J.C. et al.: A comparison of platelet production methods suitable for a service-oriented blood donor center. Transfusion 15:39, 1957.

58. Krevans, J.R., Jackson, D.P.: Hemorrhagic disorder following massive whole blood transfusions. JAMA 159:171, 1955.

59. Lackner, H.: Hemostatic abnormalities associated with dysproteinemias. Semin. Hematol. 10:125, 1973.

60. Lawler, S.D., Shatwell, H.S.: Are Rh antigens restricted to red cells? Vox. Sang. 7:488, 1962.

61. Lewis, J.H., Draude, J., Kuhns, W.J.: Coating of 'O' platelets with A and B group substances. Vox. Sang. 5:434, 1960.

62. Liebert, M., Aster, R.H.: Expression of HLA-B12 on platelets, on lymphocytes and in serum: A quantitative study. Tissue Antigens 9:199, 1977.

63. Lim, R.C. Jr., Olcott, C.IV, Robinson, A.J.: Platelet response and coagulation changes following massive blood replacement. J. Trauma 13:577, 1973.

64. Lohrmann, H., Bull, M.I., Decter, J.A. et al.: Platelet transfusion from HL-A compatible unrelated donors to alloimmunized patients. Ann. Intern. Med. 80:9, 1974.

65. McKenna, R., Bachmann, F., Whittaker, B. et al.: The hemostatic mechanism after open heart surgery. J. Thorac. Cardiovasc. Surg. 70:298, 1975.

66. McKenzie, F.N., Dhall, D.P., Arfors, K.E., et al: Blood platelet behaviour during and after open heart surgery. Br. Med. J. 2:795, 1969.

67. Mielke, C.H. Jr., Kaneshiro, M.M., Maher, I.A. et al.: The standardized normal Ivy bleeding time and its prolongation by aspirin. Blood 34:204, 1969.

68. Miller, R.O., Robbins, T.O., Tong, M.J. et al.: Coagulation defects associated with massive blood transfusion. Am. Surg. 174:794, 1971.

69. Mittal, K.K., Rider, E.A., Green, D.: Matching of histocompatibility (HLA-A) antigens for platelet transfusion. Blood 47:31, 1976.

70. Mittal, K.K., Terasaki, P.I.: Serological crossreactivity in the HLA system. Tissue Antigens 2:146, 1974.

71. Moriau, M., Masure, R., Hurlet, A. et al.: Hemostasis disorders in open heart surgery with extracorporeal circulation. Vox. Sang. 32:41, 1977.

72. Morrison, F.S.: The effect of filters on the efficiency of platelet transfusion. Transfusion 6:493, 1966.

73. Murphy, S., Koch, P.A., Evans, A.E.: Randomized trial of prophylactic vs. therapeutic platelet transfusion in childhood acute leukemia, abstracted. Clin. Res. 24:379a, 1976.

74. Murphy, S., Sayar, S.N., Abdou, N.L. et al.: Platelet preservation by freezing. Use of dimethylsulfoxide as cryoprotective agent. Transfusion 14:139, 1974.

75. Nagasawa, T., Kim, B.K., Baldini, M.G.: Temporary suppression of circulating antiplatelet alloantibodies by the massive infusion

of fresh, stored, or lyophilized platelets. Transfusion 18:429, 1978.

76. Nakamoto, S., Kolff, W.J.: Hemorrhagic diathesis in uremia and the avoidance of bleeding problems during dialysis. Ann. N.Y. Acad. Sci. 115:348, 1964.

77. Nusbacher, J., Scher, M.L., MacPherson, J.L.: Plateletpheresis using the Haemometics Model 30 Cell Separator. Vox. Sang. 33:9, 1977.

78. Opelz, G., Terasaki, P.I.: Improvement of kidney-graft survival with increased numbers of blood transfusions. N. Engl. J. Med. 299:799, 1978.

79. Pfisterer, H., Thierfelder, S., Stich, W. et al.: ABO Rh blood groups and platelet transfusion. Blut 17:1, 1968.

80. Rabiner, S.F.: Uremic bleeding. Prog. Hemostas. Thromb. 1:233, 1972.

81. Roy, A.J., Jaffe, N., Djerassi, I.: Prophylactic platelet transfusions in children with acute leukemia: A dose response study. Transfusion 13:283, 1973.

82. Schiffer, C.A. (ed.): Platelet Physiology and Transfusion. Washington DC, American Association of Blood Banks, 1978.

83. Schiffer, C.A., Aisner, J., Wiernik, P.H.: Platelet transfusion therapy for patients with leukemia. The Blood Platelet in Transfusion Therapy. New York, Alan R. Liss Inc., pp. 276-279, 1978.

84. Schiffer, C.A., Aisner, J., Wiernik, P.H.: Frozen autologous platelet transfusion for patients with leukemia. N. Engl. J. Med. 299:7, 1978.

85. Schiffer, C.A., Buchholz, D.H., Wiernik, P.H.: Intensive multiunit plateletpheresis of normal donors. Transfusion 16:321, 1976.

86. Schiffer, C.A., Lichtenfeld, J.L., Wiernik, P.H. et al.: Antibody response in patients with acute leukemia. Cancer 37:2177, 1976.

87. Schiffer, C.A., Weinstein, J.H., Wiernik, P.H.: Methicillin associated thrombocytopenia. Ann. Intern. Med. 85:338, 1976.

88. Schiffer, L.M., Atkins, H.L., Chanana, A.D. et al.: Extracorporeal irradiation of the blood in humans. Effects upon erythrocyte survival. Blood 27:831, 1966.

89. Sheldon, G.F., Lim, R.C.Jr., Blaisdell, F.W.: The use of fresh blood in treatment of critically injured patients. J. Trauma 15: 670, 1975.

90. Shulman, N.R.: Immunological considerations attending platelet transfusion. Transfusion 6:39, 1966.

91. Shulman, N.R., Marder, V.J., Hiller, M.C. et al.: Platelet and leukocyte isoantigens and their antibodies: serologic, physiologic and clinical studies. Prog. Hematol. 4:222, 1964.

92. Shulman, N.R., Watkins, S.P. Jr., Itscoitz, S.B. et al.: Evidence that the spleen retains the youngest and hemostatically most effective platelets. Trans. Assoc. Am. Physicians 81:302, 1968.

93. Silvergleid, A.J., Hafgleid, E.B., Harabin, M.A.: Clinical value of washed-platelet concentrates in patients with non-hemolytic transfusion reactions. Transfusion 17:33, 1976.

94. Simon, T.L., Henderson, R.: Coagulation factor activity in platelet concentrates. Transfusion 19:186, 1979.

95. Simpson, J.G., Stalher, A.L.: The concept of disseminated intravascular coagulation. Clin. Haematol. 2:189, 1973.

96. Simpson, M.B.: Platelet function and transfusion therapy in the

surgical patient. Platelet Physiology and Transfusion. Washington, DC, American Association of Blood Banks, p. 51-67, 1978.

97. Slichter, S.J.: Selection of compatible platelet donors. Platelet Physiology and Transfusion. Washington, DC, American Association of Blood Banks, pp. 83-92, 1978.

98. Solomon, J., Bentler, E., Bofenkamp, R. et al.: Indication for the administration of platelet transfusions during remission induction therapy of acute leukemia, abstracted. Blood 50(suppl.):210, 1977.

99. Spector, J.I., Yarmala, J.A., Marchionni, L.D. et al.: Viability and function of platelets frozen at 2 to 3C per minute with 4 or 5 per cent DMSO and stored at -80°C for 8 months. Transfusion 17: 8, 1977.

100. Stefanini, M.: Studies on the hemostatic breakdown during massive replacement transfusions. Am. J. Med. Sci. 244:298, 1962.

101. Stern, K., Davidson, I., Masartis, L.: Experimental studies on Rh immunization. Am. J. Clin. Pathol. 26:833, 1956.

102. Stuart, M.J., Murphy, S., Oski, F.A. et al.: Platelet function in recipients of platelets from donors ingesting aspirin. N. Engl. J. Med. 287:1105, 1972.

103. Svejgaard, A., Kissmeyer-Nielsen, F.: Crossreactive human HLA iso-antibodies. Nature 219:868, 1968.

104. Svejgaard, A., Kissmeyer-Nielsen, F., Thorsby, E.: HL-A typing of platelets. Histocompatibility Testing 1970. Copenhagen, Munksgaard, p. 160, 1970.

105. Szymanski, I.O., Patti, K., Kliman, A.: Efficacy of the Latham Blood Separator to perform plateletpheresis. Transfusion 13:405, 1973.

106. Technical Manual, ed. 7. Washington, DC, American Association of Blood Banks, p. 240, 1977.

107. Thorsby, E., Hegelson, A., Gjendal, T.: Repeated platelet trans-fusions from HLA compatible unrelated sibling donors. Tissue An-tigens 2:397, 1972.

108. Tomasulo, P.A.: Management of the alloimmunized patient with HLA-matched platelets. Platelet Physiology and Transfusion. Washington, DC, American Association of Blood Banks, p. 69-81, 1978.

109. Tosato, G., Applebaum, R., Deisseroth, A.B.: HLA-matched platelet transfusion therapy of severe aplastic anemia. Blood 52:846, 1978.

110. Tosato, G., Appelbaum, F.R., Trapani, R.J. et al.: Use of in vitro assays in selection of compatible platelet donors. Transfusion 20: 47, 1980.

111. Valeri, C.R.: Hemostatic effectiveness of liquid-preserved and previously frozen human platelets. N. Engl. J. Med. 290:353, 1974.

112. Valeri, C.R.: Circulation and hemostatic effectiveness of platelets stored at 4C or 22C: Studies in aspirin-treated normal volunteers. Transfusion 16:20, 1976.

113. Van der Weerdt, C.M.: Platelet Antigens and Isoimmunization. Thesis, Drukkerij Aemstelstad, Amsterdam, 1965.

114. Van Eys, J., Thomas, D., Olivos, B.: Platelet use in pediatric on-cology: A review of 393 transfusions. Transfusion 18:169, 1978.

115. Van Rood, J.J., Van Leeuwen, A., Keuning, J. et al.: The serologic recognition of the human MLC determinants using a modified cyto-toxicity technique. Tissue Antigens 5:73, 1975.

116. Wiener, A.S., Sonn Gordon, A.B.: Simple method of preparing anti-Rh serum in normal male donors. Am. J. Clin. Pathol. 17:67, 1947.

117. Weiss, H.J., Aledort, L.M.: Impaired platelet/connective tissue reaction in man after aspirin ingestion. Lancet 2:495, 1967.
118. Weiss, H.J., Rogers, J.: Correction of the platelet abnormality in Von Willebrand's disease by cryoprecipitate. Am. J. Med. 53: 734, 1972.
119. Weiss, H.J., Aledort, L.M., Kochwa, S.: The effect of salicylates on the hemostatic properties of platelets in man. J. Clin. Invest. 74:2169, 1968.
120. Wu, K.K., Hoak, J.C., Koepke, J.A. et al.: Selection of compatible platelet donors: A prospective evaluation of three cross-matching techniques. Transfusion 17:638, 1977.
121. Wu, K.K., Hoak, J.C., Thompson, J.S. et al.: Use of platelet aggregometry in selection of compatible platelet donors. N. Engl. J. Med. 292:134, 1975.
122. Yankee, R.A., Graff, K.S., Dowling, R. et al.: Selection of unrelated compatible platelet donors by lymphocyte HL-A matching. N. Engl. J. Med. 760, 1973.
123. Yankee, R.A., Grumet, F.C., Rogentine, G.N.: Platelet transfusion therapy: the selection of compatible platelet donors for refractory patients by lymphocyte HL-A typing. N. Engl. J. Med. 281:1208, 1969.
124. Zaroulis, C.G., Spector, J.I., Emerson, C.P. et al.: Therapeutic transfusions of previously frozen washed human platelets. Transfusion 19:371, 1979.

CRYOPRESERVATION OF PLATELET CONCENTRATE: A COMPARISON OF DMSO AND GLYCEROL SYSTEMS

H. Von Bartheld, F. Arnaud, P.C. Das and C. Th. Smit Sibinga

INTRODUCTION

The concept of specific blood component therapy is a comparatively young discipline. The demand for support for thrombocytopenic patients with platelet concentrates has increased considerably, especially in leukemia and oncology units. Routinely prepared platelets have 2-3 days shelf life. The preserved platelets from compatible donors for alloimmunized patients or patients before undergoing treatment, or when they are in remission (autologous platelets) for a longer period of time would be of considerable importance. With this in mind we conceived a platelet freezing program.

METHODS

Two approaches are available:
1. DMSO as freezing solution as practiced in Schiffers' laboratory (5).
2. Glycerol as freezing solution, as practiced in Germany and Sweden and described by Pert and his colleagues (1,4).

Both methods follow a somewhat common pathway (Fig. 1):
1. Blood (450 ml CPD) is gently centrifuged at room temperature (1200 g for 9 min.) to obtain platelet rich plasma (PRP). In the glycerol method this is acidified to pH 6.5 (10 ml per 100 ml PRP). Platelet concentrate (PC) is obtained (1400 g at room temperature for 30 min.) and the supernatant platelet poor plasma (PPP) deep frozen for subsequent use.
2. The platelet concentrate is transferred to a special freezing bag, and the cryopreservative solution added. For 10 ml of platelet concentrate 10 ml of 10% DMSO is added over 7 min. with continuous agitation to dissipate heat. The Pert method uses 5 ml platelet concentrate and 5 ml glycerol added over 2 min.
3. The bag is put into a hard board metal cassette and frozen and stored in the vapor phase of nitrogen for DMSO system, or frozen in the liquid phase and stored in the vapor phase of the nitrogen for the glycerol system.
4. Thawing in the DMSO system was at 37°C for 10 min., then

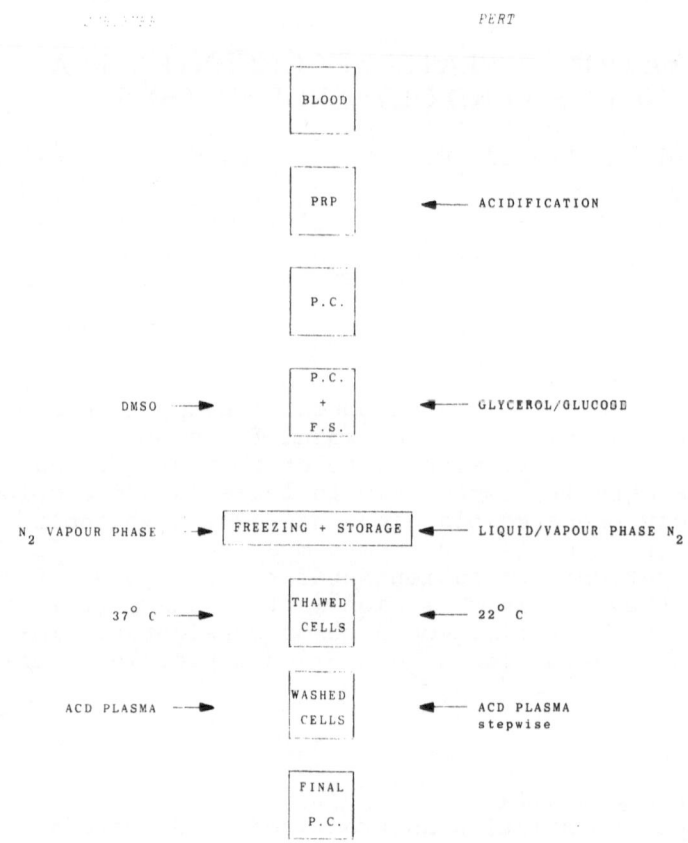

Fig. 1. Comparison of freezing protocol DMSO vs. glycerol.

20 ml of plasma was added over 7 min. while the bags
were gently shaken. The platelets were transferred to a
giving bag centrifuged for 30 min. at room temperature,
the supernatant plasma removed and fresh plasma at volume
of 15 ml added. In the glycerol system thawing was done
at 22°C for 10 min. Then at 15 min. intervals 10 ml, 20
ml and another 20 ml of plasma was added.

Following a final rest period of 30 min. the bag is centrifuged and the supernatant plasma removed leaving about
15 ml plasma with the platelets.

In both systems platelets are allowed to stand one hour
at room temperature before being re-suspended.

ASSESSMENT

Functional study of platelets is like an impressionist painting, never finished. We have arbitrarily chosen 3 systems:
hypotonic shock response (HSR), aggregation by ristocetin
and 3 hours clot retraction - all presented as percentages

TABLE I. Platelet function (%) in cryopreservation; DMSO vs. glycerol

	DMSO system			Glycerol system		
	Mean (SD)		N	Mean (SD)		N
Before freezing						
H.S.R.	62.1 (10.9)		30	52.3 (11.1)		7
Aggregation	81.2 (12.1)		27	71.7 (20.6)		7
Clot retraction	66.3 (11.6)		26	63.5 (7.4)		7
After thawing						
H.S.R.	20.6 (12.3)		20	3.9 (8.3)	*	8
Aggregation	59.7 (12.5)		18	26.9 (25.6)	*	8
Clot retraction	49.6 (16.1)		18	17.3 (7)	*	8

* significant difference ($p < 0.05$)

(Table I). Of these three test systems, hypotonic shock response seems to be a robust test indicating overall platelet membrane functions and is about 60% in fresh control platelets. Platelet count was done by Coulter counter and by phase contrast microscopy, and morphology by light and electron microscopy. The yield of platelets after freezing in DMSO and glycerol is about 70%. The electron microscopy picture suggest at least 50% of the platelets suffer freeze damage to some extent. As expected, the functional parameters do not show any significant difference before freezing in both systems. But after freezing all the three functional parameters are significantly higher in DMSO indicating better preservation (Table I). So far we have concentrated on routine platelets, harvested manually from ordinary blood donations and pooled. We next collected platelets by machine apheresis (cell separator machine: Hemometics model 30). The end results show that apheresis concentrates could also be effectively frozen (Table II). However, since the anticoagulants are different for both collection techniques, we looked at the different steps in some detail. Compared to CPD the pH of the ACD machine collected platelets was lower but never below 6.7 (Fig. 2). The HSR activity follows a parallel curve (Fig. 3). The reduction of aggregation during handling occurs at a rate very similar in CPD and ACD anticoagulants (Fig. 4).

For in vivo study, frozen platelets were tagged with ^{51}Cr. Since very little information is available on labelling of frozen platelets, we also labelled fresh non frozen platelets as control, left both at room temperature and followed them for 5 days. This in vitro experiment shows (Fig. 5) that over 24 hours 90% activity is retained in fresh compared to 81% in the frozen platelets, although the percentage of radioactivity in the cells was low.

Graphically, it demonstrates that activity diminishes in the test tubes more easily for frozen platelets but, of course, the active platelets immediately after labelling at

TABLE II. Platelet function (%) in cryopreservation manual vs. apheresis collection

	Manual			Apheresis		
	Mean	(SD)	N	Mean	(SD)	N
Before freezing						
H.S.R.	62.1	(10.9)	30	58.9	(15.4)	9
Aggregation	81.2	(12.1)	27	86.5	(9.7)	9
Clot retraction	66.3	(11.6)	26	60.3	(16.3)	9
After thawing						
H.S.R.	20.6	(12.3)	20	17.4	(11.8)	13
Aggregation	59.7	(12.5)	18	37.1	(16.3)*	11
Clot retraction	49.6	(16.1)	18	58.1	(13)	8

*significant difference (p < 0,001)

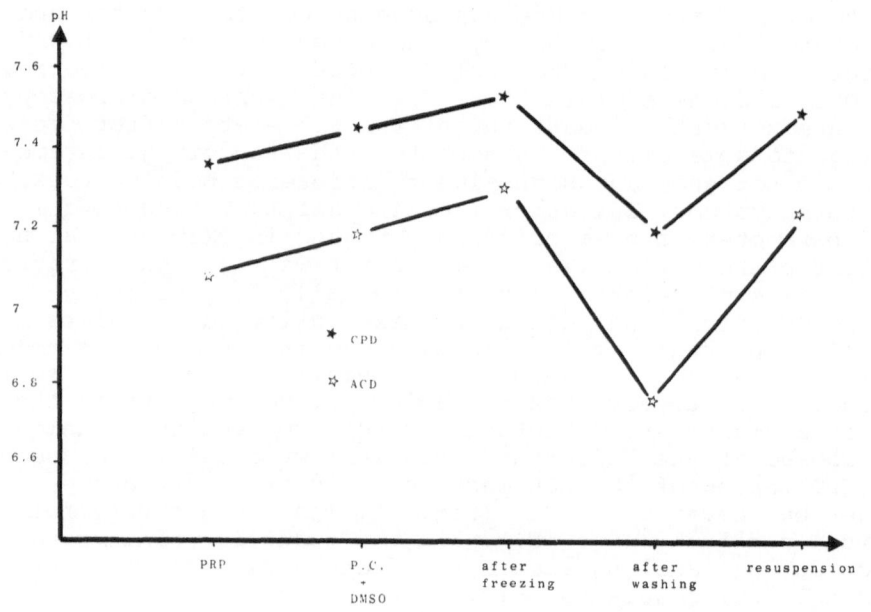

Fig. 2. Platelet function in cryopreservation pH in CPD and ACD.

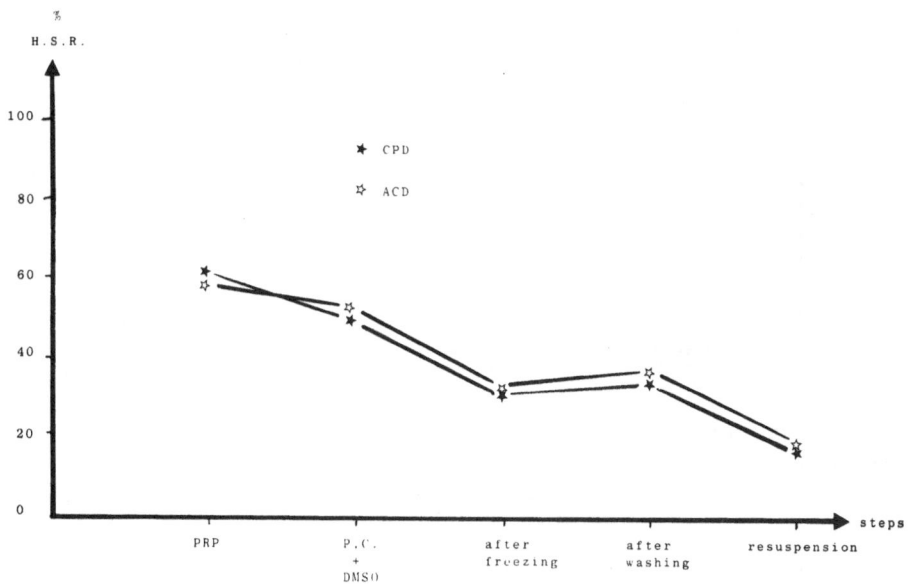

Fig. 3. Platelet function in cryopreservation H.S.R. (%) in CPD and ACD.

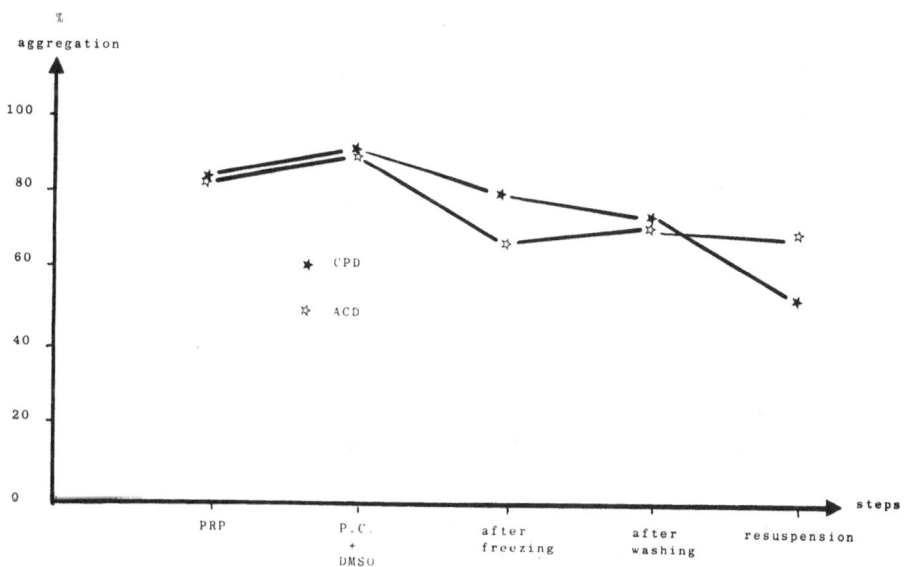

Fig. 4. Platelet function in cryopreservation aggregation (%) in CPD and ACD.

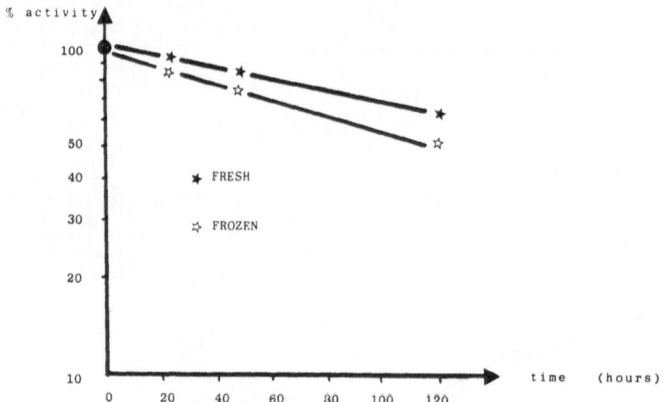

Fig. 5. Comparison of labelling between fresh and frozen platelets presented in % of activity.

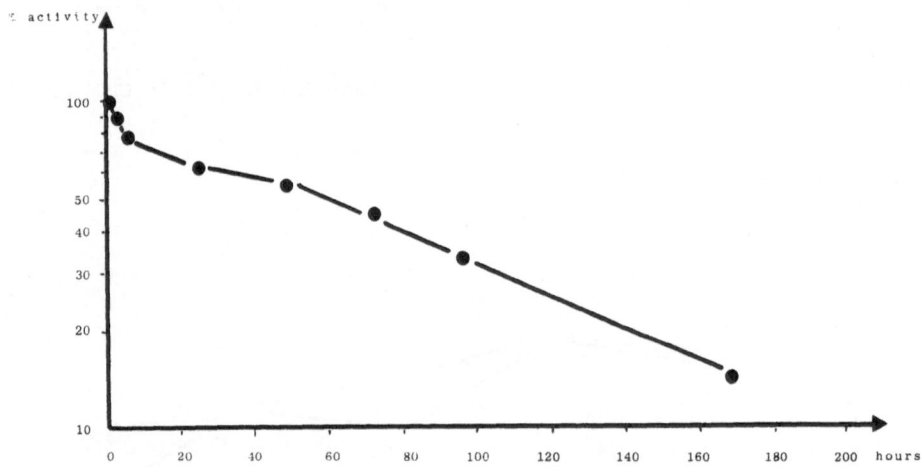

Fig. 6. In vivo survival of frozen platelets presented in % of activity experiment 1.

0 hour, would be used for in vivo experiments. Platelets from two healthy individuals, after freezing and storage for 6 weeks and 3 months, were used, and after labelling autologously given for in vivo survival studies. Samples were taken for 5 days and activity was analyzed as percentage activity (Table III and Fig. 6) and count per minute. In the experiments this represented a half life of 3.7 days or about 8 days of platelet life span. This compares favorably with fresh platelets showing 7-10 days of circulating life span. No untoward reaction or unpleasant smell of DMSO was noted.

TABLE III. In vivo survival of frozen platelets % of activity

Time	Experiment 1	Experiment 2
3 min.	-	-
30 min.	100	100
2 hr	87.5	96.1
4 hr	76.6	87
24 hr	61.5	68.7
48 hr	54	58.3
72 hr	42.6	51
96 hr	33.1	50.9
120 hr	-	47.4
144 hr	-	-
168 hr	14.3	40.3

CONCLUSION

Of the two methods investigated, DMSO seems to provide a better cryoprotectant for platelets. The yield of 70% after thawing is only a platelet count, it does not indicate their viability. For clinical efficacy we have used frozen platelets in a neonate with iso-immune thrombocytopenia and a leukemic adult. The frozen platelets derived from the mother had immediate clinical effect with excellent one hour post infusion platelet rise in the child. In the multitransfused refractory adult, however, the results were marginal; this was not unexpected since the frozen platelets collected from siblings were not completely HL-A matched.

We are concentrating our work on the in vivo recovery of frozen platelets by stock-piling platelets from leukemic patients who are in a remission phase. The platelet freezing story is by no means over, and still remains an impressionist painting requiring more colors and more lights.

REFERENCES

1. Dayin, C., Rowe, A.W.: Cryopreservation for human platelets for transfusion, a glycerol-glucose, moderate cooling procedure. Cryobiology 13:1, 1976.
2. Kahn, R.A., Staggs, S.D., Miller, W.V., Heaton, W.A.: Recovery, life span and function of C.P.D.-adenine platelet concentrates stored for up to 72 hours at 4°C. Transfusion 20:498, 1980.
3. De Maat, C.E.M.: De biologische halveringstijd van met Cr51 gemerkte bloedplaatjes. Ph.D. thesis, University of Utrecht, 1969.
4. Pert, J.M.: A simplified method for freezing human blood platelets in glycerol glucose using a statically controlled cooling rate device. Transfusion 19:253, 1979.
5. Schiffer, C.A. et al.: Frozen autologous platelet transfusion for patients with leukemia. New Engl. Med. 299:7, 1978.
6. Scott, E.P., Slichter, S.J.: Viability and function of platelet concentrates stored in CPD-adenine. Transfusion 20:489, 1980.

Discussion

Moderator: R.A. Kahn

R.A. Kahn, St. Louis, USA:

I want to ask dr. Ten Cate a question regarding the Hammerstein syndrome you described. Apparently this was treated successfully by the administration of aspirin, which suggests that the patient had an abnormal or continuous release reaction in the platelets. Do you have any electron microscope studies of these platelets and perhaps any studies on the molecular mechanism of the disorder?

J.W. Ten Cate, Amsterdam:

Indeed we did some more studies in order to define and correct the defect. We did not attempt to count the granules in cells in order to detect depletion. Serotonin contents were normal, the plasma BTG was increased, corrected also during aspirin therapy. After interruption of the aspirin it increased again. Anyhow, it reveals an enormous interaction and reactivity of the platelets with the vessel wall.

W.G. Van Aken, Amsterdam:

Can anyone comment on the clinical significance or physiological significance of the beta-thromboglobulin? More specifically, I would be interested to know if it really is dangerous or not for the organism when a high level of this protein is present.
Dr. Cobert told us that platelet transfusions with high amounts of beta-thromboglobulin are probably given by most of us. I would be interested to know whether perhaps beta-thromboglobulin affects for instance vessel wall function, as has been indicated in the past.

B.L. Cobert, New York, USA:

The actual function of BTG is not known. So one can only speculate on whether high levels are bad or not. If you look at it as a marker of the release reaction for continuous platelet aggregation, one might be very worried in a patient who had had for example myocardial infarction and 5 months later would still have elevated aggregation or release reaction as measured by BTG. I think in any disease state in which platelet aggregation and release reaction is suspected to play a role, not necessarily causitive it would be potentially useful in looking at BTG levels.

J.W. Ten Cate, Amsterdam:

I remember an abstract where interference of BTG with the PGI-2 production of endothelial cells was reported. When that is correct then that could answer in some way your question: it could eventually increase the arterial thrombotic process, just by inhibition of production of this physiological so important platelet aggregation-inhibitor. Secondly, I believe it is a reflection of release and during release all kinds of substances are thrown into the circulation including all kinds of potentially damaging compounds.

C. Vermijlen, Leuven:

Dr. Silvergleid mentioned in his presentation the use of Aspirin as a real platelet killer. Aspirin is a European trademark. Salicylic acid is present in a lot of drugs. It wonders me that all the time Aspirin is named and made responsible for killing the platelets. If we make a questionnaire to our donors, whether they have taken Aspirin, most of them say they have not. If we determine at random in the plasma or in the blood from regular blood donors or plasmapheresis donors salicylates, we do find them at least in 8% of the cases, while the donors answered that they did not take any drug at all.
Dr. Silvergleid stated that the increase of the number of platelets in the peripheral blood 1 hr after transfusion is a good parameter for hemostatic function. I agree completely, but I think that this is just the case when you are transfusing platelets for prophylactic purposes, because I hope that when you transfuse them for an acute bleeding, they have disappeared after 1 hr, and are consumed into the bleeding sites. Therefore I think, that the best test to assess platelet function is to perform 15 min after transfusion the bleeding time, because then you have the real hemostatic function of the perfused platelets. If you are transfusing fixed platelets, there will be a normal survival after 1 hr.

A.J. Silvergleid, San Bernardino, USA:

Thank you for the comments. Certainly someone who is experiencing an acute bleed and transfused with platelets, I think you have better parameters than 1 hr platelet count. You can see the arrested hemostasis, which is a lot better and more important than doing a 1 hr count. I agree with your comment about salicylates. It is quite commonly found. We did a study on patients having hip surgery and were going to give them Aspirin in prophylaxis and 50% of them said, they never had taken Aspirin. We had to eliminate 25% of all the patients because they all had an Aspirin level. A good study by Stewart has shown that you only need 15 to 20% of your platelet pool to be normal in order to have normal hemostasis. So an individual who is totally Aspirinated with acetyl-salicylic acid has a normal bleeding time after 1 or 2 days, and will have normal platelets. In addition, if you are going to transfuse patients with platelets, you usually will give 4 to 6 or 8 units of platelets and since at least one or two of those are going to come from donors who have taken Aspirin, it does not make sense to eliminate donors who have taken Aspirin from making platelet concentrates.

C. Vermijlen, Leuven:

I am from the Red Cross Bloodbank in Belgium, and I have nothing to do with the Bayer concern, but what is the reason for using a trademark like Aspirin as a platelet killer and not the other drugs containing salicylic acid?

A.J. Silvergleid, San Bernardino:

You are correct. It is acetyl-salicylic acid, where it really is the acetylgroup that is responsible for the damage.

J.G. Jolly, India:

Most of the bloodbanks are storing platelets for a period of 72 hrs at room temperature. Attempts are being made storing the platelets at 4°C after giving treatment. Is there any functional utility for such platelets?

A.J. Silvergleid, San Bernardino:

There is now an extensive amount of data on storage conditions for platelets. I think that most people would agree that storage below 20°C is deleterious to platelet function. In fact in the United States now 4°C stored platelets can only last 48 hrs of storage. We have to store them for 48 hrs, we cannot store them for 72 hrs anymore. This November at the American Association of Blood Banks Meeting, an excellent group in Milwaukee presented data where they had stored platelets at 21°, 19.5° and 18°C, and showed that storage under 20°C caused significant impairment of platelet function and survival[*]. I would suggest that 4°C is not an appropriate temperature to store platelets.

[*] Gottschall, J.L. et al., Transfusion 1981, 21, 619.

J.J. Van Loghem, Amsterdam:

Dr. Silvergleid mentioned many times the importance of all
kinds of antigens and antibodies in regard to platelets.
I think we agree that A and B antigens are not very important, and that probably more important are HL-A antigens and antibodies. However, the most important are the
platelet specific antigens and antibodies. To recognize
these, I think you can do of course a test in vivo to see
how the function is, but more important even is to do a
proper cross-match procedure or any other method, in order
to recognize allo- and auto-antibodies against platelets.
Many methods have been described in the past. As far as
the experience goes in the Central Laboratory of the Bloodtransfusion Service in Amsterdam the test with the immunofluorescent method is the most sensitive to be used for
recognition of all kinds of platelet specific antibodies.
My question to you is: have you done any studies in this
regard? Have you studied this from a point of immunology?
Did you look for a more specific test to recognize antibodies in allo- and auto-immunisation?

A.J. Silvergleid, San Bernardino:

I quite agree that ultimately when you find a patient who
is refractory to platelet therapy, platelet specific antigens are probably the best explanation. From the clinical standpoint it is the very rare patient, however, that
reaches that particular stage where you cannot provide
platelets that give an adequate rise in platelet counts.
So that it is ultimately the best way to assess whether
you are going to get a rise in platelet count, still most
patients can be managed by providing them with type compatible platelets, type specific platelets, HL-A matched
platelets. I myself have not been doing any platelet specific tests. The most popular one in the United States at
this time and the one you are probably familiar with, is
platelet associated IgG by various techniques. This now is
considered an extremely sensitive test for determining
whether or not there are specific antibodies to platelets.
For the selected patient who is not able to be managed with
HL-A typed, or HL-A compatible platelets, one of these
platelet specific tests are certainly indicated. That is
the only way we can do it. With ITP for years, people have
tried to find the antibody. A good test for the antibody
has yet to be developed, that everybody agrees on, although
now platelet associated IgG is considered a good test. I
agree, a platelet specific test is necessary, but I don't
do one. There are laboratories who do each test available.
Each laboratory is convinced that they have the best test.

R.A. Kahn, St. Louis, USA:

We do quite a number of platelet antibody tests on all

kinds of patients. There are quite a number of assays one might use. Some, like your laboratory has developed the immunofluorescent test, are relatively easy compared to the platelet associated IgG test. On the other hand, they all seem to have one major problem. When you think of a cross match test, you think of a test being done prior to transfusion between the donor and the recipient. In this situation, we have a patient who is refractory to random donor platelets, and we wish to get an apheresis donor in. Well, the apheresis donor shows up at the laboratory and you get a sample of blood. They go on the machine and collect these platelets. All of these tests take a long time to perform. Some are in the order of 3 to 5 hours at least. At that time the procedure is over and you are left with the platelet concentrate in your hand, the apheresis concentrate and find out that it is a positive cross match. What are you going to do? Are you going to call an other apheresis donor, since that patient needs the platelets that day, so this will be another delay, or do you take your chances that it might be a false positive? We have taken our chances and given the unit. So it may be true that there is a platelet antibody. One of the unfortunate things of these tests is that they can not discriminate at this point between platelet specific antibodies and HL-A antibodies. The major problem, however, is that you cannot use them in a traditional cross-match setting. You use them more after the fact, as it is a great tool for proving that the platelets did not work, but not necessarily for selecting the best donor.

J.J. Van Loghem, Amsterdam:

The cross-match is of course not always possible and it takes a lot of time. I speak especially about the recognition of allo- and auto-antibodies in patients. For instance in patients with neonatal thrombocytopenia, in all cases you find specific antibodies against the platelets.
There is only one test which is really useful and that is the immunofluorescence test. There is no doubt that all the others are less sensitive. This is not just a remark, this is the result of a study of more than 5 years in our institute. We have compared all these tests. Again I want to say that this is an important test to apply for auto- and allo-antibodies if you want to make diagnostic procedures. There are more than 35 tests described, but only the one I mentioned, is the real good one.

R.A. Kahn, St. Louis:
That is an unbiased endorsement of a test.

C. Vermijlen, Leuven:

I agree that platelet compatibility plays an important role in prophylaxis. That means that for profylactic purposes transfused platelets should stay as long as possible in the circulation.
I think the situation is completely different when you need to have platelets for an acute bleeding. Even if you have at that moment HL-A or platelet antigen incompatibility, the half life of your platelets can be 10 minutes, can be 20 minutes, can be 30 minutes. I think the mechanism whereby the platelets are involved in hemostasis only takes 1 minute, and so the interference with the antibody, which takes several minutes, has nothing to do with the direct impact of platelets on hemostasis.

A.J. Silvergleid, San Bernardino:

I would agree with that comment partially. If you try to correlate the transfusion of someone who is refractory and is hemorrhaging, give platelets and you do not see either response in rising platelet count or decrease in hemorrhage then you can assume that they have been ineffective.
On the other hand, there is good evidence from some studies that suggest that one can overwhelm that response. Some people have transfused large numbers of platelets, blocking the RE system, followed by another transfusion achieving hemostasis.

III. Shock and massive blood loss

PATHOPHYSIOLOGY OF HEMORRHAGIC SHOCK: CLINICAL AND THERAPEUTIC IMPLICATIONS

J.A. Collins

Hemorrhage has been well described as an event that not only stops the machine, but wrecks the machinery. This idea of hemorrhage as a systemic disease with widespread and lasting deleterious effects is important. It implies that the therapeutic focus must be a broad one; the criteria for optimal treatment include much more than the restoration of the circulation to 'normal'. Much of what we know about the effects of hemorrhage and its treatment is based on controlled studies in animals, but studies in humans have revealed aspects of the problem not characteristic of changes that are seen in other species. Careful analysis of the data in fact reveals significant differences in response among the experimental species used for research. The most extensively studied species is the canine, but this is also perhaps the large mammalian species most differ   in response from the human. Much has been learned from these studies but the application to clinical conditions is often not as simple as is sometimes inferred. The differences in survival resulting from the use of different fluids in controlled studies do raise interesting questions however (Table I).

Some basic principles have been deduced, however, that almost certainly are directly applicable to man. Lack of perfusion is more than simply lack of oxygen, and is more rapidly destructive of cells, tissue, and organs than is anoxia alone. Stated another way, anoxic or hypoxic perfusion is vastly preferable to no perfusion. The reasons probably are based on the ability to maintain cellular integrity longer if waste products are removed and perhaps if non-oxygen components are delivered. In clinical terms, the first priority for resuscitation from exsanguinating hemorrhage is to restore perfusion, and secondarily to restore the delivery of oxygen. Volume is initially more important than oxygen-delivering capacity, fluid more important than hemoglobin. Oxygen is required, however, and even perfusion cannot maintain mammalian life in the sustained absence of oxygen at the cellular level.

The other basic principles that apply clinically are that the complications of hemorrhage are related to the degree of hemorrhage, the duration of hypoperfusion, the other (abnormal) conditions existing at the time of

TABLE I. Mortality in hemorrhaged rats treated with various fluids[*]

Groups	Number dead/ number treated	Ratio
Sham shock	0/47	.00
Blood	3/40	.08
Rbc + saline	4/32	.13
Lact. Ringer's 2.5X	10/51	.20
Hydroxyethyl starch	8/33	.24
Lact. Ringer's, equal vol.	9/36	.25
Dextran 70	8/32	.25
Dextran 40	7/22	.32
Plasma	12/38	.32

[*]From Collins, J.A., Braitberg, A., Butcher, H. Surgery 73:401, 1973.

TABLE II. Responses to hemorrhage[*]

Blood loss	Vascular response	Metabolic response	Signs and symptoms
Small (15% of blood volume)	Contraction of great veins; recruitment of ECF	Slight	Mild and transient
Moderate (30%)	Above marked; arteriolar constriction in carcass; perhaps tachycardia, reduced cardiac output	Mild hyperglycemia, mobilization of lipids, slight increase in lactate; decreased urinary sodium and water; hyperventilation, hypocarbic alkalemia	Thirst, apprehension, weakness, orthostatic hypotension, cool skin, pallor
Large (45%)	All above marked; hypotensive, severely reduced cardiac output	Severe lactic acidosis, oliguria, mixed venous PO$_2$ below 30 ton	Unobtainable blood pressure; severe air hunger; panic, agitation, loss of consciousness

[*]Collins, J.A. See Reference 6.

hemorrhage, and the details of treatment. Subsequent challenges to the organism are more than usually damaging the sooner they occur after severe hemorrhage. Derangements caused by the hemorrhage can persist long after restoration of blood volume and blood flow.

The intrinsic responses to hemorrhage are proportional to the extent of hemorrhage and are ordered (Table II) in sequence (6). Loss of about 15% of blood volume is not life-threatening and usually does not cause persistent hypotension. The great veins (compliance system) contract, allowing perfusion to persist unchanged with a smaller blood volume. Interstitial fluid is shifted into the intravascular space, and preformed albumin is more gradually transferred to the intravascular fluid from extravascular sites of storage. There is some retention of salt and water by the kidneys, mediated by small increases in production of aldosterone and antidiuretic hormone, and a small increase in production of erythropoietin begins the process of restoring the mass of red cells to normal. Production of protein by the liver, especially of albumin, is increased and the rate of destruction of albumin is decreased. Various stress-related hormones, including some coagulation factors, may be raised to above-normal concentrations for several days. The full stress response is not expressed, as there is minimal increase in 17-hydroxy steroids and catecholamines, and little alteration in the body's handling of its fuels.

With a more severe degree of hemorrhage, about 30%, hypotension usually results but life is not endangered unless other conditions are also present. As compared with lesser hemorrhage, the responses are greater in intensity and new responses occur. Perfusion to certain tissues and organs is restricted, generally preserving visceral perfusion. The force and rate of myocardial contraction increases, at least partially preserving the rate of delivery of oxygen to the peripheral tissues but at the cost of increased work by the heart. The 'stress' hormones are released with concomitant alterations in body composition and fuel metabolism, respiration increases producing a mild hypocarbic alkalemia, and urinary output is markedly reduced. If the subject is awake, there is increased alertness and apprehension, and perhaps palpitations and dyspnea. There may be sweating and cold skin. Somatic pain associated with the injury decreases. Less acutely, 2,3 diphosphoglyceric acid increases in the erythrocytes, platelet count usually transiently decreases but the granulocyte count may increase.

If half the blood volume is lost rapidly, life is seriously threatened. The circulation and volume-related responses are greatly surpassed. Perfusion falls sharply to most of the body, including the viscera, with perfusion of the heart and brain the best preserved. Blood pressure is very low or unobtainable, respiration rapid, and the patient may be terrified or confused but usually agitated. Loss of consciousness in a supine patient is a grave sign because loss of perfusion of the brain is often a sign of breakdown of the most rigorously defended responses. Severe lactic acidosis is characteristic and in some species hypoglycemia occurs, but this does not seem to happen commonly in man. Death from hemorrhage during the acute phase probably occurs when the central aortic pressure and consequent coronary blood flow are insufficient to maintain the paradoxically increasing demands of the heart. Once the central pump begins to fail, a viscious circle is entered which rapidly worsens.

Most patients can correct and repair the loss of 30% of their blood volume and perhaps more without external, i.e. medical, help. With losses approaching half a blood volume, however, hypoperfusion may persist long enough without treatment to produce secondary systemic complications. The ability to withstand hemorrhage is much less at the extremes of age, and major pre-existing diseases also reduce the ability to withstand hemorrhage.

In the following sections we will briefly consider some of the complications of hemorrhage, and how these may be changed by specific types of treatment. The principle already inferred, that early and complete restoration of perfusion diminishes complications, applies to all these considerations.

HEART, CIRCULATION, OXYGEN DELIVERY

Persistent damage to and impaired function by the heart is not a common complication of severe hemorrhage except in certain circumstances. In some experimental models, ultrastructural changes have been found in myocardial fibers after fatal hemorrhage (18), but this has been difficult to correlate with functional changes. Nevertheless, the human heart is particularly vulnerable to damage during hemorrhage and legitimate questions have been raised about certain details of treatment as they relate to myocardial function. The heart responds differently to hemorrhage than most of the other organs. Its work-load increases as a result of the compensatory effort to maintain circulation in the face of a decreasing filling pressure and volume of blood. Initially, its oxygen requirements increase. If hemorrhage continues and systemic blood pressure falls, the oxygen requirements of the heart are still increased relative to the amount of oxygen it is pumping via the blood to the systemic circulation. This is because the heart becomes driven by increasing sympathetic neural and hormonal stimulation. The blood supply to the heart flows mainly during diastole and primary as a result of diastolic pressure in the supravalvular aorta. Both time and pressure in diastole decrease with severe hemorrhage, however, at the very time that oxygen requirements increase. The human heart has very limited ability to work at a lower mixed venous tension; relatively small decreases in coronary sinus oxygen tension are associated with decreased performance by the left ventricle. This set of circumstances, some of which are unique to the heart, places great importance on the ability of the coronary arteries to dilate during hemorrhage. The response to sympathetic hormonal stimulation, in fact, is vasodilatation in the coronary vessels and vasoconstriction in most other vascular beds. Coronary atherosclerosis is quite common in industrialized societies, however. Clinical experience indicates that patients with

coronary atherosclerosis tolerate hemorrhage very poorly.
Clinical practice dictates that operation to control hemorrhage be carried out sooner in such patients in spite
of the increased risk of anesthesia and operation. In another form of increased demand, that produced by exercise,
many patients with coronary atherosclerosis who have normal left ventricular function at rest develop deterioration of left ventricular function during exercise in the
form of increased end diastolic volume and decreased ejec-
tion fraction. This abnormality can be completely reversed
by surgically bypassing the coronary arterial block, indicating that the cause is circulatory and is not intrinsic
to the heart muscle (20). Case, Berglund and Sarnoff performed some highly pertinent experiments 25 years ago,
which have still not been surpassed (2). Isolated, working
canine hearts performed well when the hematocrit of the
blood perfusing the coronary vessels was reduced moderately. When the coronary vessels were banded, however, so
that they could not dilate, every decrease in hematocrit
produced a decrease in left ventricular function. These
studies indicated that when coronary perfusion is limited,
the performance of the left ventricle is dependent on the
oxygen-delivering properties of the blood perfusing it.
The clinical equivalent is found in patients with coronary atherosclerosis and chronic anemia, many of whom
have a rather narrow range of hematocrit above which they
are asymptomatic and below which they experience angina
or even overt congestive heart failure. There are certainly patients in whom heart failure can be treated by the
cautious transfusion of red blood cells. If we accept this
as true for anemia, why should the same not be true for
the functional properties of red cells? It is equally as
consistent and logical. The implication is that the functional properties of the red cells used to treat patients
with coronary atherosclerosis are clinically important,
especially in the special circumstances that apply during
hemorrhage. Several investigators have tried to extend the
observations of Case et al. to oxygen-delivering properties other than the quantity of hemoglobin. One experiment
seemed to demonstrate the same phenomenon for exposure to
carbon monoxide (1) but the heart as well as the red cells
were exposed to the carbon monoxide. Another used red cells
with varying concentrations of 2,3 DPG, but adequate controls were lacking (13). Several clinical studies have
dealt directly with the 2,3 DPG content of the blood used
to treat patients with coronary atherosclerosis. One such
experiment compared patients after the coronary block was
corrected, however, and the results in the control group
seemed unusually poor for the model used (11). In another
different kind of red cells were used but the groups of
patients also differed in that those getting functionally
superior blood underwent elective operations while the
others were operated upon after severe hemorrhage (23).
This study did demonstrate, however, that severe left ven-

TABLE III. Survival of rats (ratio living/total) exchanged transfused, hemorrhaged, then transfused with the blood indicated (A), or exchange transfused with three week old blood at hematocrit 25%, then hemorrhaged and transfused with the blood indicated[*]

Hematocrit	Fresh blood	Old blood
	A	
15-20	.63	.24
21-30	.65	.47
30	.59	.57
	B	
20	.75	.90
50	.72	.50

[*]From Collins, J.A. and Stechenberg, L.: Surgery 85:412, 1979.

tricular dysfunction is very common after severe hemorrhage in patients presumed to have coronary atherosclerosis. In spite of the lack of convincing direct demonstration either clinical or experimentally, I find the reasoning compelling and the available evidence supportive. It is highly likely that the functional properties of the red blood cells transfused are clinically important in treating severe hemorrhage in patients with coronary atherosclerosis. In CPD, reasonably good functional properties are maintained in the red cells through the first week of storage, when most of the blood is used. With adenine added, however, most red cells are significantly different from normal in the ability to deliver oxygen at the time of transfusion. Some day this may not be acceptable for the treatment of serious hemorrhage in patients with known or suspected coronary artery disease.

As stated earlier, death during hemorrhage is probably most often due to inadequate delivery of oxygen to the heart. Serious questions have been raised about the use of red cells with impaired function to treat massively hemorrhaging patients even if the coronary circulation is normal. Many efforts to demonstrate impaired survival in controlled experiments have yielded little such evidence, and many of these experiments have gone unreported. All of the evidence on both sides cannot be reviewed in the space allowed (5), but two recent sets of experiments deal with hemorrhage and the effect on survival of the oxygen delivering properties of the blood used for resuscitation. We found that in rats treated for hemorrhage with relatively normally functioning red cells, there was no impairment of survival (Table III) when hematocrit was reduced to half normal (9). In the same model, when red cell function was impaired by nearly complete depletion of 2,3 DPG, survival was similarly unchanged when blood of near-normal hematocrit was used for treatment. When the blood contained red cells in reduced concentration that were also impaired by depletion of 2,3 DPG, however, survival was significantly worse. The pattern suggested that the oxygen-delivering properties of blood could be reduced by half without impairing the survival of hemorrhaged and treated animals, but that reduction below that level caused increasingly higher mortality. This is consistent with a large number of other experimental models, especially those using various kinds of hemodilutional resuscitation. Very similar experiments were subsequently reported by Malmberg and Woodson with slightly different results (16,17). They found some impairment of survival when red cells depleted of 2,3 DPG were used even at normal hematocrits. There were differences in the details of the experiments that might explain the results, however. The time allowed for recovery after exchange transfusion and before hemorrhage was twice as long in our experiments, thus more likely avoiding problems of persisting high levels of citrate. The results are similar enough in any case to suggest that the conclusions have been confirmed in the species tested. Man is not a rat, but similar experiments would be impossible to perform clinically. It seems prudent to assume that hemodilution should not be combined with use of functionally impaired red cells in bleeding patients, but that reduction of the oxygen-delivering capacity of the blood of some extent can be tolerated by the bleeding, but otherwise normal, patient.

LUNGS

Pulmonary impairment after hemorrhage has received considerable attention in the past decade. Indeed, the term 'shock lung' became something of a cliche. A detailed review has been published elsewhere and only a summary can be included here (4). There is very little experimental evidence supporting the concept that hemorrhage alone produces serious impairment of pulmonary function. What little there is consists of variable morphologic changes in canine lungs, with little functional derangement. Similarly, there is surprisingly little clinical evidence to support the idea of 'shock lung'. Some bleeding patients do develop pulmonary insufficiency, but another explanation can usually be found. Often this is a manifestation of left ventricular failure in patients with coronary atherosclerosis, as discussed above. Sometimes it represents aspiration pneumonitis in patients with hematemesis. Often pulmonary insufficiency is the result of overtransfusion or overinfusion in a difficult situation of varying and unknown rates of hemorrhage. One of the few instances in which pulmonary insufficiency can be causally linked to hemorrhage occurs when a severe coagulopathy such as disseminated intravascular coagulation develops. This probably results from diffuse hypoperfusion and probably signals the activation of a number of circulating inflammatory mediators, some of which probably increase pulmonary capillary permeability.

There are two questions which have been rather intensely debated regarding the relationship between the treatment for hemorrhage and the development of pulmonary insufficiency. One involves the use of non-blood, non-colloid containing fluids for resuscitation, especially simple salt solutions. This involves complex physiologic relationships, and fortunately pertinent and solid clinical data have been obtained.

The other relationship is that between transfusion of stored blood and the subsequent development of pulmonary insufficiency. The greatest attention has recently been paid to the possible role of microembolization and its prevention by the use of specially designed filters. There is supportive evidence for such a relationship in dogs, but it has not been found in other species. The clinical studies have all been flawed and are not convincing (15). In addition to microembolization, there are numerous other mechanisms whereby transfusion might cause pulmonary insufficiency. These have been discussed elsewhere (7). Studies on combat casualties in Vietnam yielded conflicting results regarding the relationship between transfusion and pulmonary insufficiency. We reviewed retrospectively the data gathered by the first three surgical research teams of the U.S. Army in Vietnam to see if we could answer this seemingly simple question (Table IV) (7).

TABLE IV. Arterial oxygen tensions (means) in combat casualties before (Pre) and following operation for injuries, according to site of injury and amount of blood transfused; numbers of patients in parentheses[*]

Transfusion range (units)	No. units (mean)	Pre	Day 1	Day 2	Day 3
			Peripheral injuries		
None	-	83(18)	77(18)	80(18)	78(6)
1-5	3.2	87(24)	85(24)	84(21)	82(11)
6-10	7.9	88(12)	77(12)	80(12)	76(7)
10	24.5	87(18)	75(16)	77(17)	80(13)
			Abdominal injuries		
None	-	81(9)	79(8)	78(9)	75(4)
1-5	3.2	86(16)	78(16)	78(14)	72(12)
6-10	7.8	85(10)	76(10)	81(7)	82(9)
> 10	25.2	87(10)	76(10)	72(10)	72(9)
			Thoracic injuries		
None	-	72(24)	72(24)	77(15)	73(16)
1-5	3	70(31)	71(26)	70(27)	71(26)
6-10	7.9	71(14)	63(14)	64(14)	69(13)
> 10	21.4	72(13)	59(12)	59(12)	65(12)

[*]From Collins, J.A., James, P.M., Bredenberg, C.E., Anderson, R.W., Heisterkamp, C.A. and Simmons, R.L.: Ann. Surg. 188:513, 1978.

We found that there was no apparent relationship between transfusion and pulmonary insufficiency in casualties studied before they were given anesthesia. In the postoperative period (3 days), no relationship was found in those whose wounds were limited to the limbs, even when transfused very large volumes of blood. For those with injuries to the abdomen, there was a suggestion of more severe hypoxemia in those most heavily transfused, but it was not statistically significant. In those wounded in the chest, there was a statistically significant, dose-related relationship between transfusion and hypoxemia on the first two postoperative days. Thus, in the same study we found evidence for and against the relationship. It is possible that the effects of transfusion were subclinical unless another form of pulmonary damage was present, in this case the direct thoracic injuries. This seemed unlikely, however, in view of the very large amounts of blood transfused rapidly to significant numbers of casualties with wounded limbs. We prefer to think that in those with thoracic injury, both the hypoxemia and the need for extensive transfusion shared a common cause. Typically, these casualties had been hit with multiple or single large high velocity missiles. Their wounds were extensively destructive and required extensive operative debridement. The injury to the pulmonary parenchyma was more severe and typically this pulmonary contusion produced the worst hypoxemia on the first and second postoperative days. Thus we believe that the data on combat casualties in Vietnam do not support the concept of transfusion-induced pulmonary insufficiency. These kinds of studies had the advantages of large numbers of patients without associated medical abnormalities. In addition, the blood used was almost invariably in the third week of storage (in ACD), fine filters were not available, and indeed in these settings even the gross filters were not changed until they became grossly clogged with clot. The disadvantage is that the subjects were in such excellent physical condition that it is difficult to extrapolate to patients with pre-existing disease.

HEMOSTASIS

The breakdown of hemostasis that sometimes occurs in hemorrhaging, transfused patients is one of the most distressing clinical complications encountered because it seems to lead into a vicious circle of more bleeding, more transfusion, and worse hemostasis, and because the outcome is so often fatal. Many studies have been done in this area, but the results are not clear (3). Our studies on combat casualties in Vietnam (22) plus a few similar studies in relatively large numbers of heavily transfused patients led us to the conclusion that the acquired coagulopathy was often disseminated intravascular coagulation or something like it, and was related to the injury, not the transfusions. The reasons for the latter conclusions were that the deficits in various specifically measured hemostatic factors were greater than could be accounted for by exchange transfusion, there were severe deficits in factors (especially fibrinogen) that should not have been depleted by transfusion but would be depleted by consumption, split products and complexes could often be detected, and the measurable disorders often worsened when transfusion stopped and improved somewhat when transfusion was resumed. Since these studies, two other important studies have been reported. A group of heavily transfused patients were grouped according to the duration of hypotension. The degree of abnormality in various tests of coagulation correlated with the duration of hypotension, not with the quantity of blood transfused (12). This important study reinforces the idea that the breakdown in hemostasis that sometimes occurs is related to the hypoperfusion and not to the transfusions. A recently reported study dealt with various measures of hemostasis in multiple transfused patients, and documented the expected range of changes in such patients (10). It can be used to rationally plan prospective replacement therapy during massive transfusion, but neither this study nor any other yet reported gives a clear answer to the questions of whether, when, or how much component therapy is needed during massive transfusion to protect hemostatic function. If there is a message, it is that the sooner perfusion is restored, the less likely there will be a breakdown in hemostasis.

METABOLIC STATUS

The metabolic abnormalities of hemorrhage are well known: lactic acidosis, a mild hyperkalemia, and an uncertain hypoglycemia. The acidosis of hemorrhage has probably been overemphasized. It is much easier to produce in anesthetized dogs than in conscious man, and it is doubtful that acidosis itself becomes a mechanism of disease except in special circumstances. We studied the changes in acid-base balance in combat casualties and found appreciable acidosis only in the most profoundly injured, and not always even then (8). More importantly, the acidosis that was expected to result from the transfusion of acidic blood into acidotic recipients did not develop except when the circulation could not be restored. Clearly, it was a complication of hypoperfusion, and not of transfusion. Attempts to reverse the acidosis of exsanguination by administering alkali were largely futile. Similar findings were reported by the U.S. Navy Surgical Research Team (14). If alkali is to be given during transfusion, its use should be guided by actual measurements of acid-base balance and not by assumptions. Whether it should be used is also questionable. It is far better to spend time correcting the cause, which is usually uncorrected hypovolemia. Acidosis is a doubtful cause of cardiovascular insufficiency: exercise produces significant acidosis with excellent cardiovascular performance, correction of hypovolemia without correcting acidosis in patients

with cholera restores the circulation, and the same is true
for diabetic ketoacidosis. There is evidence that newborns
and patients with pre-existing heart disease tolerate acidosis less well, but in others it is far better to treat
the cause. There may even be harm in aggressively treating
acidosis, as metabolic alkalosis is a common sequel of serious injury or massive transfusion and would be made worse
by giving exogenous alkali.

Hypoglycemia has rarely been reported as a complication
of hemorrhage in humans. Hyperglycemia is occasionally a
complication of treatment, however. Stored blood, and to an
even greater extent 5% dextrose solutions, contain concentrations of glucose well above normal. The maximum recommended rate for administration of glucose to an adult, 0.5
g/kg/h, is often exceeded during rapid infusion of blood
and fluids, and the tolerance for glucose may well be less
than normal in the seriously injured patient. Severe hyperglycemia has been reported during and after resuscitation and may be even more common than is suspected. Hyperkalemia is rarely a problem, with or without transfusion.
Experimentally, however, prolonged transfusion of whole
blood at high rates can produce significant hyperkalemia
which is rapidly reduced when the transfusion stops (19).
The clinical significance of this is unknown.

Citrate intoxication was one of the first described
complications of massive transfusion. Its clinical significance is still not clear, but with calcium-ion sensitive
electrodes it has become easier to measure the important
variable, ionized calcium, in clinical settings. Experimentally, we can regularly kill pigs with a massive transfusion model in which citrate is the lethal agent, but this
requires very rapid infusion for prolonged periods. The
effect of citrate is worsened by added potassium, and is
much worse in animals allowed to become hypothermic. Hypothermia may well, in fact, be the clinically most important
metabolic complication of massive transfusion. It occurs
commonly and it probably facilitates the development of or
intensifies hypercitratemia, hyperkalemia, acidosis, hyperglycemia, impaired coagulation, and the impaired function
of hemoglobin. It is worth some effort to prevent. One of
the unusual aspects of the studies in Vietnam was the rare
occurrence of hypothermia during transfusion because the
environmental temperature was so high.

OTHER ORGANS

Renal failure is a very serious complication of hemorrhage,
because post-traumatic renal failure still has a mortality
rate of 60-80%. We do not have time to review it in detail.
It is primarily a complication of reduced perfusion of the
kidneys. The tubules are relatively far along the perfusion
sequence in the kidneys, but they have the highest requirements for oxygen, thus making them doubly vulnerable. There
is evidence that even without the appearance of frank renal

failure, impairment of the functions of the distal nephron, concentration and acidification, can be detected rather commonly after severe hemorrhage. There is little or no evidence that transfusion increases the risk of developing renal failure, except when intravascular hemolysis occurs, which is a rather effective way of producing renal failure. Most authorities believe that early use of salt solutions helps to reduce the risk of post-traumatic renal failure even though controlled clinical trials have not been performed.

Hepatic failure is not commonly listed as a complication of hemorrhage. Overt hepatic failure is indeed an uncommon complication except in patients with cirrhosis, but some evidence of impaired hepatic function is quite common. The mild jaundice usually attributed to transfusion of abundant quantities of blood cannot in fact be accounted for on that basis. Hepatic parenchymal insufficiency is more likely. Structural studies in animals show that centrilobular damage is very common after severe hemorrhage. This probably also occurs in man, but is usually repaired without permanent impairment. Again, rapid and early resuscitation minimize its development.

Intestinal ulceration, especially gastroduodenal, is a well known complication of hemorrhage in both animals and man. Effective prophylaxis is now possible; if the pH of gastric luminal contents is kept above 4, the complication is rare (21). There is debate about the best method for doing this, but that is about detail, not effects. There is no apparent specific relationship to treatment.

ANTIMICROBIAL DEFENSES

The impairment of antibacterial defenses after serious hemorrhage is one of the main reasons for clinical failure of treatment. Death from infection is perhaps the leading cause of preventable death in seriously injured patients. This is finally beginning to receive the attention it deserves. In some unpublished studies in rats, for example, we found that susceptibility to endotoxin and to live bacteria was increased after hemorrhage, this susceptibility persisted beyond the period of apparent recovery, and the degree and duration were related to both the degree of hemorrhage and to the specific kind of treatment. The latter observation obviously has important clinical observations. Some exciting possibilities of correcting this increased vulnerability with specific component therapy will be discussed by Dr. Blumenstock.

UNANSWERED QUESTIONS

In spite of the fact that hemorrhage is a rather simple and straightforward event, unanswered questions and disagreements persist regarding details of treatment. What are the best clinical/laboratory signs for completeness of resuscitation? What are the best combinations of agents for use for resuscitation? When should whole blood, fresh blood, coagulation components, platelets, antibacterial substances be used/added and in what amount? To what extent can non-blood materials be used? How can the complications of treatment be prevented?

REFERENCES

1. Aranow, W.S., Isbell, M.W.: Carbon monoxide effect on exercise-induced angina pectoris. Ann. Intern. Med. 79:392, 1973.

2. Case, R.B., Berglund, E., Sarnoff, S.J.: Ventricular function. VII. Changes in acute coronary resistance and ventricular function resulting from acutely induced anemia and the effect thereon of coronary stenosis. Am. J. Med. 18:397, 1955.

3. Collins, J.A.: Massive blood transfusion. Clinics in Haematol. 5:201, 1976.

4. Collins, J.A.: The acute respiratory distress syndrome. Adv. Surgery 11:171, 1977.

5. Collins, J.A.: Abnormal hemoglobin-oxygen affinity and surgical hemotherapy. Biblthca Haemat. 46:59, 1980.

6. Collins, J.A.: Hemorrhage and burns. Pathophysiology and treatment. In: Clinical Practice of Blood Transfusion. Eds. S. Swisher and L. Petz, Churchill Livingstone, New York, 1982.

7. Collins, J.A., James, P.M., Bredenberg, C.E., Anderson, R.W., Heisterkamp, C.A., Simmons, R.L.: The relationship between transfusion and hypoxemia in combat casualties. Ann. Surg. 188:513, 1978.

8. Collins, J.A., Simmons, R.L., James, P.M., Bredenberg, C.E., Anderson, R.W., Heisterkamp, C.A.: The acid-base status of seriously wounded combat casualties. I. Before treatment. II. Resuscitation with stored blood. Ann. Surg. 171:595, 1970; 173:6, 1971.

9. Collins, J.A., Stechenberg, L.: The effects of the concentration and function of hemoglobin on the survival of rats after hemorrhage. Surgery 85:412, 1979.

10. Counts, R.B., Haisch, C., Simon, T.L., Maxwell, N.G., Heimbach, D.M., Carrico, C.J.: Hemostasis in massively transfused trauma patients. Ann. Surg. 190:91, 1979.

11. Dennis, R.C., Vito, L., Weisel, R.D., Valeri, C.R., Berger, R.I. and Hechtman, H.B.: Improved myocardial performance following high 2,3-DPG red cell transfusion. Surgery 77:741, 1975.

12. Harke, H., Ruhman, S.: Haemostatic disorders in massive transfusion. Biblthca Haemat. 46:179, 1980.

13. Holsinger, J.W., Salharry, J.M., Eliot, R.S.: Physiologic observations on the effect of impaired blood oxygen release on the myocardium. Adv. Cardiol. 9:81, 1973.

14. Lowry, B.D., Cloutier, C.T., Carey, L.C.: Blood gas determinations in the severely wounded in hemorrhagic shock. Arch. Surg. 99:330, 1969.

15. Lundsgaard-Hansen, P.: Symposium on microfiltration of blood and pulmonary function. Vox Sang. 39:46, 1980.

16. Malmberg, P., Hlastala, M.O., Woodson, R.D.: Effect of increased blood oxygen affinity on oxygen transport in hemorrhagic shock. J. Appl. Physiol. 47:889, 1979.

17. Malmberg, P., Woodson, R.D.: Effects of anemia on oxygen transport in hemorrhagic shock. J. Appl. Physiol. 47:882, 1979.
18. Martin, A.M., Hackel, D.B.: An electron microscopic study of the progression of myocardial lesions in the dog after hemorrhagic shock. Lab. Invest. 15:243, 1966.
19. Miller, L.W., Collins, J.A., Sherman, L., Ladenson, J.: Massive transfusion in swine. Surg. Forum 28:21, 1977.
20. Newman, G.E., Rerych, S.K., Jones, R.H., Sabiston, D.C.: Non-invasive assessment of the effects of aorta-coronary bypass grafting on ventricular function during rest and exercise. J. Thoracic Cardiovasc. Surg. 79:617, 1980.
21. Priebe, H.J., Skillman, J.J., Beishnell, L.S., Long, P.C., Silen, W.: Antacid versus cimetidine in preventing acute gastrointestinal bleeding. New Engl. J. Med. 302:426, 1980.
22. Simmons, R.L., Collins, J.A., Heisterkamp, L.A., Mills, D.E., Andren, R., Phillips, L.L.: Coagulation studies in combat casualties. I. Acute changes after wounding. II. Effects of massive transfusion. III. Post-resuscitative changes. Ann. Surg. 169:455, 1969.
23. Weisel, R.D., Dennis, R.C., Manny, J., Mannick, J.A., Valeri, R., Hechtman, H.B.: Adverse effects of transfusion therapy during abdominal aortic aneurysmectomy. Surgery 83:682, 1972.

PLASMA FIBRONECTIN: BIOCHEMICAL PROPERTIES AND CLINICAL RELEVANCE

F.A. Blumenstock, T.M. Saba and J.E. Kaplan

The reticuloendothelial system (RES) consists of a network of sessile and mobile mononuclear phagocytes which perform a variety of physiological functions with respect to host defense. Those fixed macrophages that reside in the liver and spleen and comprise the majority of the RES are uniquely located anatomically such that they can monitor the circulation and have been demonstrated to remove a variety of blood-borne toxic and particulate material of both endogenous and exogenous origin (37). These cells can selectively recognize and remove from the vascular compartment endogenously generated material including cell debris (26), denatured collagen (43), fibrin aggregates (23), and a variety of exogenous colloidal and particulate material including bacteria (4,16,34,41). Early studies involved in the evaluation of the activity of this system which is responsible for the removal of circulating particulate demonstrated that activation of the system as evidenced by an enhanced rate of removal of test particulate from the blood was associated with an increased resistance to a variety of pathophysiological situations such as traumatic injury (51), infection (34), and tumor growth (4). Conversely, depression of the clearance capacity of the system resulted in an increased sensitivity of experimental animals to the same pathological insults. Therefore, the concept that the RES was important in host defense processes became firmly established.

Once the importance of the RES in host defense was recognized, a variety of studies focused on factors that were involved in the control of RES clearance function. These investigations revealed that parameters such as liver blood flow, age, sex, species and the type of colloid or particulate used to test RE function were important aspects to consider when assessing RE clearance function (5). Other studies demonstrated that the presence of circulating factors in the blood which aid in the recognition process were also critically important in the modulation of RE clearance function (14,25). Investigation of the importance of plasma proteins in the support of RE clearance function demonstrated that antibody and complement functioned in the RE clearance of bacteria (48), while other studies revealed that another protein was involved in the clearance of 'inert' non-bacterial particulate.

Originally referred to by a number of terms such as opsonic protein, humoral recognition factor (14), aspecific opsonin (36), and opsonic alpha-2-surface binding (SB) glycoprotein (8), this factor was demonstrated to be important in the clearance of some of the test colloids used to demonstrate that the clearance capacity of the RE system was proportional to the host defense of the organism. The hypothesis was therefore presented that the maintenance of adequate levels of this protein in the plasma was necessary for the RES to be functional in host defense mechanisms. In direct support of this concept was the observation that colloid injection which induces a subsequent depression in RES clearance function can also lead to host defense deficits. This experimentally induced 'colloid blockade' has been used to depress RES function and can reverse tolerance to trauma, infection, and hemorrhagic shock, which can be achieved by activation of the RES (reviewed in 37). The demonstration that RE clearance deficits induced in animals by RE blockade was, in part, due to a decrease in the ability of the plasma from these animals to support in vitro hepatic phagocytosis, further supported the importance of the role played by this factor in normal clearance mechanisms and host defense (42). Other studies demonstrated that RES clearance deficits that occur with traumatic injury were also associated with depressed humoral support of hepatic macrophage uptake of test colloid (21).

Thus, since colloid blockade depressed normal and activated host defense mechanisms and depressed plasma support of in vitro hepatic phagocytosis occurred following colloid blockade and traumatic injury, the importance of identifying and characterizing the plasma factor responsible for supporting RES clearance of gelatinized colloid seemed evident.

OPSONIC PROTEIN AND PHAGOCYTOSIS

The evidence that RES dysfunction following traumatic injury in both man and experimental animals was associated with a depression in humoral support of in vitro hepatic phagocytosis and the fact that similar observations were made during RE depression during tumor growth (37) stimulated investigations to identify, purify and characterize this factor from plasma. Early studies documented that this factor was thermolabile, could be absorbed from plasma by gelatin-coated particles, and could be characterized electrophoretically as an α_2 globulin. Other functional studies demonstrated an elevation in female rats prior to parturition (19) and in patients during normal labor (18). The protein was distinct from complement (26) and precipitable from plasma in the cold, especially in the presence of heparin (14). Similarly, studies in the isolated perfused liver demonstrated that a plasma factor with an affinity for gelatinized particulate was important in the removal of gelatinized carbon by the intact liver in vitro and that RE dysfunction during RE colloid blockade could be due to the extraction of a circulating humoral factor in the plasma (17).

Eventual isolation and purification of this protein first from rat plasma and later from human plasma demonstrated that the protein responsible for the opsonic activity toward gelatinized test colloid is a glycoprotein, migrating as an α_2 globulin with a molecular weight of 440,000 (7-9). The protein is a disulfide-linked dimer of two nearly or completely identical monomers of 220,000. Amino acid analysis of both the human and rat protein demonstrated an amino acid analysis strangely similar to some membrane glycoproteins containing high amounts of serine and threonine as well as other hydrophilic amino acid residues. The purified protein was able to support macrophage phagocytosis in vitro, a function that could be inhibited by monospecific antibody to the opsonic protein. Other studies demonstrated that intravenous injection of the antibody to the rat protein could depress in vivo clearance of test particulate as well as drastically increase the sensitivity of these animals to traumatic injury (22).

Immunochemical quantitation of the plasma levels of the opsonic protein demonstrated fairly high circulating levels of the protein, 400-450 µg/ml in rats (10) and 300-400 µg/ml in humans (6), which was dramatically reduced following colloid blockade in rats (10) and was depressed in man after traumatic injury (45). These quantitative observations again supported the concept that the maintenance of normal circulating levels of the opsonic protein was important for normal RES function.

OPSONIC PROTEIN AND COLD-INSOLUBLE GLOBULIN (CIg)

Cold-insoluble globulin (CIg) was originally described in 1948 as a protein present in fibrinogen-rich plasma cryoprecipitate which resisted purification but somehow seemed to be involved in the cryoprecipitation of fibrinogen from citrated plasma (27). Later studies demonstrated that it was not coagulable by thrombin and thus distinct from fibrinogen. Purification of the protein from human plasma cryoprecipitate in 1970 revealed that it was a 440,000 mw glycoprotein consisting of a disulfide bond dimer with a monomer-size of 220,000 (28). The purified protein had an affinity for heparin and was cryoprecipitable in the presence of heparin and fibrinogen. At this time the biological function of CIg was unknown but subsequent studies demonstrated the molecule could be cross-linked to fibrin by factor XIIIa and was thus thought to contribute to the coagulation process (30).

Another major discovery concerning CIg that occurred at about the same time was the identification of a cell surface protein on mesenchymally derived cells in tissue culture

122

that was lost upon oncogenic transformation. This fibrous
protein, which is involved in cellular adhesion to colla-
genous substructures and termed fibronectin was identified
as being antigenically related to CIg (32). This protein
has now been identified as being important in cell-to-cell
and cell-to-substratum interactions in vivo and is an important constituent in basement membranes and connective
tissue (50). It was this demonstration of the antigenic
relationship between cell surface fibronectin and plasma
CIg that led to the term 'plasma' fibronectin as an alternative name for plasma CIg. Biochemical studies of the two
types of proteins (plasma fibronectin and tissue fibronectin) have revealed that they have similar monomeric structures and that the domain structure and function are similar but not identical (49).

We were struck by the similarities between the opsonic
protein and CIg, and through a generous gift of purified
CIg and antibody to the protein by Dr. Deane Mosher, we
were able to demonstrate the identity of the two proteins
(Fig. 1).

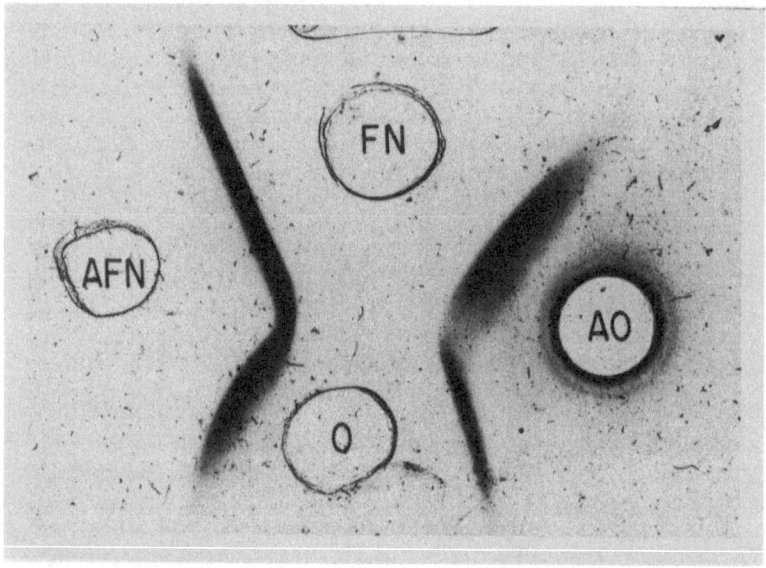

Fig. 1. Ouchterlony double diffusion of human opsonic α_2SB glycoprotein (O) and plasma fibronectin (FN) against monospecific antiserum to
plasma fibronectin (AFN) as well as to antibody to the human opsonic
protein (AO). Reproduced from Blumenstock, Saba, Weber and Laffin (16)
with permission of the Journal of Biological Chemistry.

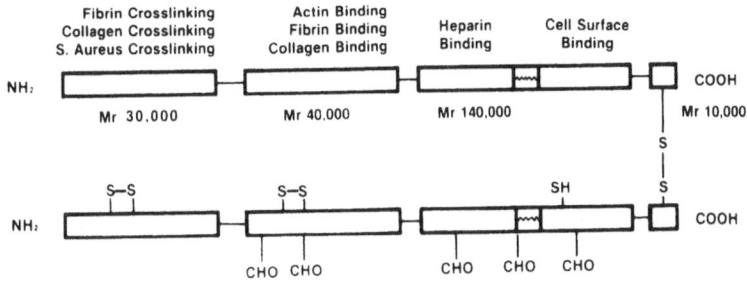

Fig. 2. Proposed domain structure of plasma fibronectin.

This discovery of the identity of the two proteins demonstrated a biological function for plasma CIg and provided
a means for the reversal of plasma opsonic deficiencies
in patients by treatment with CIg rich plasma cryoprecipitate (39,40).

Figure 2 illustrates our current understanding of the
general structure and functional aspects of the plasma fibronectin molecule although this is most likely incomplete
since some of the structural and functional aspects are
the results of studies on the cell surface form of the molecule (Review in 15). The cell surface protein is probably
the product of a different gene than the plasma form since
it is becoming more evident that the polypeptide sequence
of the plasma form is different from the cell surface form
(3).

In general, each monomer consists of 4 separate domains
which may not be separate distinct globular regions but
are probably areas of polypeptide chain separated by segments of increased flexibility and sensitivity to protease.
The N-terminal domain has been demonstrated to be the area
of the molecule where covalent cross-links to other molecules occur as catalyzed by transglutaminase enzymes. Such
cross-linking has been demonstrated to occur to fibrin,
collagen, and to the bacteria S. aureus. This domain of
Mr 30-40,000 also may have a low affinity for heparin. The
next segment of the molecules of Mr 40,000 contains the
high affinity binding sites for collagen, gelatin, actin
and fibrin. This area of the molecules also contains some
of the covalently linked carbohydrate which does not seem
to be involved in the binding properties of the molecule
but may be important in the protection of the molecule from
proteolytic degradation. The Mr 140,000-160,000 dalton segment contains areas involved with cell attachment and heparin binding. This domain of the plasma form of the molecule contains one or more free sulfhydryl groups which may
be involved with cell attachment and is certainly involved
with the polymerization of the molecule derived from the

cell surface. The last domain is involved with the inter-
molecular disulfide bridge and provides the plasma form
of the molecule with its dimeric character.

FIBRONECTIN THERAPY IN SEPTIC INJURED PATIENTS

The observations that there is a direct relationship between RES function and sensitivity to traumatic injury and
sepsis in experimental animals suggested that such a relationship might be expected to be true in man subjected
to injury such as trauma, burn or surgery. Direct assessment of RE function should be avoided especially in injured
man because intravenous injection of test colloid would be
expected to depress the host defense capabilities of the
RES (colloid blockade) whose normal protective capability
might already be compromised as a result of the previous
injury. Prior to the purification of the human protein and
production of monospecific antibody for immunochemical
quantitation of circulating fibronectin antigen, in vitro
bioassay of the opsonic activity of human serum and plasma
was used to indirectly assess the functional state of the
RES (45). Such studies documented that trauma patients who
develop organ failure and sepsis demonstrate persistent deficits in humoral support of RE function. In our studies,
mortality of these patients was directly associated with
the prolonged deficits in plasma opsonic activity (45). Injured patients who survived their injuries demonstrated a
transient decline in the plasma opsonic activity for the
first few days following injury followed by a return to
normal levels by days 3-4. Similar assessment of plasma immunoassayable fibronectin levels as well as the bioassayabl
fibronectin levels in patients suffering from severe burn
injury document similar changes (24). Immediately post-burn
there is a rapid decline in the plasma levels of the protein followed by a restoration in plasma levels by 48 hr
post-burn. It is interesting to note that a subsequent depression in the plasma levels of the protein occurs within
4-5 days at a time immediately prior to the documentation
of sepsis, indicating that the fall in plasma levels of
fibronectin might be prognostic of the beginning of the
septic episode.
   The documentation that deficits in circulating levels
of the opsonic protein correlated with sepsis, organ failure and mortality in injured man suggested that treatment
of such patients with concentrates of plasma fibronectin
(39) to restore the circulating levels to normal and con-
comitantly restore normal RES clearance function might result in an improvement in organ function, resolve the septic state and reverse mortality in such clinical situations
With the demonstration that the opsonic α_2SB glycoprotein
and CIg (plasma fibronectin) were identical, a modality
for the treatment of hypoopsonemia in the septic injured
patient became available since plasma cryoprecipitate contains 10 times more CIg (plasma fibronectin) on a weight

per volume basis than normal human plasma. Testing our
hypothesis in the initial group of patients treated with
10 units of cryoprecipitate per patient resulted in a normalization of the plasma opsonic activity and a restoration of immunoassayable levels to normal (39). In association with the increased plasma levels of the protein
there appeared to be an improvement in pulmonary function
as evidenced by a decrease in the need for positive expi-
ratory pressure (PEEP) to maintain normal oxygenation as
well as a decline in the septic state as demonstrated by
an increase in alertness, normalization of leukocyte levels
and arterial pulse as well as improvement in various hemodynamic parameters, appearance of negative blood cultures
and the alleviation of the febrile state (39).

In severely ill patients with sepsis and a focus of
tissue injury or invasive wound infection the hypoopsone-
mic state often redeveloped within 48 hours, indicating
to us that consumption of plasma fibronectin was continuing due to sequestration at sites of tissue injury and
sepsis or due to the continued release of microthrombi
into the circulation as a result of low-grade disseminated intravascular coagulation (DIC) as well as be consumed by the RES as a result of the opsonization of intravascular particulate. Other clinical studies in patients
studied in a non-longitudinal manner demonstrated that
only in patients with DIC was there a consistent finding
of depressed plasma fibronectin levels (31,47). This concept is supported by animal models of DIC where significant depression in plasma fibronectin is also observed
(29).

In order to more adequately quantitate alterations in
organ function following cryoprecipitate infusion in the
critically injured patient, a study of such patients was
initiated in the Trauma Study Unit at Albany. These studies represent a collaborative effort between surgeons,
biomedical engineers and several of the staff of the physiology department. In these studies alterations in cardiovascular, pulmonary and renal parameters were investigated following cryoprecipitate infusion into patients.
Techniques utilized in this study included assessment of
limb blood flow using venous occlusion plethysmography
and ventilation perfusion imbalance, as determined by the
multiple inert gas elimination technique (MIGET) (2, 44).
These techniques allow for quantitation of limb oxygen
consumption and the identification of the existence of
well-ventilated but non-perfused regions (physiological
dead space) of the lung as well as perfused but non-venti-
lated areas (shunt). Evaluation of renal function was performed using the endogenous creatinine clearance techniques (2). Infusion of cryoprecipitate consisted of the administration of 10 units of the concentrate over a period
of 60 minutes. Cryoprecipitate infusion was associated
with a decrease in shunt fraction and dead space which resulted in an improvement of the ventilation-perfusion ra-

tio. There was an increase in both the normal and post-ischemic limb blood flow which was associated with an increase in limb oxygen delivery and consumption. An elevated creatinine clearance occurred only after 14-20 hr and remained elevated for 3 days following the initial rise.

These initial studies seemed to indicate that some beneficial effects can be obtained by cryoprecipitate infusion into septic patients of the type described in these studies. There were several patients who did not demonstrate an improvement in their pulmonary status. These patients were on high dose heparin therapy and demonstrated very low plasma levels of fibronectin (40-50 µg/ml) prior to cryoprecipitate infusion. Since heparin has a documented affinity for the molecule and can enhance the rate of binding of fibronectin to gelatinized particulate (20), the lack of improvement might have occurred as a result of an enhancement in the aggregation of circulating opsonized microthrombi by heparin which might be expected to embolize in microvascular beds and result in a worsening of the clinical situation.

We are now proceeding with a double-blind prospective study in the Trauma Study Unit at Albany to confirm our original observations with respect to the beneficial effects cryoprecipitate treatment might have on host defense and organ function. Confirmatory support for our initial observations in injured man treated with cryoprecipitate have been provided by other investigators indicating that indeed cryoprecipitate therapy may provide an important modality of therapy in clinical situations associated with sepsis and multiple organ failure (11,33).

Many factors are probably involved in the development of opsonic fibronectin deficiency following injury and in association with bacterial sepsis. Major contributors may be tissue injury since fibronectin with its multiple affinities would be expected to bind to exposed collagen and would be closely associated with altered platelets and fibrin that would be deposited in areas of injury. Fibronectin would also be utilized in the RES clearance of microaggregates and tissue debris such as actin, platelet microaggregates and fibrin microthrombi. Thus, plasma fibronectin deficiency may result from an 'overloading' of the system with particulate resulting in an endogenously generated 'colloid blockade' plus extravascular sequestration by binding to damaged tissue. Contributing to the deficit would be dilutional effects as a result of fluid therapy, while transfusion of stored blood that is improperly filtered to remove microaggregates would also produce transient deficiencies in plasma levels of the protein (46). Nutritional deprivation in the later post-injury period may further contribute to fibronectin deficiency (13). Regardless of the factors involved in the induction of plasma opsonic fibronectin deficiency, RES clearance function would be expected to be inefficient.

In addition, fibronectin deficiency might lead to enhanced fibrin microthrombi formation since fibronectin enhances solubility of fibrin monomer while inhibiting fibrin-collagen interaction (Table I). Consequently, plasma fibronectin deficiency may lead to an increase in circulating particulate load further endangering the tissue microcirculation.

TABLE I. Effect of plasma fibronectin on fibrin-fibrin and fibrin-collagen interaction

System tested	% Insoluble fibrin after incubation with plasma fibronectin (μg/ml)			
	0	50	100	400
Fibrin-fibrin	53.3±1.5	29.0±1.5	5.6±1.0	0.89±0.51
Fibrin-collagen	83.5±2.4	59.5±2.1	8.0±2.2	2.36±1.2

I^{125} labelled fibrin monomer (400 μg/ml) alone or fibrin in the presence of collagen (1 mg/ml) were incubated with various concentrations of plasma fibronectin at 37°C for 30 minutes prior to centrifugation to determine the fraction of counts pelletable after incubation. The % of the I^{125} labelled fibrin that was pelletable represents insolubilized fibrin. Non-pelletable fraction does not represent proteolysis since protein inhibitors did not effect the amount of pelletable counts.

COMMENTS AND CAUTIONS

The use of plasma cryoprecipitate for the treatment of host defense deficits in septic injured patients manifesting low plasma fibronectin levels is based upon sound scientific reasoning. However, interpretation of the observed clinical and physiological improvement of these patients as being solely due to the restoration of circulating opsonic fibronectin levels would be premature and unjustified until further studies are completed. Cryoprecipitate contains a variety of concentrated plasma proteins besides fibronectin, including fibrinogen and Factor VIII that may participate in the observed response to cryoprecipitate therapy. Until purified opsonically active fibronectin is available for clinical trials so that verification of the results obtained with cryoprecipitate can be identified as being solely due to the restoration of circulating levels of fibronectin, we must guard against over-enthusiasm. To consume a blood product so necessary for the routine treatment of Factor VIII deficient patients until efficacy is proven should be avoided if possible. If treatment is considered, it is important to document that there exists a sustained deficiency in fibronectin levels in the patient. Experimental evidence in animal models has demonstrated that raising the concentration of plasma fibronectin to excessive levels actually inhibited RES clearance function (12). There is commercially available an immunoturbidimetric assay (Biodynamics-BMC, Indianapolis, IN, USA) that can be used for the rapid (10 min) quantitation of fibronectin that correlate exceedingly well with the standard but time consuming Laurell assay (38). This assay procedure can be used routinely when or if opsonic fibronectin therapy has been demonstrated to be of utility in the treatment of the septic injured patient. It may also be of prognostic value in the determination of the efficacy of standard therapy on the clinical course of the critically injured patient.

ACKNOWLEDGEMENTS

Supported by NIH Grants GM-21447 and AI-17635. Clinical studies were performed in the Albany Trauma Center, GM-15426. The authors wish to acknowledge the secretarial assistance of Mrs. Maureen Davis for her invaluable assistance in the preparation of this manuscript.

REFERENCES

1. Allen, C., Saba, T.M., Molnar, J.: Isolation, purification and characterization of opsonic protein. J. Reticuloendothelial Soc. 13:410, 1973.
2. Annest, S.J., Scovill, W.A., Blumenstock, F.A., Stratton, H.H., Newell, J.C., Paloski, W.H., Saba, T.M., Powers, S.R.: Increased creatinine clearance following cryoprecipitate infusion in trauma and surgical patients with decreased renal function. J. Trauma 20:726, 1980.
3. Atherton, B.T., Hynes, R.O.: A difference between plasma and cellular fibronectins located with monoclonal antibodies. Cell 25:133 1981.
4. Biozzi, B., Stiffel, C., Halpern, B.M., Manton, D.: Etude de la fonction phagocytaire du SRE au cours du développement de tumeurs expérimentales chez le rat et la souris. Ann. Inst. Pasteur. 94: 681, 1958.
5. Biozzi, G., Benacerraf, B., Halpern, B.N.: Quantitative study of the granulopectic activity of the reticuloendothelial system. II. A study of the kinetics of the granulopectic activity of the RES in relation to the dose of carbon injected. Relationship between the weight of the organs and their activity. Brit. J. Exp. Path. 34:441, 1953.
6. Blumenstock, F.A., Saba, T.M.: Purification of alpha-2-opsonic glycoprotein from human serum and its measurement by immunoassay. J. Reticuloendothelial Soc. 23:119, 1978.
7. Blumenstock, F.A., Saba, T.M., Weber, P., Cho, E.: Purification and biochemical characterization of a macrophage stimulated alpha-2-globulin opsonic protein. J. Reticuloendothelial Soc. 19:157, 1976.
8. Blumenstock, F.A., Saba, T.M., Weber, P., Laffin, R.: Biochemical and immunological characterization of human opsonic alpha-2-SB glycoprotein; Its identity with cold-insoluble globulin. J. Biol.

Chem. 253:4387, 1978.

9. Blumenstock, F.A., Weber, P.B., Saba, T.M.: Isolation and purification from rat serum of an alpha-2-opsonic glycoprotein. J. Biol. Chem. 252:7156, 1977.

10. Blumenstock, F.A., Weber, P., Saba, T.M., Laffin, R.: Electroimmunoassay of alpha-2-opsonic protein during reticuloendothelial blockade. Am. J. Physiol. 232:R80, 1977.

11. Brodin, B., Bergham, L., Frigerg-Nielson, S., Nordstrom, H., Schildt, B.: Fibronectin in the treatment of septicemia - a preliminary report. Excerpta Medica. 7th World Congress of Anesthesiology. Hamburg, 1980, p. 504.

12. Dillon, B.C., Saba, T.M.: Starvation-induced hepatic phagocytic depression: Role of opsonic fibronectin and neutrophils in the distribution of blood-borne *Staphylococcus aureus*. Abstracts of Association for Academic Surgery, 1981, p. 68.

13. Dillon, B.C., Saba, T.M., Cho, E., Lewis, E.: Opsonic fibronectin deficiency in the etiology of starvation induced reticuloendothelial phagocytic dysfunction. Exp. and Molec. Path. 36 (in press), 1982.

14. Di Luzio, N.R.: Macrophages, recognition factors and neoplasia. In: RES System. International Academy of Pathology Monograph. Baltimore, MD, Williams and Wilkins, 1975, p. 49.

15. Engel, J., Odermatt, E., Engel, A., Madri, J.A., Furthmayer, H., Rohde, H., Timpl, R.: Shapes, domain organization and flexibility of laminin in fibronectin. Two multi-functional proteins of the extracellular matrix. J. Molec. Biol. 150:97, 1981.

16. Filkins, F.P.: Detoxification of endotoxin by leukocytes and macrophages. Proc. Soc. Exp. Biol. Med. 137:1396, 1971.

17. Filkins, F.P., Chase, R.E., Smith, J.J.: Characteristics of a plasma factor governing carbon phagocytosis in the isolated perfused rat liver. J. Reticuloendothelial Soc. 2:287, 1965.

18. Graham, C.W., Blumenstock, F.A., Saba, T.M., Gotoff, S.: Labor modulates alpha-2-opsonic protein (α_2OP) for fixed macrophages. J. Reticuloendothelial Soc. 24:31a, 1978.

19. Graham, C.W., Saba, T.M.: Opsonin in reticuloendothelial regulation during and following pregnancy. J. Reticuloendothelial Soc. 14:121, 1973.

20. Jilek, F., Hormann, H.: Fibronectin (cold-insoluble globulin). VI. Influence of heparin and hyaluronic acid on the binding of native collagen. Hoppe-Seyler's Z. Physiol. Chem. 360:597, 1979.

21. Kaplan, J.E., Saba, T.M.: Humoral deficiency and reticuloendothelial depression after traumatic shock. Am. J. Physiol. 230:7, 1976.

22. Kaplan, J.E., Saba, T.M., Cho, E.: Serological modifications of reticuloendothelial capacity and altered resistance to traumatic shock. Circ. Shock 3:203, 1976.

23. Kaplan, J.E.: The role of the reticuloendothelial system in control of hemostatic and thrombotic mechanisms. In: Pathophysiology of the Reticuloendothelial System. eds. B.M. Altura and T.M. Saba. Raven Press, New York, 1981, p. 111.

24. Lanser, M.E., Saba, T.M., Scovill, W.A.: Opsonic glycoprotein (plasma fibronectin) levels after burn injury: Relationship to extent of burn and development of sepsis. Ann. Surg. 192:776, 1980.

25. Manwaring, W.H., Coe, H.C.: Endothelial opsonins. J. Immunol. 1:401, 1916.
26. Molnar, J., McLain, S., Allen, C., Laga, H., Gava, A., Gelder, R.: Specificity of a non-complement related opsonic protein. Biochem. Biophys. Acta 493:37, 1977.
27. Morrison, P.R., Edsall, J.T., Miller, S.G.: Preparation and properties of serum and plasma proteins. XVIII. The separation of purified fibrinogen from fraction I of human plasma. J. Am. Chem. Soc. 70:3103, 1948.
28. Mosesson, M.W., Umfleet, R.A.: The cold-insoluble globulin of human plasma. I. Purification, primary characterization and relationship to fibrinogen and other cold-insoluble fraction components. J. Biol. Chem. 245:572 8, 1970.
29. Mosher, D.F.: Changes in plasma cold-insoluble globulin concentration during experimental Rocky Mountain Spotted Fever infection in rhesus monkeys. Thromb. Res. 9:37, 1976.
30. Mosher, D.F.: Cross-linking of cold-insoluble globulin by fibrin stabilizing factors. J. Biol. Chem. 250:6614, 1976.
31. Mosher, D.F., Williams, E.M.: Fibronectin concentration is decreased in plasma of severely ill patients with disseminated intravascular coagulation. J. Lab. Clin. Med. 91:729, 1978.
32. Ruoslahti, E., Vaheri, A.: Interaction of soluble fibroblast surface antigens with fibrinogen and fibrin. Identity with cold-insoluble globulin of human plasma. J. Exp. Med. 141:497, 1975.
33. Robbins, A.B., Doran, J.E., Reese, A.C., Mansberger, A.R.: Cold-insoluble globulin levels in operative trauma: Serum depletion, wound sequestration and biological activity. Am. Surg. 46:663, 1980.
34. Rogers, B.E.: Host mechanisms which act to remove bacteria from the bloodstream. Bact. Rev. 24:50, 1960.
35. Saba, T.M.: Physiology and pathophysiology of the reticuloendothelial system. Arch. Intern. Med. 126:1031, 1970.
36. Saba, T.M.: Aspecific Opsonins. In: Proc. of 4th Internat. Convocation on Immunology. In: Immune System and Infectious Diseases. S. Karger Co., Basel, 1975, p. 489.
37. Saba, T.M., Antikatzides, T.G.: Humoral mediated macrophage response during tumor growth. Brit. J. Cancer 21:471, 1975.
38. Saba, T.M., Albert, W.H., Blumenstock, F.A., Evanega, G., Staehler, F., Cho, E.: Evaluation of a rapid immunoturbidimetric assay for opsonic fibronectin in surgical and trauma patients administered cryoprecipitate. J. Lab. Clin. Med. 90:473, 1981.
39. Saba, T.M., Blumenstock, F.A., Scovill, W.A., Bernard, H.R.: Cryoprecipitate reversal of opsonic alpha-2-surface binding glycoprotein deficiency in septic surgical and trauma patients. Science 201:622, 1978.
40. Saba, T.M., Blumenstock, F.A., Weber, P., Kaplan, J.E.: Physiologic role for cold-insoluble globulin in systemic host defense: Implications of its characterization as the opsonic α_2SB glycoprotein. Ann. N.Y. Acad. Sci. 312:43, 1978.
41. Saba, T.M., Di Luzio, N.R.: Kupffer cell phagocytosis and metabolism of a variety of particles as a function of opsonization. J. Reticuloendothelial Soc. 2:437, 1965.
42. Saba, T.M., Di Luzio, N.R.: Reticuloendothelial blockade and recovery as a function of opsonic activity. Am. J. Physiol. 216:197,

1969.

43. Saba, T.M., Jaffe, E.: Plasma fibronectin (opsonic glycoprotein): Its synthesis by vascular endothelial cells and role in cardio-pulmonary integrity after trauma as related to reticuloendothelial function. Am. J. Med. 68:577, 1980.

44. Scovill, W.A., Saba, T.M., Blumenstock, F.A., Bernard, H., Powers, S.R.: Opsonic alpha-2-surface binding glycoprotein therapy during sepsis. Ann. Surg. 188:521, 1978.

45. Scovill, W.A., Saba, T.M., Kaplan, J.E., Bernard, H.R., Powers, S.R.: Disturbances in circulating opsonic activity in man after operative and blunt trauma. J. Surg. Res. 22:709, 1977.

46. Snyder, E.L., Mosher, D.F., Hezzey, A., Golenwski, G.: Effect of blood transfusion on in vivo levels of plasma fibronectin. J. Lab. Clin. Med. 98:336, 1981.

47. Stathakis, N.E., Fountas, A., Tsianos, E.: Plasma fibronectin in normal subjects and in various disease states. J. Clin. Pathol. 34:504, 1981.

48. Stossel, T.P.: Phagocytosis. New Engl. J. Med. 290:717, 1974.

49. Yamada, K.M., Kennedy, D.W.: Fibroblast cellular and plasma fi-bronectin are similar but not identical. J. Cell. Biol. 80:492, 1979.

50. Yamada, K.M., Olden, K.: Fibronectin: Adhesive glycoproteins of cell surface and blood. Nature 275:179, 1978.

51. Zweifach, B.W. Benacerraf, B., Thomas, L.: Relationship between the vascular manifestation of shock produced by endotoxin, trauma and hemorrhage. II. The possible role of the RES in resistance to each type of shock. J. Exp. Med. 106:403, 1957.

DISSEMINATED INTRAVASCULAR COAGULATION AND ITS IMPACT ON BLOOD TRANSFUSION

C.A.M. Haanen

Disseminated intravascular coagulation (DIC) represents a spectrum of disease with a variable degree of inappropriate blood clotting in response to a variety of stimuli. It implies widespread deposition of altered fibrinogen and/or platelets, with concurrent obstruction of the microcirculation and desintegration of the hemostatic mechanism. The processes involved in DIC are triggered by an underlying pathological state and the sequences of DIC aggravate the clinical condition of the patient to such an extent that one may consider DIC as an intermediary mechanism of disease to death and as such as a really life-threatening complication.

Under normal conditions, there exists a precisely balanced dynamic equilibrium between a continuous low grade activation of clotting factors and blood platelets and a neutralization of the activation products in the circulating blood. The blood stream causes dilution of the activated factors and prevents further interaction; potent humoral inhibitors of the activated factors bind and inactivate them; labile activation products deteriorate spontaneously and the stable activation products are effectively cleared by the reticuloendothelial system. Normal endothelial cells produce prostacyclin, a potent inhibitor of platelet adhesion and aggregation (7). Emboli of platelet aggregates desintegrate and fibrin deposits are lysed by a fibrinolytic system. All these mechanisms keep the activation of the hemostatic system under control and when it presents to a minor extent, it results only in a local thrombus formation or a hemostatic plug (Fig. 1).

A massive or longer standing intensive activation of the hemostatic mechanism may result in a failure of this equilibrium: if the resultant activated clotting factors overcome normal humoral inhibition and are not cleared by the reticuloendothelial system, clotting is initiated and coagulation factors and blood platelets are consumed. Altered fibrinogen and platelet-clumps persist in the streaming blood and obstruct the microcirculation, causing extensive ischemic damage to the tissues. Additionally secondary triggered fibrinolysis generates fibrinogen/fibrin degradation products that in various ways interfere with platelet function and fibrin polymerization. One end of these processes

LOCAL   adherence of platelets
                  secondary aggregation   < seconds
             activation coagulation factors
                  extrinsic pathway   seconds
                  intrinsic pathway   minutes
             activation fibrinolytic system   hours
BLOOD STREAM
             dilution   < seconds
             inhibition by humeral factors   seconds
             deterioration labile clotting factors   minutes
CAPILLARIES
             fibrinolysis of fibrin deposits   hours
             desaggregation of platelet clumps   minutes
RETICULOENDOTHELIAL SYSTEM
             $t_{\frac{1}{2}}$ of activated clotting factors   minutes to
                                                                   hours

Fig. 1. The function and time-relationships of different mechanisms, which under normal conditions prevent dissemination of the local processes, leading to hemostasis or thrombosis.

is the so-called consumption coagulopathy in which bleeding becomes the major clinical manifestation. The other end result is a clinical picture characterized by ischemia of various tissues due to generalized obstructions in the microvasculature. The clinical picture includes thrombotic and bleeding phenomena with variable pictures depending from a wide range of precipitating factors and individual abilities in the reaction and defense mechanism.

PATHOPHYSIOLOGY

It is generally assumed that in DIC procoagulant materials, ordinarily not in contact with blood, gain access to the circulation. Activation of the coagulation system may occur along an intrinsic pathway by activation of the contact factors F XII and F XI through negatively charged surfaces or collagen fibres. It is suggested that absorption of HF warp the molecule as to expose buried hydrophobic groups necessary for its action, leading to kinin formation, fibrinolysis activation, activation of the first component of complement and enhanced vascular permeability. Two additional factors participate in this reaction namely prekallikrein and high molecular weight kininogen (HMWK).

The extrinsic pathway is triggered when tissue fluid get access to the circulation. Tissue thromboplastin activates factor VII, which in turn activates the further cascade of clotting factors. The interaction of clotting factors IX, VIII and of X, V is enhanced by the presence of phospholipids, which are released by platelets when they adhere to altered endothelial lining or when triggered by traces of thrombin (Fig. 2).

When the activation of clotting factors or platelets

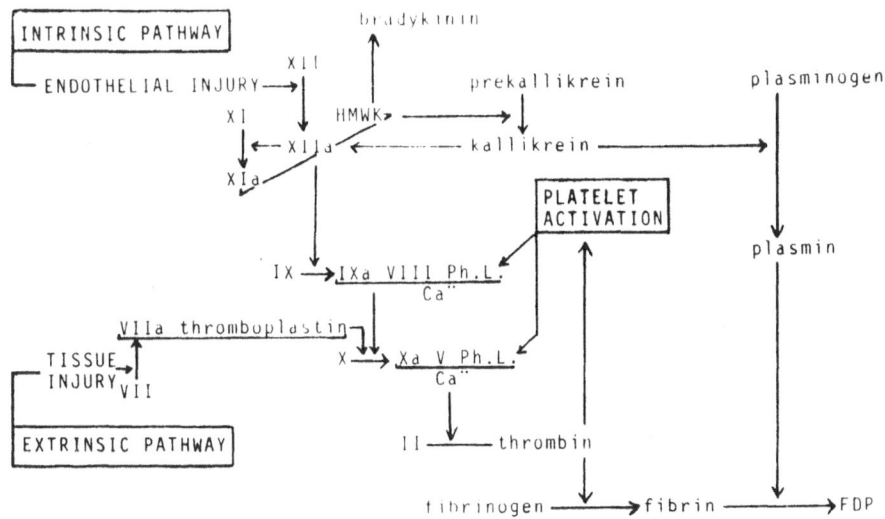

Fig. 2. Activation of the coagulation system by the intrinsic or extrinsic pathway in relation with platelet function.

surpasses certain limits the blood stream velocity is not sufficiently high enough to dilute the activated material; the reticulo-endothelial system becomes saturated and the plasma inhibitors are consumed. In such situations the activated material remains in the circulating blood and leads to alteration of fibrinogen and platelets. A great variety of disease processes leads to leakage of clotting activating material into the circulating blood (Table I), or is characterized by widespread endothelial damage (Table II), giving rise to massive intravascular activation of the coagulation mechanism. A special entity of DIC is characterized by platelet consumption (disseminated intravascular platelet aggregation). In these cases thrombocytopenia predominates with clinical signs of fluctuating progressive multifocal neurological disturbances, complicated by micro-angiopathic hemolytic anemia (Moschcowitz syndrome). The underlying cause of this syndrome is unknown but is related with the functionality of the platelets and the endothelial cells (Table III). There is circumstantial evidence that suggests the existence of a plasma factor that is abnormal or lacking in these patients (5,6,10,15).

As a result of the deposition of fibrin or platelets in the microvasculature, local endothelial plasminogen activator is released and diffuses into the fibrin deposits. Resultant plasmin activity leads to circulating soluble fibrin degradation products. The circulating fibrin fragments may inhibit platelet aggregation, polymerization of fibrin monomers and thrombin action, and thereby intensify the hemorrhagic diathesis.

DIC, when fully expressed is a catastrophic clinical

TABLE I. Clinical conditions which may trigger DIC predominantly by activation of the extrinsic system

extensive surgery
obstetrical complications
massive tissue injury
mucinous carcinoma
tumor cell embolism
intravascular hemolysis
intravascular proteolysis
liver cirrhosis
arsine, carbon tetrachloride
Gram-positive sepsis

TABLE II. Clinical conditions which may trigger DIC, predominantly by activation of the intrinsic clotting system

Gram-negative sepsis
viral infections
Rickettsiosis
fungal infections
protozoal infections
mycoplasma sepsis
immune complexes
giant hemangioma
dissecting aneurysm
cyanotic congenital heart disease (?)
extracorporeal circulation

TABLE III. Clinical conditions which may trigger disseminated intravascular platelet aggregation (DIPA)

thrombotic thrombocytopenic purpura (Moschcowitz syndrome)
hemolytic uremic syndrome (?)
obstetrical complications, toxicosis
oral contraceptives
malignant hypertension (?)
generalized vasculitis
immune complex disease
viral infections (?)
Rickettsiosis
kidney allograft rejection (?)
unknown

syndrome manifested by <u>bleeding</u> due to depletion of platelets and coagulation factors; by organ <u>ischemia</u> consequent to deposition of fibrin and platelets in the microcirculation and by occult or overt <u>hemolytic anemia</u> caused by traumatic red cell destruction in the altered microvasculature. A large proportion of DIC episodes is minor in nature, remains occult but still may have clinical importance. These cases may present real diagnostic problems and are often overlooked.

CLINICAL CONDITIONS

The clinical symptoms of DIC can be arranged in four categories:
1. The symptoms of the underlying disease-state which triggers DIC
2. The clinical signs of organ dysfunction due to the obstruction of the microvasculature
3. The consequences of mechanical red cell lysis
4. The hemorrhagic diathesis due to consumption of hemostatic factors and secondary fibrinolysis

1. From a diagnostic and therapeutic point of view it is important to distinct the precipitating events according to the modes of triggering the intravascular coagulation, that means resulting in acute or chronic DIC.

The clinical features of acute DIC develop over a period of a few hours to days. Disease states leading to acute forms of DIC are summarized in Table IV. The patient is usually critically ill and the symptoms of organ dysfunction due to obstruction of the microcirculation prevail next to a bleeding diathesis that ranges from oozing to life-threatening hemorrhage. The mortality is high ranging from 50-70%.

TABLE IV. Clinical conditions which may precipitate acute forms of DIC

---

extensive surgery
abruptio placentae
amniotic fluid embolism
shock, anoxia, anaphylaxis
trauma, burn, frost bite
hyperpyrexia, heat stroke
fat embolism
acute liver failure
intravascular hemolysis
acute pancreatitis, snake bite
Gram-negative sepsis
viral infections
Rickettsiosis
purpura fulminans

The manifestations of chronic DIC wax and wane over periods of weeks to months. The patient is usually not critically ill. While episodes of bleeding occur, thrombotic complications (phlebitis, embolism) dominate. The disease processes which can lead to chronic DIC are summarized in Table V.

TABLE V. Clinical conditions which may be complicated by chronic
forms of DIC

---

      retention of dead fetus
      ecclampsia
      malignancies
      essential thrombocytosis
      splenomegaly
      liver disease
      peritoneal-venous shunt
      generalized vasculitis
      dissecting aneurysm
      giant hemangioma
      necrotizing enterocolitis
      thrombotic thrombocytopenic purpura

---

2. The generalized obstructions in the microvasculature
cause signs and symptoms of dysfunction of multiple organs.
It is often difficult to decide whether the dysfunctions
are related to DIC or to the underlying diseases. The situations where organ dysfunction appears related to DIC
include the early symptoms: hypertension, respiratory distress syndrome, cardiogenic shock, neurologic syndromes,
renal insufficiency, infarcted skin syndrome and adrenal
infarction (Table VI).

TABLE VI. Early symptoms which occur during DIC

GENERALIZED MICROVASCULAR OBSTRUCTION

     - insufficient tissue oxygenation
     - shock

MICROCIRCULATORY DAMAGE IN VARIOUS ORGANS

     - myocardium: arrhythmia, shock
     - lung: respiratory distress
     - CNS: tachypneu, fever, convulsions
     - kidney: renal insufficiency
     - skin: infarctions of the skin
     - adrenals: shock (Waterhouse-Friederichsen)

CONSUMPTION OF COAGULATION FACTORS AND PLATELETS

     - generalized bleeding tendency

When the patient survives the acute episode, the late results of organ damage may come to attention, like chronic
renal insufficiency, liver dysfunction, microangiopathic
hemolytic anemia, non-bacterial endocarditis, pulmonary
hypertension, sinus thrombosis and other complications as
summarized in table VII.

TABLE VII. Late sequelae of DIC

ORGAN DYSFUNCTION

Frequent
- kidney: uremia
- liver: jaundice
- red cells: microangiopathic hemolysis

Rare
- heart: thrombotic endocarditis
- lung: pulmonary hypertension
- CNS: sinus thrombosis, hypopituitarism
- kidney: renal vein thrombosis
- liver: portal thrombosis
- extremities: acrocyanosis, erythromelalgia, gangrene

---

3. In some patients DIC is complicated by a more or less intensive intravascular red blood cell lysis. This hemolytic component is most pronounced in the so-called hemolytic-uremic syndrome often occurring in neonates and children related to gastrointestinal infections or vaccination. In adults concomitant hemolysis is seen especially in disseminated platelet aggregation with pronounced thrombocytopenia and fluctuating neurological symptoms due to obstruction of the cerebral vasculature (Moschcowitz syndrome).

Classical symptoms of hemolytic anemia, like jaundice, reticulocytosis, increased LDH and low haptoglobin are accompanied by the presence of schistocytes, helmet cells and burr cells in the circulating blood.

4. The consumption of coagulation factors and platelets is manifested by an overt hemorrhagic diathesis. This bleeding tendency is amplified by secondary fibrinolysis and generalized capillary fragility due to local anoxia. Symptoms vary from oozing and bleeding from venipuncture sites to hematemesis, severe intestinal bleeding, generalized purpura (purpura fulminans) to adrenal infarction with irreversible shock (Waterhouse-Friederichsen syndrome).

DIAGNOSIS

The presence of DIC is usually suspected on the basis of several factors such as the clinical setting, bleeding or thrombotic manifestations, unexplained neurological disturbances, respiratory distress, oliguria, jaundice or circulatory failure.

The laboratory manifestations of DIC are related to:
1. Depletion of coagulation factors and platelets due to consumption faster than they can be replaced
2. The presence in the circulation of products of clotting such as soluble fibrin monomer complexes or activated clotting factors

3. Activation of fibrinolysis and the presence of fibrin
   degradation products (FDP)
4. Consequences of endothelial damage in the microcirculation such as microangiopathic hemolytic anemia.

For the primary routine diagnostic screening are most
important: a low platelet count; a prolonged thrombin and
reptilase time; decreased fibrinogen and clotting factors
II, V and VIII; positive protamin paracoagulation or al-
cohol-gel test, which detects soluble fibrin monomer complexes and semiquantitative tests for FDP (Table VIII).

TABLE VIII. Diagnostic criteria which are in favor of the diagnosis
of DIC

DEPLETION OF COAGULATION FACTORS AND PLATELETS

     - low fibrinogen, thrombocytopenia
     - decreased factor VIII, V, II
     - antithrombin-III low or absent

PRESENCE ACTIVATED OR ALTERED CLOTTING FACTORS

     - soluble fibrin monomer complexes
     - fibrinopeptide A, β-thromboglobulin in circulation
     - factor VIII elevated

ACTIVATION OF FIBRINOLYSIS

     - prolonged thrombin time, reptilase time
     - presence fibrin degradation products
     - plasminogen low or absent

MICROANGIOPATHY

     - fragmentation hemolysis
     - haptoglobulin low or absent
     - LDH increased

The detection of an acute massive DIC will not be a diagnostic problem, in subacute or chronic DIC the consumption
of clotting factors may be matched by an increased synthesis rate and no depletion occurs. In a small group of patients the fibrinolytic response may be low or inadequate
and in these the fibrin degradation products are only moderately elevated to a level which may occur during fever,
pneumonia, deep vein thrombosis, normal parturation. On
occasion fibrinolysis is very marked or may persist after
DIC has ceased.

TREATMENT

The clinical picture and the hematological sequences of
DIC show great variability related to the triggering cause,
the individual abilities in the reaction mechanism, and
the time relation and speed of the processes. With that

fact in mind each patient with DIC has to be treated individually although some general outlines can be formulated.

1. Prevention of conditions which favor the occurrence of DIC

It has been recognized that circulatory stasis, hypoxia, shock and acidosis may promote the occurrence and severity of DIC. This must be kept in mind when critically ill patients need large doses of blood. When the transfused red cells have a low 2,3 DPG content the oxygen dissociation is diminished. In ACD blood the 2,3 DPG level drops to 20% by storing blood for five days.

2. Identification and treatment of the underlying disease state

Identification and treatment of all precipitating factors is the keystone of the management of DIC. The many ways in which DIC can be triggered are broadly classified in the Tables I, II and III. In clinical practice the most common causative agent is likely to be infection.

Whereas Gram-negative sepsis may represent the most frequent triggering infection, other micro organisms have also been clearly implicated, including viruses, fungi, Rickettsia and others. The mechanism of clotting activation is complex and may involve interaction with granulocytes, platelets, clotting factors and endothelium. Additional factors are shock with sluggish blood flow and reticuloendothelial system blockade. Antibiotics must be chosen with care and preferably with expert advise. Strenuous efforts must be made to treat shock. It is advisable to avoid the use of plasma expanders such as dextrans and gelatins as these may exacerbate the bleeding tendency; 5% human albumin and fresh red blood cells are preferable. When microcirculatory blockade in the lungs or central nervous system dominates some form of artificial ventilation may be indicated. Other DIC triggering situations may be seen in treatment modalities like irradiation or chemotherapy in malignancies; surgical treatment of dissecting aneurysm; termination of pregnancy in dead-fetus syndrome; immune suppression in vasculitis, and others.

3. Effective blockade of further intravascular activation of the coagulation mechanism

Since the diagnosis of DIC is based on laboratory findings it has been recognized that a large proportion of DIC episodes is minor in nature and may have various clinical importance ranging from temporarily minor disturbances to life-threatening shock or bleeding, and irreversible damage of vital organs and tissues. A number of therapeutic approaches adapted to circumscribed clinical situations and individual patients are discussed briefly:

a. Expectation and symptomatic therapy

In a number of cases of DIC there may be good evidence that the triggering episode has ended at the time that the diagnosis is made. In such conditions there is no rational to start with anticoagulant therapy.

A good example is DIC which has occurred in an obstetrical emergency and is diagnosed when the fetus and placenta have been delivered. All therapy can be best directed symptomatically. No anticoagulant therapy carries with it the risk of continuing defibrination, but is often the best choice if it appears that the clotting is over or will end shortly with the control of the underlying disease

b. Heparin-therapy

The role of heparin in the management of DIC remains controversial arising from the fact that this disease state is heterogeneous in cause and severity. At present time still no controlled clinical trial is documented about the effectiveness of heparin in DIC. The anticoagulant action of heparin needs the presence of antithrombin III in the patients circulation. Unfortunately in DIC antithrombin III may be diminished or absent (1). If antithrombin III is present then heparin effectively blocks further continuing of intravascular clotting factor activation, but, of course, it may make the bleeding worse. Heparin is also best withheld if there are obvious open wounds and risk of massive bleeding. A further complication is the recently discovered heterogeneity of heparin activity within and between batches.

If there are good reasons to assume that consumption of coagulation factors continues and the clinical situation aggravates progressively then heparinization may be indicated. This is begun cautiously by a loading dose of 50-75 mg and a continuous intravenous infusion 5 mg/hr for 3 hrs and increased to 10 mg/hr if no improvement in fibrinogen values occurs and there is no exacerbation of the bleeding. Effective heparinization includes a concentration of 5-10 µg/ml and a 2-2.5 fold increase of the whole blood clotting time or partial thromboplastin time. Failure of heparin therapy may be related to antithrombin III deficiency. In such situations additional transfusion of fresh heparinized plasma or concentrated antithrombin III may be indicated (11).

c. Fresh plasma infusions or plasmapheresis

The question has been raised if the mechanisms responsible for DIC are much more complex than hitherto appreciated. Certainly heparin does not influence the release and migration of leukocytes, the activation of complement and kininogens neither the functional abilities of the endothelial cells. Moreover the precipitation of soluble fibrin monomer complexes is not prevented by heparin and the clearing capacity of the reticulo-endothelial system is unaffected. These considerations and the disappointing results of heparin therapy suggest that new approaches are required for the management of DIC. The currently available continuous flow separators have made intensive 'washout' plasmapheresis feasible. Most successful results with this technique were obtained in thrombotic thrombocytopenic purpura in which 80% of the patients dies within three months after onset (14).

Bukowski et al. (2) obtained with plasma exchange transfusion complete remissions in 6 out of 13 patients. Pisciotta et al. (9) achieved with plasma exchange 7 remissions out of 9 cases with T.T.P. Plasmapheresis has been used in combination with anti-platelet drugs by Mijers et al. (8) who achieved complete remissions in 8 out of 9 patients with such a combined treatment.

Byrnes and Khurana and Upshaw (4,12) reported remissions in T.T.P. with use of massive plasma infusions without exchange providing evidence of a factor present in normal plasma that reverses platelet consumption and microangiopathic hemolysis. During the last years we had the opportunity to study 9 patients with T.T.P.; seven of them were seen the last four years.

Four out of six patients who have been treated by massive plasma infusions recovered. Two patients who only received symptomatic therapy and one, who underwent but a few courses of plasmapheresis died. At this moment one can only speculate about the possible mechanism of action. Remuzzi et al. (10) have suggested that in T.T.P. plasma a factor is lacking which stimulates the formation of prostacyclin by the endothelial cells, which is a potent endogenous inhibitor of platelet aggregation. Plasma infusions and plasmapheresis may be life-saving in T.T.P. and has to be continued for weeks, even months before a definite remission is obtained. The significance and value of plasmapheresis in DIC is not yet evaluable but is at best of importance as replacement therapy and does not offer the final solution.

d. Antiplatelet drugs

Platelet consumption plays a role in a number of DIC patients such as thrombotic thrombocytopenic purpura, probably also in the hemolytic uremic syndrome, in generalized vasculitis, in virus and Rickettsial infections, and immune complex disease. Favorable effects are reported from dextran therapy, from dipyridamole (300-600 mg/day), sulfinpyrazone (800-1600 mg/day) and acetylsalicylic acid (0.5-1.5 g/day). In most reports anti-platelet drugs are given in combination with heparin or other therapeutic measures and their real usefulness in DIC treatment remains to be demonstrated.

4. Replacement of depleted factors

Replacement therapy of depleted factors can be given in the form of fibrinogen, plasma, platelet-concentrates and factor VIII-rich cryoprecipitate. The replacement may have the unwanted side-effect to add fuel to the fire and allow further clotting. Replacement has to be considered only after careful weighing of the advantages against the risks. Fibrinogen replacement and administration of factor II, VII IX and X concentrates carry the risk of hepatitis. If replacement therapy is nevertheless indicated then it seems advisable to give this in combination with heparin.

5. Treatment of the clinical sequelae of DIC

Severe blood loss as a consequence of the hemorrhagic diathesis or severe microangiopathic hemolysis have to be
corrected by freshly packed cells or fresh whole blood.
DIC may be complicated by renal insufficiency and oliguria.
Often this complication can be prevented by adequate prevention or treatment of hypotension and metabolic acidosis and additional administration of diuretics. Hemodialysis may be indicated if renal failure is pronounced. In
cases of severe hypotension and if adrenal infarction is
suspected, treatment with steroids may be necessary. Yamada et al. (16) have reported that respiratory distress
after DIC may improve after administration of α-blocking
agents. Infarctions of skin, extremities, segments of the
intestines and other organs may need surgical correction.

REFERENCES

1. Braunstein, K.M., Eurenius, K.: Minimal heparin co-factor activity in disseminated intravascular coagulation and cirrhosis. Am.J.Clin. Pathol. 66:488, 1976.
2. Bukowski, R.M., Hewlett, J.S., Harris, J.W.: Exchange transfusions in the treatment of thrombotic thrombocytopenic purpura. Semin. Hematol. 13:219, 1976.
3. Bukowski, R.M., King, J.W., Hewlett, J.S.: Plasmapheresis in the treatment of thrombotic thrombocytopenic purpura. Blood 50:413, 1977.
4. Byrnes, J.J., Khurana, M.: Treatment of thrombotic thrombocytope-nic purpura with plasma. N. Engl. J. Med. 297:1386, 1977.
5. Lian, E.C.Y., Harkness, D.R., Byrnes, J.J., Wallach, H., Nunez, R.: Presence of a platelet aggregating factor in the plasma of patients with thrombotic thrombocytopenic purpura (T.T.P.) and its inhibition by normal plasma. Blood 53:333, 1979.
6. McIntyre, D.E., Pearson, J.D., Gordon, J.L.: Localisation and stim-ulation of prostacyclin production in vascular cells. Nature 271: 549, 1978.
7. Moncada, S., Higgins, E.A., Vane, J.R.: Human arterial and venous tissues generate prostacyclin (prostaglandin X), a potent inhibitor of platelet aggregation. Lancet 1:18, 1977.
8. Myers, I.J., Wakem, C.J., Ball, E.D., Tremont, S.J.: Thrombotic thrombocytopenic purpura: combined treatment with plasmapheresis and antiplatelet agents. Ann. Int. Med. 92:149, 1980.
9. Pisciotta, A.V., Garthware, T., Darin, J., Aster, R.: Treatment of thrombotic thrombocytopenic purpura by exchange transfusion. Am. J. Hematol. 3:73, 1977.
10. Remuzzi, G., Marchesi, D., Mecca, G., Misiani, R., Livio, M., De Gaetano, G., Donati, M.B.: Haemolytic uraemic syndrome: deficiency of plasma factor(s) regulating prostacyclin activity? Lancet 2:871, 1978.
11. Schipper, H.S., Jenkins, C.S., Kahlé, L.H., Ten Cate, J.W.: Anti-thrombin III transfusion in disseminated intravascular coagulation. Lancet 1:845, 1978.
12. Upshaw, J.D.: Congenital deficiency of a factor in plasma that re-verses microangiopathic hemolysis and thrombocytopenia. N. Engl.

J. Med. 298:1350, 1978.
13. Weick, J.K.: Intravascular coagulation in cancer. Semin. Oncol. 5:203, 1978.
14. Wenz, B., Barland, P.: Therapeutic intensive plasmapheresis. Sem. Hemat. 18:147, 1981.
15. Wiles, P.G., Solomon, L.R., Lawler, W., Mallick, N.P., Johnson, M.: Inherited plasma factor deficiency in haemolytic uraemic syndrome. Lancet 1:1105, 1981.
16. Yamada, K., Shirahata, A., Meguro, T.: The effects of an alpha blocking agent on the respiratory distress syndrome with disseminated intravascular coagulation in the newborn infants and experimental animals. Thromb. Res. 8:179, 1976.

COLLOID OR CRYSTALLOID IN THE RESUSCITATION OF HEMORRHAGIC SHOCK: A CONTROLLED CLINICAL TRIAL*

G.S. Moss, R.J. Lowe, J. Jilek and H.D. Levine

In 1977 we reported the results of a randomized prospective trial in which 137 patients who underwent laparotomy for trauma were initially resuscitated with either Ringer's lactate solution (RL) or 4% human serum albumin (HSA) in RL (3). We found no differences between these groups in mortality rate, pulmonary function, or requirement for prolonged mechanical ventilation.

A criticism of this study was that the majority of patients were not in shock upon admission and therefore could be expected to do well regardless of the type of fluid used in resuscitation (7). Furthermore, patients with concomitant thoracic injuries were studied but deliberately excluded from that report. The combination of thoracic injury and shock necessitating volume resuscitation might result in pulmonary dysfunction.

The objective of this article is to describe the results of fluid resuscitation in trauma victims in shock requiring laparotomy whose volume replacement consisted of either HSA or RL. This report includes those patients in shock who were excluded from the first report because of concomitant thoracic injuries.

METHODS AND MATERIAL

Criteria for entry into the study**. Patients were defined as being in shock and included in this study if they met *either* of the following criteria:

1. Systolic arterial pressure of equal to or less than 80 mm Hg upon admission or prior to operation.

2. Transfusion of 5 or more units of washed red cells prior to operation.

Randomization. When the patient was admitted an envelope indicating either RL or HSA was drawn. In the HSA group 50 g of a 25% solution of HSA was added 'piggyback' to each liter of RL.

* Supported in part by a contract with the U.S. Army Medical Research and Development Command.
** Informed consent was obtained in accord with institutional and federal requirements set forth in Sections 46.9 and 46.10 of Title 45 of the Code of Federal Regulations.

Resuscitation. Initial volume expansion was performed with either test fluid until the clinical signs of satisfactory volume expansion were achieved. These signs included a pulse rate less than 100, a urine output greater than 30 ml/hr, and an increase in systolic arterial pressure above 80 mm Hg. Washed red cells were given to maintain the hematocrit equal to or greater than 30%.

In those patients who were hemodynamically unstable after operation, a flow-directed pulmonary artery catheter was inserted and used to guide further fluid therapy.

Pulmonary function data and other studies. After operation patients were extubated according to well-established criteria, including P_{CO_2} equal to or less than 45 and pH equal to or greater than 7.30. Pulmonary function studies were performed daily for 5 days. These studies (3) included respiratory rate, tidal volume, vital capacity, A-a D_{O_2} (FI_{O_2} = 1.0), intrapulmonary shunt (where $P\bar{v}_{O_2}$ was available), and V_D/V_T. In addition blood was drawn to obtain serum total protein levels.

Statistical analysis. The box and whiskers technique (9) was used to display fluid infusion volumes and red cell transfusion volumes. This technique is useful in representing data that are not normally distributed. The data points for each patient are plotted along the Y-axis, as in a histogram. The median is represented by a heavy bar. The upper and lower quartiles are represented by lighter bars. The space between the upper and lower quartiles, therefore, represents that half of the data points in the center and is delineated by a box drawn between the quartiles. The extremes of the data points are the 'whiskers' that extend above and below the box.

The significance of differences in the pulmonary function data were determined by the use of a Mann-Whitney test (8).

RESULTS

During the study period, 137 patients required laparotomy for abdominal trauma. Forty patients met the criteria for shock; four died intraoperatively. The study population comprised the remaining 36 patients. Twenty were assigned to the RL group and 16 to the HSA group.

Patient profile. Table I shows that the two groups were comparable in age, sex, number with chest injuries, and number with gastrointestinal injuries. In Table II the mechanism of injury is shown. The majority of patients in both groups sustained penetrating injuries.

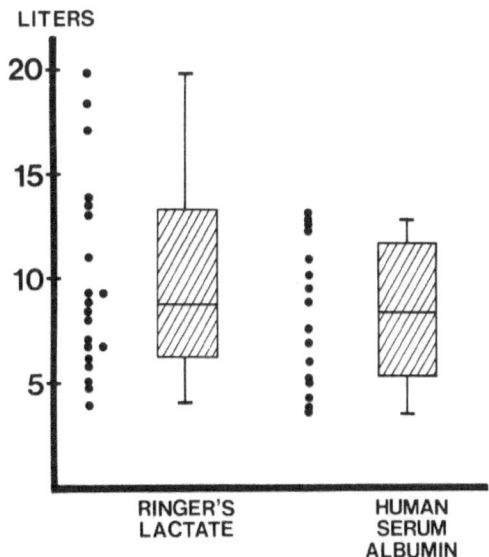

Fig. 1. Volume of test fluid infused. Each point represents an individual patient. See text for explanation of box and whiskers.

Resuscitation volumes. Fig. 1 shows the distribution of fluid volumes infused. The median volume, 8 L, is the same for both groups. A difference in the pattern of infusion volumes is best illustrated by the box and whiskers, which illustrates the tendency toward greater volumes in the RL group.

Fig. 2 shows the distribution of number of units of washed red cells transfused. The pattern is similar in both groups. The median value for the RL group was 5.5. It was 7 for the HSA group.

Mortality rate. There was one death in the 36 patients (Table III). This patient, assigned to the RL group, sustained a gunshot wound to the right colon and died of overwhelming sepsis on the third postoperative day.

Mechanical ventilation. Two patients in each group required mechanical ventilation for longer than 24 hours (Table III). No patient developed overt pulmonary edema.

Pulmonary function data and other studies. Table IV shows the results of serial pulmonary function studies performed daily for 5 days after operation. Although many of the variables are abnormal, there are no important differences between the groups on any day of the study.

The changes in plasma total protein and base deficit levels are shown in Fig. 3. Total protein was significantly reduced ($P < 0.05$) in the RL group on day 1 as compared to the HSA group. There was no difference between the groups in base deficit values.

150

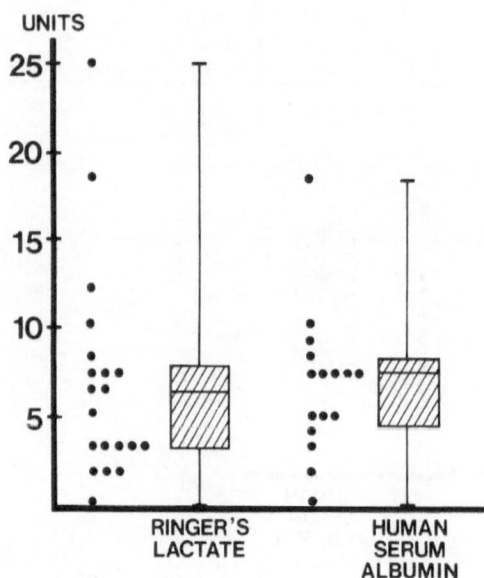

Fig. 2. Number of units of red cells transfused. Each point represents an individual patient. See text for explanation of box and whiskers.

TABLE I. Patient profile

Group characteristics	RL group	HSA group
No. patients	20	16
Age (yr)	29 ± 3 SEM	31 ± 4 SEM
Sex: male	15	14
female	5	2
Chest injuries	5	7
Gastrointestinal injuries	10	8

TABLE II. Mechanism of injury

Type of injury	RL group	HSA group
Gunshot wound	9	7
Stab wound	10	6
Blunt trauma	1	3

TABLE III. Mortality rate

	RL group	HSA group
No. patients	20	16
Mortality rate	1	0
No. requiring ventilation support > 24 hours	2	2

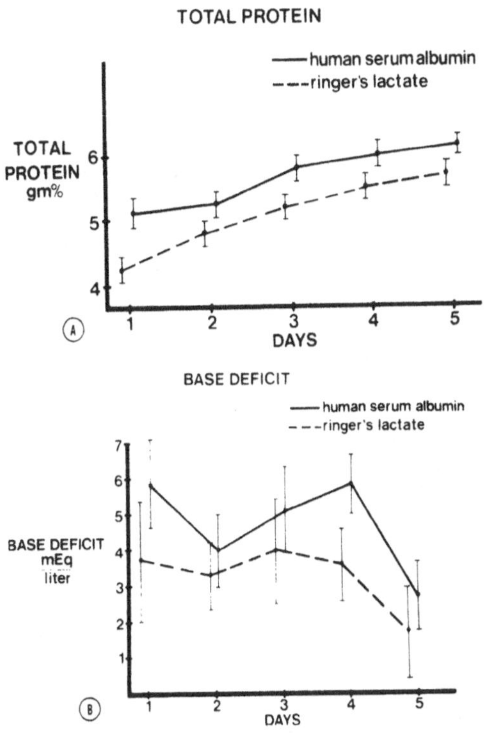

Fig. 3. Mean values (± SEM) for serum total protein: A, and base deficit: B, in the two groups.

DISCUSSION

In this study we examined a group of 36 young patients who entered the hospital hypovolemic as a result of trauma. They were initially resuscitated with either RL or HSA to physiologic end points. The median volume for both groups was 8L of fluid. Patients in the RL group received no HSA at all during their hospital stay. If important differences develop between groups of patients resuscitated with or without HSA, these differences should be seen in severely injured patients, such as these, who require large infusion volumes. We found no differences in mortality rate, requirement for prolonged mechanical ventilation, or in a battery of pulmonary function tests.

An unexpected result of this study was the similarity in the volume of infused fluid in the two groups. In studies of subhuman primates, substantially greater volumes of RL were required compared to HSA (5). Similar results were noted in patients who underwent elective vascular surgery (10). The fact that in our patients the infusion volumes were similar might indicate that either the RL patients were undertreated or the HSA patients were overtreated. This does not appear to be a good explanation for the

TABLE IV. Results of serial pulmonary function studies

Study	Variable	Day 1		Day 2		Day 3		Day 4		Day 5	
		RL	HSA	RL	HSA	RL	HSA	RL	HSA	RL	HSA
Resp. rate (breaths/min)	$\bar{X}$	28	24	25	23	26	20	25	21	26	22
	SEM	3	2	2	1	1	1	2	1	2	1
	N	12	10	14	15	17	14	14	15	14	15
Tidal vol. (ml)	$\bar{X}$	346	386	457	418	403	515	432	460	441	473
	SEM	29	38	44	34	49	35	45	38	57	39
	N	12	10	14	15	17	14	14	15	14	15
Vital cap. (ml)	$\bar{X}$	1,019	992	1,123	1,141	1,380	1,401	1,518	1,413	1,613	1,816
	SEM	84	101	116	148	130	227	224	227	138	293
	N	10	11	15	15	16	15	13	15	13	15
A-a DO$_2$ (mm Hg)	$\bar{X}$	344	297	329	312	295	307	273	278	251	259
	SEM	24	30	16	29	21	26	21	21	22	26
	N	15	11	17	15	19	14	16	15	16	15
Shunt (%)	$\bar{X}$	19	19	24	26	21	20	22	22	21	20
	SEM	2	2	2	4	2	5	3	5	5	3
	N	7	6	6	5	8	3	7	3	3	2
V_D/V_T	$\bar{X}$	0.44	0.43	0.44	0.44	0.41	0.47	0.38	0.42	0.45	0.41
	SEM	0.03	0.04	0.04	0.03	0.03	0.03	0.03	0.03	0.02	0.03
	N	12	10	13	15	17	13	14	15	14	15

following reasons:
  1. Base deficit values were normal in both groups immediately after initial resuscitation.
  2. Pulmonary edema was not seen in any patient in the study.
  3. Only one of 36 of these severely injured patients died.

A similar observation concerning infusion volumes for trauma victims resuscitated with or without extra HSA were reported by Lucas et al. (4). Both treatment groups in that study received a total of 10 L of test fluid before and during surgery. Carey, Lowery and Cloutier (2), in a report from Vietnam, did not note greater infusion volumes in combat casualties resuscitated with salt solution plus whole blood as compared to 5% HSA and whole blood. In all these studies, only small differences in serum protein values were noted between patients treated with or without HSA. It is possible that in trauma patients, substantial amounts of infused HSA leaks into the injured tissues, drawing water along and thereby increasing the total infusion volume requirement. Another possibility is that in the trauma studies the physiologic end points for volume replacement were clinical criteria and therefore varied, of necessity, over a broad range of 'normal'. In the laboratory studies, as in Virgilio's elective surgical studies in humans, fluid replacement was titrated against left ventricular filling pressure and/or cardiac output, and the allowed range of these variables was much more narrow than in our study or that of Lucas.

The principal objection to resuscitation with RL is that the infusion of protein-free fluid will dilute the recipient plasma protein level, which may lead to pulmonary edema. Several experimental and clinical studies do not substantiate this concern. For example, baboons resuscitated with protein-free fluid and packed red cells did not demonstrate any evidence of pulmonary edema despite a 50% reduction in serum protein values and a 10% gain in body weight (5). In a randomized prospective study of patients undergoing elective vascular surgery (10), either RL or HSA was given during operation plus packed red cells. Patients in the RL group developed a 50% reduction in serum protein level, whereas no change was seen in the HSA group. There was no correlation noted between reduced serum protein level and deranged pulmonary function in these patients. In fact, the two patients who did develop pulmonary edema had normal serum protein levels. Pulmonary edema in these patients was associated with unexpected elevations in left atrial pressure related to inadvertent overinfusion of HSA. In our present study, as well as our previous report of the entire group of 137 patients, we also found no relationship between the type of infusion fluid and pulmonary dysfunction. The literature now contains controlled studies in our younger trauma patients in shock and studies in older patients undergoing elective vascular surgery.

Combining these two studies yields an aggregate of 35 patients resuscitated with RL and red blood cells and 30 patients resuscitated with HSA and red blood cells. No differences other than weight gain and slightly decreased serum protein levels exist between the two groups. Thus these two studies demonstrate that blood volume can be effectively restored and maintained without HSA and without resulting in pulmonary dysfunction.

Why does hypoproteinemia during resuscitation or elective operation not lead to pulmonary edema? The best explanation lies in the newly understood relationship concerning albumin and water movement across pulmonary capillary membranes. Studies of pulmonary lymph in sheep (1) and baboons (11) have shown that albumin normally exists in the lung interstitium at levels only slightly lower than plasma levels and is not largely excluded from the lung interstitium as was previously believed. Further studies in baboons (11) have shown that a reduction in serum albumin levels is associated with a simultaneous reduction in pulmonary interstitial albumin levels. Thus hypoproteinemia does not necessarily alter the balance of forces at the pulmonary capillary membrane favoring water movement into the lung interstitium.

Finally, costs should also be considered in deciding whether HSA should be used for resuscitation. In the present study, 8L of test fluid was the median volume used during resuscitation and operation. Since 50 g of HSA costs approximately $ 130, the price of resuscitation in this group was $ 1,040 per patient. In contrast, a liter of RL costs approximately $ 1, and the price of resuscitation was therefore only $ 8 per patient. On the national level, the plasma industry reports a volume of $ 230 million in 1978, a 12% increase over the previous year (6). By 1983 it anticipates growth to $ 400 million. Albumin represents approximately 75% of this market.

It has been shown that the circulating blood volume of severely traumatized patients can be restored by use of an inexpensive colloid-free regimen of RL and red cell concentrates without incurring pulmonary dysfunction.

REFERENCES

1. Brigham, K.L., Wolverton, W.C., Blake, H.L.: Increased sheep lung vascular permeability caused by pseudomonas bacteremia. J. Clin. Invest 54:792, 1974.
2. Carey, L.C., Lowery, B.D., Cloutier, C.T.: Hemorrhagic shock. Curr Prob. Surg. 8:2, 1971.
3. Lowe, R.J., Moss, G.S., Jilek, J., Levine, H.D.: Crystalloid vs. colloid in the etiology of pulmonary failure after trauma: A randomized trial in man. Surgery 81:676, 1977.
4. Lucas, C.E., Weaver, D., Higgins, R.F., Ledgerwood, A.M., Johnson, S.D., Bouwman, D.L.: Effects of albumin vs. non-albumin resuscitation on plasma volume and renal excretory function. J. Trauma

18:564, 1978.

5. Moss, G.S., Siegel, D.C., Cochin, A., Fresquez, V.: Effects of saline and colloid solutions on pulmonary function in hemorrhagic shock. Surg. Gynecol. Obstet. 133:53, 1971.

6. Randolph, H.B.: PLasma, its derivatives and market. Plasma Quarterly 1:74, 1979.

7. Shoemaker, W.C., Hauser, C.J.: Critique of crystalloid vs. colloid therapy in shock and shock lung. Crit. Care Med. 7:117, 1979.

8. Siegel, S.: Nonparametric statistics for the behavioral sciences. New York, Mc Graw-Hill, p. 116, 1956.

9. Tukey, J.W.: Exploratory data analysis. Reading, Mass, Addison-Wesley, p. 39, 1977.

10. Virgilio, R.W., Rice, C.L., Smith, D.E., James, D.R., Zarins, C.K., Hobelmann, C.F., Peters, R.M.: Crystalloid vs. colloid resuscitation: Is one better. Surgery 85:129, 1979.

11. Zarins, C.K., Rice, C.L., Peters, R.M., Virgilio, R.W.: Lymph and pulmonary response to isobaric reduction in plasma oncotic pressure in baboons. Circ. Res. 43:925, 1978.

LIVER TRANSPLANTS: FACING THE FACTS OF MASSIVE BLOOD LOSS

D.E.F. Newton, H. Wesenhagen and C.R. Stoutenbeek

Liver transplantation in man has been a practical possibility for over a decade.

For a number of technical reasons man appears to give greater problems in implantation than experimental animals of a similar size. While the immunological problems are less than with other organs, the general condition of patients in end stage liver disease contributes both anatomical and hematological difficulties during surgery and the postoperative period.

Initial series in both the USA (1) and England (3) have demonstrated that the problems of surgical implantation and clinical immunology have to a large extent been overcome. Based on this large experience: 170 plus in Denver and 100 plus in Cambridge, a study of the literature, and personal contacts have enabled the liver transplantation team in the University of Groningen to set up a program within a relatively short space of time (4). Essentially the principal problems have been organizational, the setting up of interdisciplinary contacts, the assembly and training of a team containing over 20 medical staff and the arrangement of fast and extensive laboratory services. This end necessitated the writing of a comprehensive perioperative protocol which, now updated, runs to 70 pages.

This paper outlines the perioperative anesthetic problems of liver transplantation, and concentrates on the measures taken to maintain circulating blood volume and the clotting mechanism.

The clinical details of the 12 patients so far transplanted are summarized in Table I.

The first patients were of necessity in a poor preoperative condition, and this is reflected in the ASA anesthetic score as well as the perioperative mortality. Progressive improvement in patient selection as well as operative technique has resulted in a fall in the complication rate, especially from massive blood loss.

For a clear understanding of the anesthetic problems to be met during liver transplantation it is necessary to outline the sequence of events and phases of the procedure. These are summarized in Table II.

During the perioperative period the anesthetic team has two separate tasks, the first to set up all the monitoring

TABLE I. Liver transplant operations, Groningen 1979-1981

No.	Date	Age	F/M	Diagnosis	ASA	Fate
1.	12/3/79	23	F	Primary biliary cirrhosis	4	DOT
2.	16/4/79	45	F	do	3	Home
3.	31/10/97	42	F	Primary hepatoma	2	Home
4.	4/12/79	56	F	Primary biliary cirrhosis	4	dd
5.	4/3/80	54	F	do	4	Home
6.	6/5/80	54	F	Chronic hepatitis	4	dd
7.	14/10/80	55	M	Primary biliary cirrhosis	3	Home
8.	14/1/81	50	F	do	3	Home
9.	18/3/81	43	F	do	3	dd
10.	5/7/81	58	F	do	3	Home
11.	14/9/81	49	F	do	3	Home

TABLE II. Liver transplant operations, sequence of events

1. Preoperative preparation	-	Correction of biochemical, hematological and cardiopulmonary problems
2. Surgical preparation	-	Dissection and removal of diseased liver
3. Anhepatic phase	-	Implantation of donor liver
4. Recirculation		
5. Biliary reconnection		
6. Hemostasis and closing		

anesthetic and transfusion apparatus, and to ensure that the full range of IV fluids and blood products are assembled, and second when necessary to correct hematological and circulatory disturbances before surgery can take place. To this end it is essential that detailed clotting investigations are made by the physicians throughout the period when the patient is waiting for a liver to become available Of the 12 patients transplanted 9 had clotting functions within normal limits, and the remainder required preoperative correction.

During operation, apart from replacement of lost blood and coagulation defects the anesthetist has to face the following problems: a decrease in body temperature due to poor liver metabolism, massive exposure during the anhepatic phase, and transplantation of a cooled liver; a high risk of air embolism from the inferior vena cava; citrate acidosis and serum Ca decrease due to massive blood transfusion; lactic acidosis due to the anhepatic period, and recirculation of the lower body area, disturbances in glu-

cose metabilism in the anhepatic period and during the re-
function of the new liver, and consequently progressive hypokalemia as the function of the new liver improves.

These problems notwithstanding, the principal problem
remains the replacement of blood loss and the control of
bleeding. The magnitude of which is illustrated by the extent of blood replacement given in this series of patients
(Fig. 1).

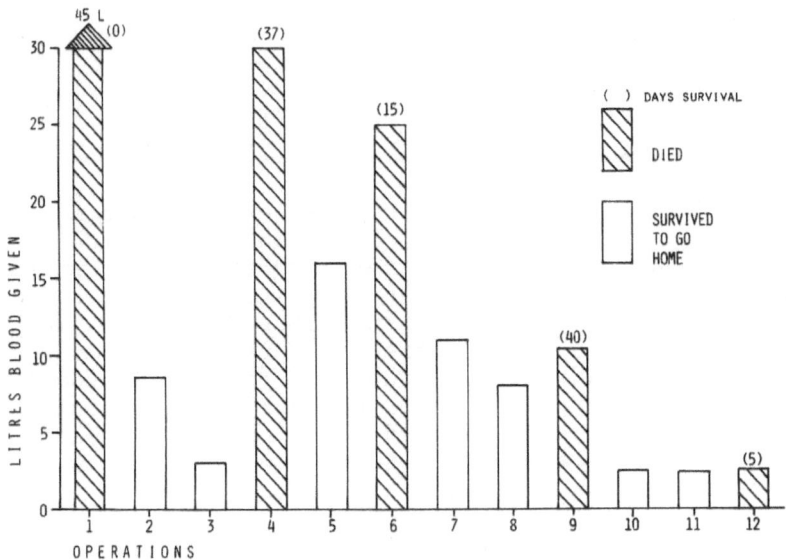

Fig. 1. Preoperative blood requirements during liver transplantation.

From the block diagram it can be seen that there has
been an enormous variation in the volume needed, and that
the trend, with improving selection and surgical technique
is to smaller losses. It is, however, too early to predict
when massive bleeding may occur, and it is therefore necessary for the moment to continue with the techniques that
we have up to now found so useful.

With such drastic disorders of the production, loss and
breakdown of clotting factors that could be expected in
these patients, it is unfortunate that preoperative clotting investigations have turned out to be of little help
both because of the time needed for the investigation, and
the rapid progress of surgical events, and when making a
retrospective assessment. So far the best guide still appears to be the appearance of the surgical field, and the
response to clotting factors given according to an agreed
protocol.

After the 8 transplants a protocol was set up (Table III)

TABLE III. Protocols for correction of clotting factors during liver transplantation

A. Patients with clotting problems before operation:
1. Preoperative: 2 FFP; cryoprecipitate; 2 Proplex; 12 units platelets.
2. Every 30 min during operation: 6 units platelet suspension; 8 units cryoprecipitate; 2 units FFP.
3. After implantation: the use of relatively 'fresh' blood.

B. Patients with no preoperative clotting abnormalities:
1. Preoperative correction of platelet deficit.
2. Administration of 12 units platelet suspension; 8 units cryoprecipitate; and 2 units FFP before recirculation of the liver.
3. After implantation: the use of relatively 'fresh' blood.
4. Reversion to protocol A at the first sign of surgical oozing.

for the regular empirical administration of clotting factors at various stages of the operation. This, albeit costly exercise has resulted in a definite subjective improvement in the operative field, and may in some part have contributed to the reduction in blood loss during the later cases. Recently, in a few patients, further decreases in blood loss have made strict adherence to this protocol, not only unnecessary, but hemodynamically undesirable because of the high colloid fluid load imposed. Supplementation has in these cases been limited to thrombocyte suspensions, and fresh frozen plasma as required.

The experience from other centers (2) fails to suggest that this satisfactory state of affairs is likely to continue indefinitely. Less fit patients (generally and consequently hematologically) will of necessity be presented for surgery with the attendant blood loss and coagulopathy

When severe hemorrhage during liver transplantation occurs it is necessary to be able to transfuse up to one liter per minute in order to maintain an adequate circulation Various methods have been employed to overcome this problem autotransfusion with attendant heparinization has resulted in uncontrollable bleeding, as has partial cardiopulmonary bypass. Strunin (5) suggested the use of an autotransfuser pump as a means of rapidly infusing stored, rather that reclaimed blood and it is this method that we have found life saving.

Before beginning liver transplantation it is thus necessary to assemble both the apparatus and a store of blood products appropriate to the various phases of the operation (Table IV).

This follows a logical sequence, both to maintain clotting function, and to make the best possible use of the blood available (Table V).

Three large infusion cannulas are inserted in peripheral arm veins before surgery commences, and are used as 'normal infusions until the critical phases of the operation are

TABLE IV. Blood and blood products available during liver transplantation

---

15 units 'old' whole blood
15 units 'fresh' whole blood
10 units packed cells

4 units FFP
8 units cryoprecipitate   } ordered 1 hour before needed
2 x 6 unit packs platelet suspension

10 x 500 ml human albumin 5%
5 x 100 ml human albumin 20%

TABLE V. Protocol for blood administration during liver transplantation

---

A. Preparation stage: 'old' whole blood.

B. Anhepatic phase: 'old' whole blood and in emergency, 'fresh' whole blood or RBC's + human albumin 5%.

C. Post recirculation: 'fresh' whole blood and then RBC's as indicated.

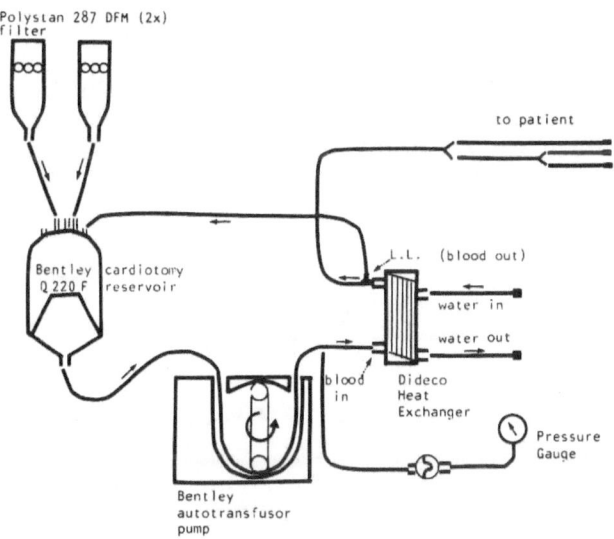

Fig. 2. Infusion pump assembly for use during massive surgical hemorrhage.

reached. Meanwhile the infusion pump assembly is set up as shown in Figure 2.

A Bentley Q220F cardiotomy reservoir is set up and connected via a roller pump (Bentley autotransfuser) to a heat exchanger (Dideco). When not infusing the blood is recirculated slowly to prevent sludging. During the operation blood loss is measured in suction reservoirs placed directly in front of the anesthetist controlling the transfusion.

Transfusion proceeds both in accordance with the measured blood loss, and according to the values of venous, pulmonary arterial, and radial arterial pressure continuously displayed. Although adequate filling pressures are necessary to maintain cardiac output, relative overtransfusion increases pressure on the caval venous anastomoses and can provoke unnecessary bleeding during the critical reconnection phase. Against this has to be set the need to maintain a positive pressure in the vena cava above the liver in order to prevent air embolus.

Using this technique we have been able with the cooperation of our blood bank to meet surgical blood losses of up to 16 liters with a perioperative survival.

The various clotting factors are of course infused separately via another peripheral line.

The methodology outlined makes it possible to infuse rapidly large quantities of properly warmed fluid without recourse to armies of helpers blowing up pressure bags, batteries of blood warmers etc.

The hemodynamic consequences of temporary venacaval disconnection are interesting in that there is on the arterial side a vast capacitance via the descending aorta to the lower body from which blood can only slowly through collaterals return. Without significant blood loss the transfusion system can give essential support until a steady state is reached (Fig. 3).

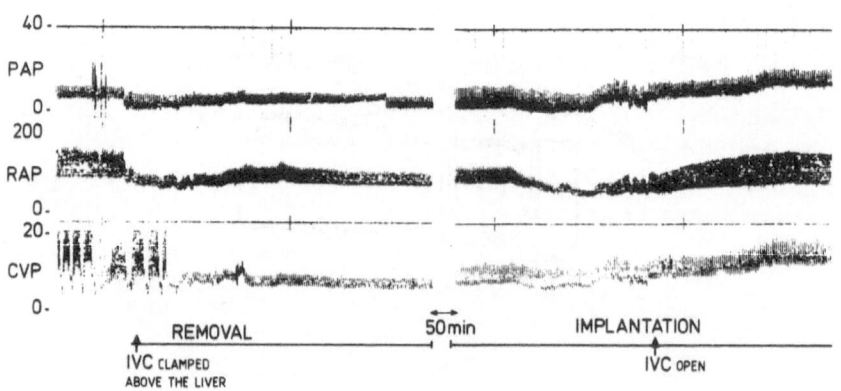

Fig. 3. Hemodynamic changes during the anhepatic phase of liver transplantation.

For the majority of the patients the immediate post-operative care on the ITU proceeds at a more leisurely pace, and it is then possible to investigate the clotting function in depth, and make the necessary corrections. As can be expected the least changes are found in patients in which satisfactory hepatic function establishes itself.

Liver transplantation throws a heavy load on a wide range of facilities in the hospital, not least the blood transfusion service. The operating team, together with the clinical hematologist carry the heavy ethical responsibility of regulating the extensive use of donor services for one patient and have to make together the decision when to stop. We have no evidence as to the toxic effect of huge amounts of donor blood in these patients, as certainly transfusions of up to 16 liters are compatible with survival. The decision, therefore, rests on two main factors, the likelihood of a successful surgical outcome, and the availability of blood without threatening the service to other patients....

REFERENCES

1. Aldrete, J.A., LeVine, D.S., Gingrich, T.F.: Experience in anaesthesia for liver transplantation. Anesth. Analg. Curr. Res. 48:802, 1969.
2. Farman, J.V.: Personal communication. 1979.
3. Farman, J.V., Lines, J.G., Williams, R.S., Evans, D.B., Samuel, J.R., Mason, S.A., Ashby, B.S., Calne, R.Y.: Liver transplantation in man. Anaesthesia 29:17, 1974.
4. Krom, R.A.F., Gips, C.H., Kootstra, G., Newton, D.E.F.: Zes lever-transplantaties te Groningen verricht. Ned. T. Geneesk. 125:22, 1981.
5. Strunin, L.: The liver and anaesthesia. W.B. Saunders Co., 1977, p. 121.

TRANSFUSIONAL PREVENTION OF THE MASSIVE TRANSFUSION SYNDROME

M. Gueguen, B. Genetet, M. Tanguy and C. Saint-Marc

INTRODUCTION

In many cases, especially those encountered in intensive care units, patients are transfused massively with blood components to compensate the consequences of blood loss (hypoxemia, hemostasis disorders for example).

Sometimes during the transfusion, we notice the so-called iatrogenic 'massive transfusion syndrome' (MTS), namely coagulation disorders (DIC) (7,8) metabolic disorders (5) affecting calcium, potassium (11), acid-base balance (10), hypothermia (4), pulmonary disorders: respiratory insufficiency by circulatory overload, micro-emboli, pulmonary edema (6).

Is there a means of ensuring massive transfusion without causing MTS?

PATIENTS AND METHODS

Although the definitions of massive transfusion (MT) would vary, for our purpose we have defined it as at least one total exchange transfusion in less than 24 hours.

Patients

Our study was carried out on 75 patients hospitalized in an intensive care unit, with the following clinical picture:

- Severe trauma   53
  (essentially road accidents)
- Surgery   13
- Digestive hemorrhages   6
- Obstetrical coagulopathies   3

Products

We have used the following products:
1. Six day old packed red cells collected into CPD (Hct = 0.72 ± 0.03), CPD-adenine (Hct = 0.72 ± 0.03) or into CPD-SAG (Hct = 0.57 ± 0.02) anticoagulants.
2. Fresh frozen plasma
3. Usual plasma expanders: Ringer's lactate, dextran
4. Platelet concentrates in 10 patients
5. Neither albumin, nor whole blood was used.

166

The special feature of this study lies in the way these products were administered: whole blood was reconstituted by mixing the packed red cells and fresh frozen plasma just before transfusion (3). No warming-up system was used.

The aim of this study is the analysis of possible complications, and their eventual correlations with MT.

Evaluations had been made at the end of the MT; that is after 24 hours.

RESULTS

Figure 1 shows that all the patients corresponded to the definition: they received 13.5 liters in less than 24 hours

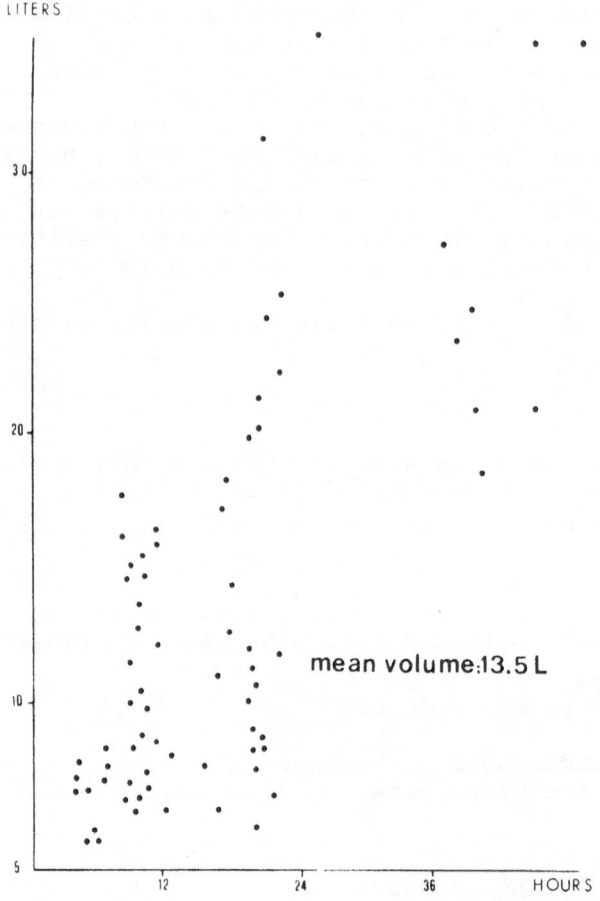

Fig. 1. Volume and time relationship.

Mortality

28 deaths occurred out of 75 patients due to:
- infectious shock (n=11) with identified germs
- acute hypovolemia (n=8): the patients were bleeding so much that it was impossible to compensate for the loss
- skull trauma (n=3) with irreversible coma
- chest injuries (n=3): the pulmonary complications were not due to MT, but to the trauma itself
- hepatic failure (n=1)

There were two cases with a possible MT etiology:
1. One refractory hypoxemia, with a pulmonary edema and left ventricular failure; but it was a 86-year-old man with a chest trauma and a history of pulmonary disorders.
2. One porta-caval shunt, with diffuse bleeding and coagulation disorders; but the complications may be due to the surgery.

Hemostasis disorders

We noticed a drop in platelets (Fig. 2) according to the transfused volumes as reported earlier in the literature (9). Prothrombin time (Table I) was maintained over 40% in 66 cases, who did not receive less blood than the others. The observed disorders are not linked to the administered volume.

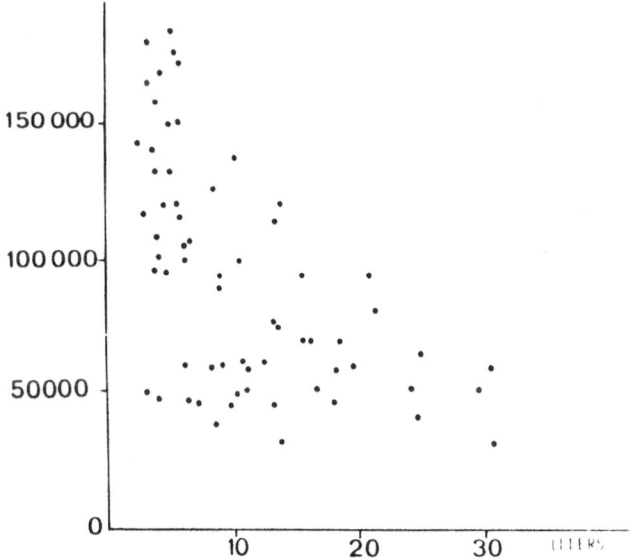

Fig. 2. The effect on circulating platelets.

TABLE I. Prothrombin time

	n	mean volume	ratio:	$\dfrac{FFP}{total\ perfused\ volume}$
> 60%	35	13.2 1		
40 → 60%	31	13.6 1		0.45
< 40%	9 (7 death)	14 1		0.28

In addition all the patients with a correct PT, showed a higher ratio of 0.45 calculated by the quantity of FFP in the total perfused volume. The nine others were not given enough plasma (ratio=0.28) and among them seven died. Two patients who are still alive had a ratio of 0.4 and 0.42 respectively.

We observed no death due to DIC.

Metabolic disorders

- We noticed a slight hypothermia about 36°C (2 cases at 34°C) without any consequence.
- Almost all the patients have hypocalcemia (= 2.4 mmole in 96% of the cases) with no cardiac impairment.
- We noticed a hypokalemia (Fig. 3), especially when the transfusion was above 10 liters; it is thought that the perfused red cell acted as potassium sponge; and there was no fatal outcome.

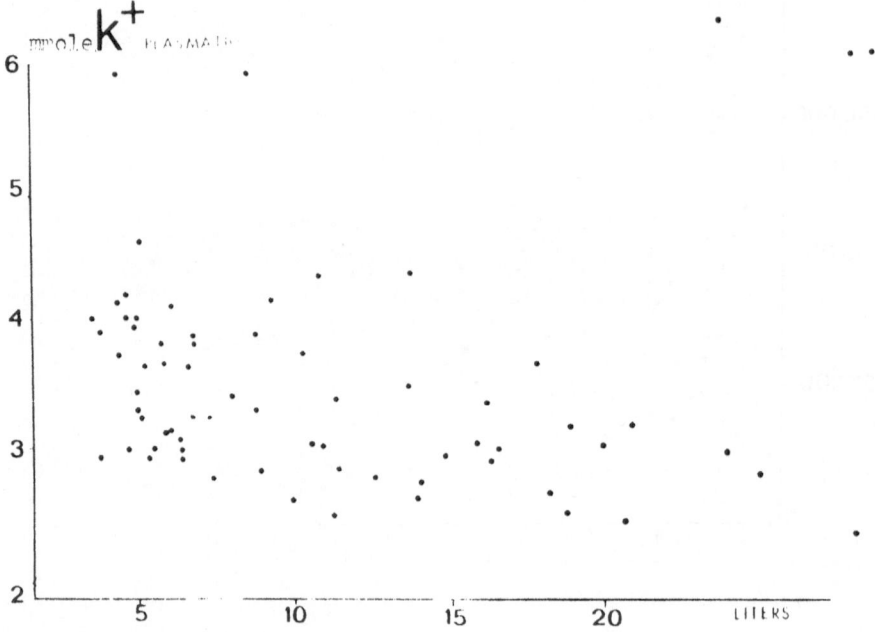

Fig. 3. Plasma potassium levels.

TABLE II. pH changes: 70% alkalosis

	n	Ventilated	Non ventilated
CO2 alkalosis	24	23	1
Metabolic alkalosis	28	17	11
Acidosis	8		
pH normal	15		

- pH changes (Table II)
  a frequent alkalosis is noticed, essentially metabolic
  alkalosis, even in the ventilated patients (2,12).
- Pulmonary complications:
  24 cases had hypoxemia, including 14 deaths, due to:
  chest injuries, infectious shock, lesional coma and acute
  hypovolemia.
  There was no circulatory overload (due, perhaps, to the
  fact that we used no albumin).

DISCUSSION

In this study, we observed that the current disorders linked to the massive transfusion are:

- drop in platelet count
- hypocalcemia
- hypokalemia
- metabolic alkalosis

But with erythrocyte concentrates and fresh frozen plasma
used in conjunction, we have maintained a correct coagulation. Slight hypothermia and less frequent pulmonary complications were encountered.

In addition, the product was easy to transfuse in an
emergency situation; and the reconstituted whole blood
(nearly fresh blood) contains no activated or degraded
coagulation factors.

REFERENCES

1. A.A.B.B.: Massive transfusion, Washington Edt., 1978.
2. Barcenas, C.G., Fuller, T.J., Knochel, J.P.: Metabolic alkalosis
   after massive blood transfusion correction by hemodialysis. J.
   Amer. Med. Ass. 236:953, 1976.
3. Bell, R., Burns, P.A., Sullivan, J.R., Cowling, D.C.: Hypervisco-
   sity of packed red cells: additional solutions. Med. J. Aust. 5:649,
   1977.
4. Boyan, C.P., Howland, W.S.: Blood temperature: a critical factor
   in massive tranfusion. Anesthesiology 22:559, 1961.
5. Bunker, J.P.: Metabolic effects of blood transfusion. Anesthesiology 27:446, 1966.
6. Collins, J.A.: Pulmonary dysfunction and massive transfusion. Bi-

bliotheca haematol. 46:220, 1980.

7. Krevans, J.R., Jackson, D.P.: Haemorrhagic disorders following massive whole blood transfusions. J. Amer. Med. Ass. 159:171, 1955.

8. McNamara, J.J., Burran, E.L., Stremple, J.F., Molot, M.D.: Coagulopathy after major combat injury: occurrence, management and pathophysiology. Ann. Surg. 176:243, 1972.

9. Miller, R.D., Robbins, T.O., Tong, M.J., Barton, S.L.: Coagulation defects associated with massive blood transfusions. Ann. Surg. 174:794, 1971.

10. Miller, R.D., Tong, M.J., Robbins, T.O.: Effects of massive transfusion of blood on acid-base balance. J. Amer. Med. Ass. 216:1762, 1971.

11. Perkins, H.A., Smyder, M., Thacher, C., Roifs, M.R.: Calcium ion activity during rapid exchange transfusion with citrated blood. Transfusion 11:204, 1971.

12. Selding, W., Rector, F.C.: The generation and maintenance of metabolic alkalosis. Kidney Internat. 1:306, 1972.

Discussion

Moderator: M. Brozovic

L.H. Siegenbeek Van Heukelom, Alkmaar:

What does dr. Haanen think about using fresh frozen plasma in acute DIC? Is it as someone said 'adding fuel to the fire', or do you think it is necessary to give it?

C.A.M. Haanen, Nijmegen:

When there are clinical reasons to suspect that DIC is still active, you must be very hesitant to give fresh frozen plasma or other coagulation factors, unless the patient is heparinised. The exception is thrombotic thrombocytopenic purpura.
In cases with severe thrombocytopenia plus hemolytic anemia and helmet cells in the blood, fresh plasma normalizes the platelet count within 24 hours and the haptoglobin rises. The plasma must be given daily, because when you stop this daily administration of 4-6 units of plasma, the thrombotic thrombocytopenic purpura relapses. We could taper it off in some weeks.
In real active DIC I should be very hesitant.

W.G. Van Aken, Amsterdam:

Related to the findings with fibronectin, what does dr. Blumenstock think is the cause of the decrease of fibronectin, e.g. in trauma patients. Is it comsumption, is it decreased synthesis of fibronectin, a combination of the two? If it is consumption, do you have an idea where the fibronectin is going?
If we are going to administer fibronectin in these patients, what can we expect from the half-life of the administered product?

F.A. Blumenstock, Albany, USA:

The fibronectin is being depleted in probably two ways. Whenever there is tissue injury it will be consumed. There is a high affinity for collagen and actin in muscle tissue, one of both is consumptive. There are also trauma patients with a fairly low nutritional status. The protein seems to be very sensitive to the nutritional status. We

have some preliminary studies showing that within 24 to
48 hours in human starvation the levels go down, are depressed by 30%. We did some preliminary studies on the
half life of the protein: it is a fairly shortliving protein of about 17 to 18 hours.

W.G. Van Aken, Amsterdam:

Do you also have any idea of a comparison between fibronectin and albumin in the patients you showed us? Whether
it is a non-specific effect of fibronectin? So, if you
make a comparative study between patients treated with albumin versus fibronectin, do you see a difference between
the two?

F.A. Blumenstock, Albany:

We have not done that. However, we are now in the process
of doing and completing a prospective and double-blind
study on a series of patients where we give a control substance, which is cryo-extracted plasma. An equal volume of
cryo-extracted plasma versus the similar volume of cryoprecipitate as a control substance. We have not used albumin.

J.Ph.H.B. Sijbesma, Dordrecht:

In DIC with a very severe thrombocytopenia, there are different approaches. Some physicians are ordering very quickly thrombocytes, and give that without anything else. Others
never give thrombocytes, because they are afraid for activating DIC, and still others give thrombocytes after they
have given heparin.
What is your approach, dr. Haanen?

C.A.M. Haanen, Nijmegen:

That depends on the clinical situation. Most patients have
a thrombocytopenia that is not so severe, perhaps they also have a thrombocytopathia. In that case, you will have
to give e.g. thrombocyte concentrates.
In the clinical situation of gastrointestinal bleeding,
with bleeding times more than 10 minutes and a low platelet
count, the situation asks for platelets to be transfused.

A.J. Silvergleid, San Bernardino, USA:

I thought that dr. Moss's previous work and others have
shown that the use of crystalloid replacement generally
requires almost 3 times the volume as with colloid. The
pre-operative volumes in Moss's two groups appear to be
the same. Is there an explanation?

G.S. Moss, Chicago, USA:

You are quite right. The studies that we did in large primates or baboons show that about 3x the volume was required, which fits precisely with our understanding of dispersion characteristics of saline as compared to albumin. We were surprised to find equal volumes and worried that it represents either undertreatment in the saline-group or overtreatment in the albumin-group. However, in reviewing the results of the study we did not find differences in mortality, the evidence of resuscitation was good. So we are left with the observation that in trauma in man the differences between albumin and Ringer's are not as great as they are in the experimental study.

B. Gullbring, Stockholm:

Dr. Moss, did you make after this study - I think it was published in 1977* - a standardised program with physiological parameters, or do you have a mixed program where you follow certain physiological parameters?
Do you have a standardised program without albumin and with a larger volume of crystalloid solutions?
This question is important because when using red cells in a 'SAG' solution, there are no plasma proteins given.

G.S. Moss, Chicago:

The data I presented today were just published**. The 1977 paper* was about the 180 randomized patients. There was a criticism: one would not expect to find differences if the patients were not sick. So we studied a group of sick patients. The answer to the question is that the criteria that we used to determine the volume of fluid, given for resuscitation, was based on bed-side clinical signs. In other words, we did not feel it was ethical to put a Swan-catheter and a radial-artery catheter in a trauma-patient, because we knew from my previous experience that we could manage them quite well with simple tests: blood pressure, urine output, skin temperature, level of consciousness, etc. So we used those indices during resuscitation and in the postoperative period, unless the patient became ill and developed unexplained changes in the circulation. At that time he had a radial-artery catheter and a pulmonary catheter inserted. The endpoints of resuscitation, as defined by us, were when the patient's pulse became slow, pressure came up, urine output became adequate, skin became warm and dry, and insomnia normalised.
Postoperatively, patients just received maintenance fluids as would any other post-operative patient, except no pa-

* Lowe, R.J. et al., Surgery 1977, 81, 676.
** Moss, G.S. et al., Surgery 1981, 89, 434.

tient received albumin. About the 'SAG', I do not believe
that would be a very proper solution to use for initial
resuscitation, because I do not believe that the patient
needs red cells during initial resuscitation. The patient
should be resuscitated without any red cells, and when he
is stable, he should get carefully cross-matched red cells.

P.C. Das, Groningen:

About the study that you mentioned, dr. Collins, in rats
with old blood and fresh blood: in our information of the
human CPD blood*, 2.3 DPG levels increased after the donation for 3 days to about 120%, and at 5 days they were
80%. My question to you: when you say 'old' blood and
'fresh' blood, how old is the old and how fresh is the
fresh?

J.A. Collins, Stanford, USA:

Fresh blood is a day old, old blood was 20 days old. To
control the plasma we use relatively fresh plasma for
both of them. So we tried to change the red cell fraction.
The red cells in rats are different from humans. In spite
of some political connotations, to the contrary, man is
not a rat. The magnitude of the shift in the red cells is
very comparable. With storage the human red cell goes
from a P_{50} of 27 down to about 18, and almost complete
disappearance of 2.3 DPG. The rat over the same period
of time also looses 2.3 DPG, but the shift in the position of the hemoglobin curve is from the high 30's to the
low 20's. So it is proportionately almost exactly the
same percentage shift, but from a different starting point
to a different ending point.

---

*Lamers, M. Project report, Red Cross Bloodbank Groningen-Drenthe,
Groningen 1980.

IV. Hemophilia home care: Practical experience

INTRODUCTION

E.J.M. Sjamsjoedin-Visser

In recent years an increasing interest has developed with
respect to Home Treatment both for patients and their parents and also by people who are involved with treating
hemophilia.

Also in the Netherlands, a small country with a high
standard of medical care, it proved to be possible and
successful to organize a home treatment program. About
35% of the potential candidates are on Home Treatment. It
became evident that a theoretical instruction is even more
important than a technical training such as instructing
the patients how to treat, when to treat, when to consult
their doctor etc.

In 1980 a study was undertaken in our national hemophilia center, the Van Creveld Clinic in Bilthoven. We asked
the patients who were potential candidates why they were
not on home treatment. We found then that there were several patients, but also quite a number of physicians who
still were not familiar with the possibility of home treatment and were reluctant to accept the responsibility. Also
some patients found it quite easy to go to the hospital
near their homes for treatment. On the other hand, we found
that all the patients on home treatment wanted to stay on
home treatment. There were no failures and everybody was
happy with the free and independent way of life.

In consequence of the development of this type of therapy, a good control system appears to be necessary. Firstly
for the patient to support the management of his treatment
and secondly, to give the medical staff the possibility to
collect data about the different aspects of relevance in
this type of treatment, for example, the degree of arthropathy, hospitalization, absence from school and work, costs,
social development and others.

With this information it is possible to teach other
people and plan for the future.

A team of people, the so-called 'comprehensive care
team', can be very helpful to organize such a program.
These first two papers deal with both aspects, that is to
say, the need for a control system and the functioning of
a team.

HOME CARE: THE NEED FOR CONTROL

P. Jones

When he prescribes home therapy for a patient the doctor
bears the immediate and long-term responsibility for the
consequences of that prescription. When the consequences
are good the patient may question the need for continued
supervision - after all, he looks to freedom, and to independence from the ties of hospital medicine. It is the
purpose of this paper to set out the reasons for follow-up
at a center with staff experienced in the management of
hemophilia.

Among the medical indications for regular follow-up
are screening for factor antibody and for biochemical
evidence of liver disease, the diagnosis of concomitant
disorders, adjustments of dose and timing of treatment
with age and changing circumstances, and recognition of
the inappropriate use of blood products or analgesic drugs.

First, the question of factor antibodies or 'inhibitors'.
We know, from careful monitoring in the United Kingdom and
elsewhere, that some 7% of those with severe hemophilia A
will develop an antibody to extraneous factor VIII. We
know that the effects of this antibody may be overcome
successfully, but that the methods we adopt are governed
by individual patient and antibody characteristics. Thus,
whilst one hemophilic boy with a high titer factor VIII
antibody may show excellent clinical responses to a modified prothrombin complex preparation, another may be able
to live an equally active and satisfying life using intermittent low dose factor VIII.

Although we know that most of those who are going to develop antibodies will have done so before they have received their 100th treatment with blood product, we do not
know which patients are most at risk. Nor can we be sure
that the occasional antibody will not present at any stage
in a patient's treatment. Sometimes there are warning signs,
for instance failure of the expected clinical response to
treatment, or a longer than usual period of convalescence
after a major bleed. But these signs can be explained in
other ways; a batch of poor quality blood product, or concomitant subicteric hepatitis are examples. Sometimes antibodies are found only on laboratory testing. Sometimes
an equivocal result signals the need for additional checks
on the efficacy of response. Whatever the marker supervision

is vital in order to avoid complications, wasted blood product and invasive procedures on the one hand, and to reassure families about the absence of antibody on the other.

Second, liver disease. Investigation of all patients exposed to blood product concentrates of whatever origin shows intermittent evidence of disordered liver function. Further, the percutaneous biopsy of hemophilic livers reveals a plethora of histological changes which are consistent with a pathological response to repeated assaults by noxious agents, presumably viral in origin. Only regular follow-up can provide the information required to modify treatment in order to reduce the risks, and to identify those patients whose infectivity might present a hazard to others. It is only through follow-up that we will learn just what the risks are, in terms both of significant morbidity, or mortality from liver failure, and whether or not links exist between the scale of prescription of blood product and the incidence of disease.

Third, concomitant disorders. Hemophilia confers no protection against other diseases, and when the emphasis is on the treatment of acute bleeding episodes rather than on the patient himself, there is a danger that other problems will be overlooked, and it is as wrong to expect someone with hemophilia to diagnose an illness as it is with anyone else. For instance, there are many causes of jaundice. Recently a boy presented in our Center with what, on first principles, was likely to be non-A non-B hepatitis. Investigation revealed that he had a profound hemolytic anemia which would have been lethal if treatment had been delayed. We have reported adverse historical and physical findings ranging from undescended testes in adult patients to failures of immunization in childhood, findings unrecorded and untreated in 50 severely affected patients despite multiple hospital visits (1).

At present hemophilia center staff see a predominantly young age group of patients, but with advances in therapy we can reasonably expect the age distribution curve for severe hemophilia to equate with that of the normal population. With this expected increase in life expectancy hemophiliacs will inevitably develop those pathological conditions associated with advancing age - diverticulosis, prostatic hypertrophy, peripheral vascular insufficiency and malignant disease. The earlier these problems are identified the better the chances of their successful management.

Fundamental to all this is, of course, an accurate diagnosis, both in terms of specific clotting defect and in terms of severity. A man with mild hemophilia presented to a surgical unit with a swollen hand. Forgetting to mention the primary diagnosis which had been made several years previously, he was treated with Streptokinase for what was assumed to be a thrombosis. The result of this treatment was catastrophic and the patient was lucky to escape with his hand intact after eventual skin grafting in the Hemophilia Center.

Analysis of patients' records, examined at follow-up, enables recognition of bleeding patterns specific to different age groups. Individual patient variance from a particular pattern helps identify target joints, and to point to changes in work or activities, the effects of recurrent trauma or stress, inadequate doses of blood product, or product given too late, the development of synovitis or the appearance of an antibody. Excessive use of blood product, in comparison with the average used by other patients, suggests that there are problems in addition to the hemophilia. Examples of this 'inappropriate use' of factor VIII or IX seen by us have included truancy from school, financial problems within a family, hospital dependence, and analgesic abuse. The underlying cause is usually very difficult to identify because it is hidden, subconsciously or consciously, by the patient or his family. It can be found only by careful follow-up and repeated consultations.

Among the social indications for regular follow-up are prevention of handicap by prior recognition of stress points in the hemophiliac's life, and help with school, work and family problems. The establishment of good rapport between social worker, nurse and family early in an affected boy's childhood is fundamental to the success of counselling as the child develops. Adequate, skilled counselling is of vital importance to hemophilic families, and is dependent on repeated consultation in a relaxed atmosphere.

Both nuclear and distant family members should be given the chance to talk with Center staff. Mothers of hemophilic first babies, and siblings who are unaffected, often feel very isolated as the focus of attention centers on the hemophilia, rather than on normal family interactions. The maternal grandmother may feel as much remorse as her daughter when she becomes aware that she might be a carrier. Sisters and female cousins should be seen for carrier detection and counselling. Advise about activities and the promotion of good health provides the background to the more specific follow-up of the hemophiliac. Marital problems exacerbated by the stress of hemophilia result, very occasionally, in non-accidental injury to the patient or his siblings and should be recognized.

Within a hemophilia center the doctor's responsibility for the prescription of blood product is exercised through a continuous process of consultation and monitoring by a variety of people who contribute varied but complementary skills (2). This process is two-way. Hemophilic families need the sorts of medical and social support I have described. Center staff need hemophilic families in order to learn from them, to teach and to plan ahead.

REFERENCES

1. Jones, P.: Haemophilia Home Therapy. Pitman Medical, London, 1980, p. 138.
2. Jones, P.: The organisation of a haemophilia service. In: Haemostasis and Thrombosis, editors A.L. Bloom and D.P. Thomas. Churchill Livingstone, Edinburgh, 1981, p. 391.

NEW ENGLAND HEMOPHILIA CENTER: A COMPREHENSIVE HOME CARE MODEL

A.I. Cederbaum

INTRODUCTION

Successful transfusional therapy for hemophilia was reported in 1840 using whole blood. In 1923 Freissly (2) reported using citrated plasma to control bleeding in hemophilia.
In 1949 Graham et al. (3) demonstrated the feasibility of
maintaining a hemophiliac dog colony in relatively good
health by the prompt and intensive use of fresh frozen
plasma transfusions for hemorrhagic episodes. The therapy
of hemophilia in humans was limited by volume restrictions
imposed by using either whole blood or fresh frozen plasma
transfusions. The era of modern treatment was made possible
in the 1960's with the development by Poole et al. (5) of
cryoprecipitate for the therapy of Hemophilia A. This was
followed shortly by the development of a number of more
highly purified AHF concentrates that were prepared by various procedures (1). Prothrombin complex concentrates
rich in factors II, VII, IX and X, useful in the treatment
of Hemophilia B were also developed at this time (6). Thus,
by the mid 1960's, the tools were available for what is
currently regarded as optimal care of the hemophiliac patient.

The New England Hemophilia Center began in the early
1960's when Dr. Anthony Britten brought together a small
group of patients in Boston and started sending factor VIII
and factor IX concentrates to the patient's homes for self-
infusions. In 1969, Dr. Peter H.Levine inherited the direction of the clinic, and a nurse was also incorporated.
These individuals started a formal program that has grown
to the present day center. The nurse acted as a health
educator, which enabled patients to understand the pathophysiology, signs and symptoms of early hemarthrosis and
musculoskeletal bleeding, as well as recognition of the
potentially more serious bleeding episodes. She was an
advocate of the major dictum 'when in doubt, infuse', a
principle emphasized by Drs. Britten and Levine. Finally,
by being easily available to patients, she encouraged frequent contact with the clinic, yet without a feeling that
the clinic controlled the patient's life.

Despite good intentions, the clinic suffered some very
definite growing pains. Initially, a follow-up clinic met

weekly, but the number of patients attending was not
enough to sustain the interest of a full-time orthopedic
surgeon, physical therapist, or oral surgeon. Another
problem we encountered was the financial aspect. The cost
of taking care of patients was at best expensive, but
third party payers viewed home therapy as any other out-
patient medication, and it was not covered by insurance.
The hospital lost a large sum of money and was not very
supportive of the concept of a comprehensive hemophilia
clinic. Dr. Levine, with the eventual assistance of a
social worker spent a great deal of time convincing insurers that it was cost effective to pay for home therapy.
Collection of data on costs aided this effort. Once we
were able to secure adequate support from the third party
insurers, and government insurers, the clinic's viability
was guaranteed and the patient population has continued
to grow. The clinic has subsequently moved to central
Massachusetts, located in the geographic center of The
New England states, Worcester.

We presently deliver care to 240 patients. Table I illustrates some important demographic information about
these patients. In addition to the patients seen primarily
at our center, another 250 patients are treated at 5 satellite centers which we have been able to help to support
in terms of protocols, staff training, finances, and specialized clinical and laboratory back-up. This organization has been made possible by funding for regional Hemophilia Centers from the federal government.

TABLE I. Demographic data on 240 patients from the New England Hemophilia Center

1. Total number		240
2. FVIII deficient		206
Severe	65%	
Moderate	27%	
Mild	8%	
3. FIX deficient		34
Severe	45%	
Moderate	45%	
Mild	10%	
4. Home therapy		195
5. Inhibitor patients		20

Our own center and our satellite centers are dedicated
to the concept of comprehensive hemophilia care. The cor-
nerstone of this philosophy has been a basic education for
the patients in their disease process that will allow them
to intelligently meet many of their own health care needs.

The clinic provides the necessary personnel to ensure
that all of the patients' medical, orthopedic, dental and
psychosocial problems can be met with the least amount of
interference from the health care system.

The current staff and structure of the clinic is outlined below. In addition, our approach to the patient will
also be discussed.

Staffing of the Hemophilia Center

The center Director's major role is coordinating the activities of the center personnel, planning appropriate research projects and ensuring a fair share of the public
and private funding. In our center there are two additional physicians, both hematologists, who along with the
director, do all of the direct patient care, formulate
long term care plans for each patient, supervise the activities of the nurse coordinator, and are available for
all medical problems related to the care of the patient
population.

The key to our effective clinic operation is the nurse
who coordinates the day-to-day operations of the clinic
and does much of the record keeping. In addition to being
the focal point of patient contact with the clinic, the
nurse is the key person in the initial education process,
as well as the ongoing education of patients, as will be
described below.

Another important function of the nurse's role is community outreach. Together with the social worker, the
nurse interacts with schools and employers, and works as
an educator of the public and an advocate of the patient.

An Orthopedic Surgeon with an interest in hemophilia
is absolutely indispensable. The success of our clinic
can be attributed to the fact that we have a single orthopedist who sees all the patients at least once a year, is
present at all follow-up clinics, as well as being available for emergencies and elective consultation. The patients gain considerably by developing a good relation
with the orthopedist, as well as the hematologists concerned with their care. The frequent group meetings of
these individuals assure that the patient receives a single
clear opinion.

As noted earlier, with the help of our Social Worker,
we have been able to put the clinic on firm financial
ground. The social worker is crucial in the absence of
guaranteed government financing, to ensure the fiscal
well-being of our patients. In addition, the social worker
does yearly psychosocial assessments, and develops appropriate support systems for patients who need help (a consultant psychiatrist is available to assist when needed).
Our social worker has been very active in going into local communities to act as a patient advocate which again
strengthens the ties of the clinic and patient. She also
accumulates significant demographic data and has been in-

strumental in setting up an effective genetics counseling program.

An Oral Surgeon serves as a special consultant to our clinic. This individual sees every patient at the annual comprehensive clinic visit and is available to consult on our patients at other times, as well as help find appropriate care for these patients in their local community when indicated. By having an individual who understands hemophilia, and the special concerns of our patients, there is better communication with dental practitioners who are then able to take care of the bulk of our patients' needs in their own communities.

A Physical Therapist is now available at all of our clinic sessions. The therapist asssists the orthopedist in formal joint measurements. The benefits of having such an individual instructing the patient in a formal exercise program, when needed, have been dramatic. The sophistication of exercise programs has improved, as well as compliance. Again, a major function of this individual has been communicating to colleagues in the patient's local community so that our patient's special needs can be met, and allowing for less reliance on the center, as well as ensuring excellent results.

Recent funding has also allowed us to have formal genetic counseling available to all of our patients. The Genetics Associate has developed extensive family pedigrees, has done case finding, and has developed (in conjunction with our laboratory and social worker), an effective genetics counseling program.

The Hemophilia Center Secretary is an important member of our staff. She is the person to whom the patients will regularly correspond. The secretary helps the nurse maintain charts, and is responsible for coordinating the mailing out of all supplies.

In addition to the above staff people who are available on a regular basis, we have a number of consultants available to the clinic if they are needed. The most important of these are the Psychiatrist who works closely with and supplies back-up to our social worker, and the Vocational Counselor who works with our patients, and more importantly, provides expertise in dealing with government and private agencies outside of our clinic.

The staff described above has developed over a period of 11 years, as our patient population has increased from 30 to 490. The key to success has been each individual's dedication to the center and bringing their own expertise to bear in such a manner that ensures that our concept of comprehensive Hemophilia care, the main stay of which is home therapy, will indeed succeed.

Operations of the Hemophilia Clinic

The day to day operation of the center includes three major aspects of hemophilia care:

1. The introduction of new patients into the clinic;
2. The routine care that is supervised through the annual comprehensive clinic visit; and
3. Follow-up and emergency care.

First visit to the Clinic

Prior to the first visit the patient is instructed to
bring with him all members of his immediate family or
household; in the case of adults, this includes children
in the family; in the case of young men who are unmarried
but living with female companions, the companion is included. The patient is carefully instructed prior to this
visit that he may spend four to six hours in the Hemophilia
Center. At the time of the initial visit, the patient does
not attend the Comprehensive Care Clinic; instead he is
seen on a one-to-one basis by one of the hematologists
at our center, and by our nurse practitioner. The patient
is individually interviewed by the physician. A detailed
history is taken and a thorough physical examination is
performed. During this time the various family members
are being interviewed by the nurse practitioner, and are
subsequently interviewed by the physician. No patient is
ever seen with a previous understanding that he will be
placed on the home therapy program. The decision to use
home therapy as opposed to some other mode is only made
after the initial history and physical have been completed and after a battery of laboratory tests have been performed. The individuals involved in the initial assessment
then confer and make an assessment of the patient's suit-
ability for home therapy.

In recent years our criteria for excluding patients
from home therapy have become fewer and fewer. Patients
are not treated at home who have inadequate veins; this
accounts for only the very rare patient. Children of
less than three years of age are not infused at home, although the families are instructed in home care and encouraged to make therapeutic decisions (an attempt to
find a local medical facility who will abide by these decisions and then carry out infusion on this basis is also
made and usually successful). In addition, a number of inhibitor patients are now treated with non-activated Factor IX products at home. Patients with severe emotional
instability or mental retardation cannot be infused at
home. Patients who have mild hemophilia and seldom require
infusions may or may not be included in the protocol, depending on the ease with which they can receive appropriate
infusions at local hospitals on the rare occasions when
they are required.

If the decision is made in favor of home therapy, the
patient and selected family members who appear to have
the greatest comprehension and reliability are all trained
in theoretic aspects of the therapy. This phase of the
training takes approximately two hours, and does not in-

clude the technical aspects of venepuncture. Training in
the theoretical and pathophysiological aspects of hemophilia are thought by us to be considerably more important than the routine technical aspects of care. This is
emphasized to the patient and his family. Further, in the
case of children with hemophilia, we insist that the children and family all be present during the entire training
session, even though the child may not be the one performing the self-infusion. In this way, the child does not
feel that there is a 'conspiracy' between his parents and
the physician. Instead, he feels a member of the Health
Care Delivery Team.

The second visit:

The patient's two hours of instruction begin with a thorough explanation to the patient and the appropriate family members of the pathophysiology of hemophilic arthropathy. A significant amount of detail is given with regard
to the development of inflamed synovial tissue which appears to be in the final common pathway to the destruction
of cartilage and bone. The importance of recognizing hemorrhage long before the development of physical signs is
stressed. The patients begin to hear, for the first of
many times, our clinic's general rule: 'When in doubt,
infuse'.

The patients learn that there are two general categories
ries of hemorrhagic episodes, mild and severe. Mild episodes are defined by us as very early symptoms indicative
of joint and muscle bleeding, prior to the appearance of
gross physical signs such as swelling, severe limitation
of motion, discoloration or heat. For such lesions, the
patient will be taught how to calculate to raise his Factor VIII level to 30%, and his Factor IX level to 20%.
Severe episodes are defined by us as advanced joint or
muscle bleeding, any severe trauma with or without recognizable hemorrhage, signs or symptoms of intracranial hemorrhage, bleeding in the region of the tongue, neck or
pharynx, gastrointestinal bleeding, or bleeding in the re-
troperitoneum or psoas muscle. For such lesions, we infuse to achieve levels of 50 and 40% of Factor VIII or IX,
respectively.

Some of the common sites of more serious bleeding are
emphasized. For instance, the patients are taught to diagnose the femoral nerve entrapment syndrome which might
result. Other closed space bleeding which might lead to
neurologic sequelae is also discussed. The signs and symptoms of intracranial hemorrhage are described.

The patient is then given a detailed session on calculation of dose based on infusion of Factor VIII or IX concentrate in units per kilogram of body weight. The importance of immediate application of therapy is again stressed.

A detailed description of the operation of our center

is then provided. This includes a description of our Annual Comprehensive Care Clinic and the patient is asked to agree to attend such clinics as a mandatory feature of our center. This insures that adequate follow-up can be maintained and that long-term problems will not be missed. The patient is made to understand that failure to attend such clinics will mean cessation of the program and of his supply of Factor VIII or IX concentrates; a 'threat' which we never actually carried out. Attendance at our Comprehensive Care Clinics continues to be close to 100%.

All of the patients are provided with a toll-free telephone number by which they may reach us at any time of night or day at no expense from any part of New England. In this way, they are encouraged to make contact with us whenever questions should arise, but the principle of early infusion whenever in doubt is again emphasized. For this reason, the patients will frequently contact us only after they have already initiated the appropriate therapy of a hemorrhagic episode. At the present time, telephone calls are received for less than 5% of hemorrhagic episodes which occur in this group of patients.

Other clinic rules include mandatory contact with us whenever more than two infusions of Factor VIII or IX are necessary for a single episode of hemorrhage. The patient must also contact us whenever the above mentioned severe hemorrhagic episodes occur.

The patients are provided with forms for record keeping. At the time of each hemorrhagic episode they record the site of hemorrhage, product name, lot number and number of units given, the time of the day, and the therapeutic result. Patients are generally provided with enough therapeutic material to treat between four and ten hemorrhagic episodes, depending on the frequency of such episodes in a given patient. When they come to only enough residual material for one more infusion, they submit these forms to us through the mail; they are reviewed by our nurse practitioner, and, if they are approved, a new supply of Factor VIII or IX concentrate is then sent to the patient by return mail.

Finally, at the end of the session, unless complete exhaustion has set in, the technical aspects of venepuncture are taught. Following a brief introductory teaching session, the nurse practitioner has the various family members practice upon one another, which they invariably successfully do to their great amazement. Only then is venepuncture performed on the hemophilic member of the family by other family members or himself.

The third and fourth visits:

The patient has been issued the appropriate forms, Factor VIII or IX concentrate, needles and syringes. He is instructed to bring all of these with him to the Hemophilia

Center, or to our Hospital's emergency room if a hemorrhagic episode occurs during the night. In either of these settings, he then makes the appropriate dose calculation, prepares the material, and infuses it under the direct supervision of our staff in order to be sure that the techniques have been properly mastered. More important is the oral examination which the patient receives at this time. He and his family members are again questioned as to many aspects of their decision making processes. For example, he is asked to describe the signs and symptoms of intracranial bleeding, psoas hematoma, or intraabdominal hemorrhage. Dose calculation is checked. The patient is asked to recite the reasons which will require him to make immediate telephone contact with the center. After two such visits the patient is 'on his own' and needs no longer contact us in person or by telephone for his next treatment episode. In a few cases, we have extended this period of observation because of the need for further educational reinforcement or because of insecurity on the part of the patient or his family.

During the initial months of home therapy, the nurse practitioner makes frequent phone calls to the home of the patient in order to assess the progress of the program. In some instances, our social worker makes a home visit to assess what is actually taking place in the home and to observe some of the mechanics of health care delivery. Is the Factor VIII or IX concentrate being properly stored? How are other members of the family handling the new program? How is the new program regarded by the patient's school or place of employment? In many cases it is extremely helpful to have the social worker also visit the school or office in this regard.

It should also be emphasized at this point that all of our patients are treated with Factor VIII or Factor IX concentrates as opposed to cryoprecipitate or other plasma products. We have in recent years made a total departure from the use of cryoprecipitate in our home therapy program. This was based on our early experience in which we found a failure rate of approximately 20% when infusing patients with cryoprecipitate. Our calculations were made on the assumption that every bag of cryoprecipitate contained an average of 100 units of Factor VIII. In point of fact, we would often achieve in vivo Factor VIII levels of only one-fourth of what we had calculated; this almost guarantees a therapeutic failure. This reflects the fact that occasional bags of cryoprecipitate contain only 20 or 30 units per bag as opposed to the expected 100. When this happens, the result may be advanced hemorrhage and a lesion which then requires many days of continuous infusions and often hospitalization. Furthermore, cryoprecipitate or fresh frozen plasma cannot be easily sent through the mail, cannot be taken to work or school, cannot be taken on trips; and often requires an additional measure of time for preparation which is sometimes enough to discourage the patient from the treatment of a 'mild' hemorrhagic episode.

The annual Comprehensive Care Clinic:

The annual Comprehensive Care Clinic for our patients with hemophilia meets weekly from October to April. Clinics meet less frequently at other times to see delinquent patients and those needing frequent follow-up. Attendance at this clinic is mandatory for all patients on home therapy, and is optional for the other patients who are not treated in this manner. Four of our clinics are held in the evenings; the evening clinics are held in order to minimize the time lost from work by adult working men. The optimum number of patients seen at each session is six, but between five and eight may be seen at any particular session. The overall purpose of the clinic is to provide attention to all the various aspects of health care, to search for long-term problems for which a revised care plan is required, and to collect data. The flow pattern for the clinic for a typical patient is as follows. When the patient first presents at the clinic, he is met by one of the hospital volunteers. The volunteer sits at a small desk in the waiting room and assures a smooth flow of patients throughout the clinic session. She will also escort the patient to the X-ray area of the hospital or to the other distant sites which occasionally might be visited by a particular patient.

After the patient has been registered by the volunteer, he is interviewed by the clinic secretary. The secretary inquires as to the present status of third party payments and as to whether any significant medical bills are outstanding. If the patient is experiencing any difficulty in this regard, a special note is made for the social worker so that she may assist the patient. The secretary then checks the name and address of all local referring physicians to whom the patient wants subsequent records and notes to be forwarded. The secretary also checks to see that the patient has in his possession a letter of introduction from our clinic which states his diagnosis, its severity, the presence or absence of inhibitor, and the mode of therapy used. This letter also explains that the individual is entitled to carry needles and syringes; a useful precaution against the patient being mistaken for a narcotics addict.

The patient is next seen by the nurse practitioner. Her role is to check into any technical problems which may have been occurring in terms of venepuncture. She also checks that the appropriate dose calculations are being made and that the patient has not gained weight sufficient to increase his dose of Factor VIII or IX. Depending on the patient, she may also again reinforce some of the basic educational material which was taught in the initial sessions with the patient.

The patient is then placed in one of several examining rooms. The patient will remain in this room during his history and physical examination which are generally performed by one of the hematologists. In the case of young children, a pediatrician sees the patient at this point and pays special attention to whether appropriate immunizations have been received. This team then leaves the roo and is replaced by the orthopedic surgeon and physical therapist, who see the patient together.

The orthopedist, using a goniometer, makes precise measurements of range of motion of all of the major joint of the body which are recorded on a data collection sheet He and the physical therapist then inquire into the present functional status of the patient and make preliminary suggestions as to conservative orthopedic manoeuvres and appropriate exercises.

The patient is then brought to a separate examining room which contains a dental chair. The oral surgeon examines each patient and fills out another specific data sheet.

Members of the family are encouraged to attend the clinic along with the patient. These individuals, while in the waiting room area, are interviewed in an informal setting by the clinic social worker. In addition, the social worker is able to talk to each patient between the various clinic stations.

Following the dental examination each patient is broug to the X-ray area. The patient has carried with him throu out his series of examinations an envelope which contains a blank X-ray slip. Any physician who sees him during the session may write in any special X-rays which he wishes t have obtained. On his way back from X-ray, the patient stops at the venepuncture area where a battery of blood studies are drawn. These include complete liver function tests, complete blood count, Factor VIII or IX level, inhibitor assay, Hepatitis B surface antigen and antibody determinations, and an additional tube of blood for any on-going research project for which the patient may have signed his consent.

By the time the first few patients return from this series of evaluations, the nurse practitioner, hematologist and orthopedic surgeon will have finished examining their last patients. When the patients return from Radiology, they are allowed to carry X-rays back to the clin with them. The hematologist, nurse practitioner and orth pedic surgeon, usually along with the social worker, the sit down with the patient in a small conference room whi contains an X-ray viewbox. The X-rays are put up for all individuals to see. A management plan for the next year is then discussed in the presence of the patient and his family. The patient is thus encouraged to participate in the development of this plan and it is hoped that he wil understand the reasons which underlie it. A decision is also made as to whether the patient will be seen on any

regular basis during the coming year, or as to whether
he will only be seen at the next Annual Comprehensive
Care Clinic.

Almost all of the members of our Hemophilia Center
look forward to each year's annual clinic. Strangely, so
do most of the patients. As we see the tangible benefits
that the program has brought, the clinic becomes a very
positive experience for everyone involved.

Follow-up and emergencies:

A third major aspect of the care given our hemophilia
population relates to follow-up and emergency care. As
noted, our comprehensive clinic meets weekly seven months
a year. During this time all routine follow-up care is
done during these clinics when all of the members of the
team are available to continue delivering comprehensive
follow-up for the given problem. The other five months
the clinic meets twice a month at which time specific
follow-up patients are seen, as well as a few delinquent
patients for annual visits.

True emergencies can be handled in a number of ways.
First, the patient is urged to contact the nurse coordinator for any bleeding episode or traumatic event that he
considers out of the ordinary. The nurse, with consultation from a clinic physician, if necessary, will decide
if the patient needs to be seen, and organizes an appropriate infusion regimen for that patient. One of the clinic physicians is on call for all night and weekend emergencies.

Our patients are urged to use our emergency room if
there is any difficulty with infusion or other problems.
This is sometimes inconvenient in that many of our patients live a long distance away. If this is the case,
their local emergency facility can contact the doctor on
call. In our emergency room, there is a file with all of
our patients names and diagnoses, as well as the appropriate level of infusion. Our Emergency Room physicians
are also taught to infuse first and evaluate later. This
system of having our Emergency Room arranged to handle
our patients expeditiously has worked well. However, the
availability of a physician who is familiar with all our
patients allows us to handle an emergency at almost any
distance.

The philosophy and the functioning of the clinic have
been discussed. It is always necessary to ask pertinent
questions to see if the system is meeting the needs of our
patients and accomplishing the objectives that we have set
out for ourselves. In order to do this we have incorporated careful data collection to try and evaluate our efficacy. The goal of our program is two-fold:

1. To attempt to normalize the life style of our patients and to do this in an affordable manner;

2. To alter the natural history of the musculoskeletal

manifestations of this disease which we believe result
in the major long term morbidity for these patients. If
we can influence these two factors, we believe that the
disabling physical and social aspects of this chronic dis
ease will be minimized.

TABLE II. Benefits of Home Therapy Program in a population of 45
hemophiliacs

	Before home therapy	After home therapy	% Change
Days lost from work or school	26.3	6.8	-74%
Days hospitalized	9.8	1.0	-90%
Outpatient visits to physician	23.0	5.5	-76%
Number of infusion episodes	32.8	29.7	- 9%
Total cost of health care excluding surgery	5780	3209	-44%

In order to evaluate the above factors, we initially
reviewed the results in our first 45 patients in 1973 (4)
This data, summarized in Table II, clearly points to a
major positive influence on the factors that we looked at
and we feel that these factors reflect a better quality o
life for these patients, although this is more difficult
to assess. As our clinic grew, we have continued to updat
our data. We were concerned that with a population that
was growing, our results may not be as impressive for the
following reasons:
1. Increasing patient:staff ratio, despite federal fun
ing that has allowed us to expand services;
2. Less motivated patients, or
3. Patients who were more disabled would begin to come
to us as it was apparent that we had made a major commit-
ment to hemophilia care. We have recently updated our dat
and Table III gives the information as of October 1980 on
a clinic population now consisting of 240 patients. As
can be seen the data are similar for that generated in th
first group of patients. The increasing number of infusio
can be attributed to a significant number of patients who
health care had been so poor that they received treatment
only in the most dire circumstances and are now being tre
ted in what we would consider an appropriate manner with
infusion for our severe hemophiliac patients being given
on an average of once a week. We believe this information
supports our position that a comprehensive care setting,
with a home infusion program being the central theme, results in a normalization of life styles. It should be poi
ted out that our patients have an unemployment rate of

TABLE III. Benefits of Home Therapy Program in a population of 240 hemophiliacs

	Before home therapy	After home therapy	% Change
Days lost from work or school	12.2	4	-67%
Days hospitalized	6.4	0.9	-86%
Outpatient visits to physician	25.3	7.8	-69%
Number of infusion episodes	30.1	34.0	+13%
Total cost of health care excluding surgery	8850	5810	-34%

about 6%, which is below the rate for healthy individuals in our region as a whole. Although it is much more difficult to document, it is our feeling that our patients have far fewer psychosocial problems than we encountered prior to development of comprehensive care for hemophiliacs.

The data generated by our earlier studies and those of other centers encouraged the federal government of the United States to fund 13 regional hemophilia centers. The purpose of these centers was to see if the experience of smaller centers in improving the quality of health care to hemophiliacs could be duplicated on a larger scale. Table IV again demonstrates the vast improvement in the categories we looked at when a concerned effort is made to deliver health care.

TABLE IV. Patterns of health care at federally funded hemophilia centers

	Prior to funding	Year after funding	% Change
Number of patients receiving comprehensive care	1477	4768	+222%
Number on Home Therapy	682	2009	+203%
Average days/year lost from work or school	20-60	8.3	-58 to 86%
Average days/year in hospital	14-60	2.4	-82 to 96%
Average costs of health care	8-22,000	5252	-34 to 76%

This improvement was accomplished with very little money, but the money available made it feasible to bring together an interested core team similar to the one described for our center. This team is then able to invariably affect major changes in the health care they deliver to the hemophilia population. Once again, the general experience has been that the health care data we are able to generate is parallelled by a better quality of life for the patients.

The second major goal of comprehensive care is to alter the natural history of the musculoskeletal manifestations of hemophilia. At the inception of our clinic it was our aim to attempt to document the effect on chronic hemophilic arthropathy of a comprehensive care system whose central theme was home infusion and early infusion. Figure 1 demonstrates the form that is filled out on each patient who is seen in our clinic.

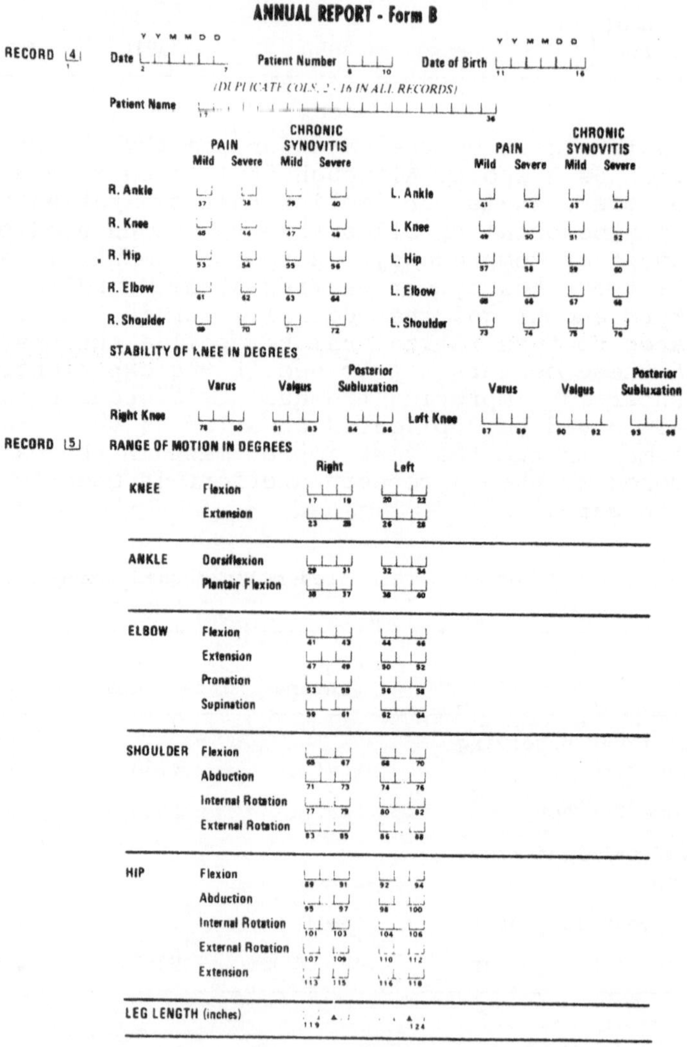

ANNUAL REPORT - Form B

RECORD 4 — Date (Y Y M M D D) — Patient Number — Date of Birth (Y Y M M D D)

(DUPLICATE COLS. 2 - 16 IN ALL RECORDS)

Patient Name

	PAIN Mild	PAIN Severe	CHRONIC SYNOVITIS Mild	CHRONIC SYNOVITIS Severe		PAIN Mild	PAIN Severe	CHRONIC SYNOVITIS Mild	CHRONIC SYNOVITIS Severe
R. Ankle					L. Ankle				
R. Knee					L. Knee				
R. Hip					L. Hip				
R. Elbow					L. Elbow				
R. Shoulder					L. Shoulder				

STABILITY OF KNEE IN DEGREES

	Varus	Valgus	Posterior Subluxation
Right Knee			
Left Knee			

RECORD 5 — RANGE OF MOTION IN DEGREES

		Right	Left
KNEE	Flexion		
	Extension		
ANKLE	Dorsiflexion		
	Plantair Flexion		
ELBOW	Flexion		
	Extension		
	Pronation		
	Supination		
SHOULDER	Flexion		
	Abduction		
	Internal Rotation		
	External Rotation		
HIP	Flexion		
	Abduction		
	Internal Rotation		
	External Rotation		
	Extension		
LEG LENGTH (inches)			

Fig. 1. Form for collection of orthopedic data completed annually by the orthopedic surgeon.

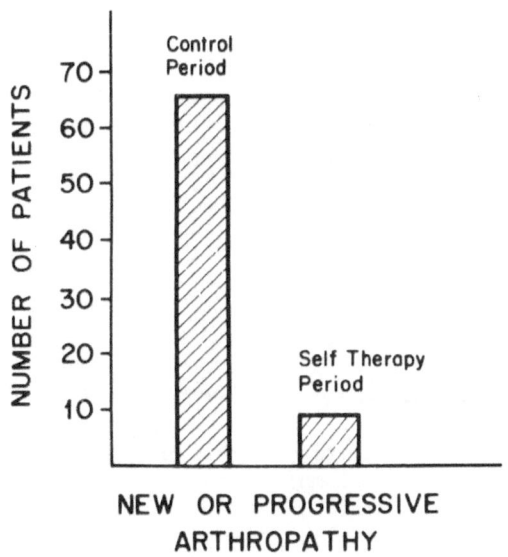

Fig. 2. Incidence of newly developed hemophilic arthropathy or progression of old lesions before and after home therapy.

Fig. 2 shows the occurrence of new hemophilic arthropathy or the significant progression of pre-existing lesions which was noted prior to and during the home therapy program. Some patients have developed chronic synovitis and must be considered failures of early infusions. We are continuing to look at this data analyzed by individual joints over a longer follow-up period to identify causes of failure. However, we are impressed by the obvious lack of progression when early and intensive therapy is appropriately applied at home. It should be emphasized that those patients who still have progression are often predictable in terms of the fact that their progression occurs in joints which are already badly diseased and unstable or that the progression can be related to the fact that the patients, many of whom are in the older age group (Fig. 3), have still not learned to infuse with an appropriate frequency and intensity (Fig. 4).

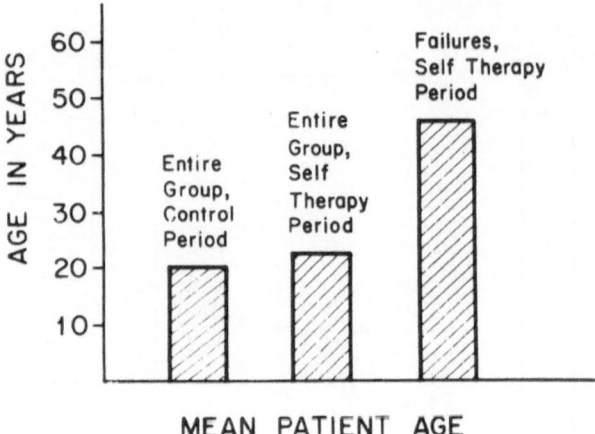

Fig. 3. Average age of patients exhibiting new or progressive arthropathy while on home therapy (third column) as compared to study group as a whole.

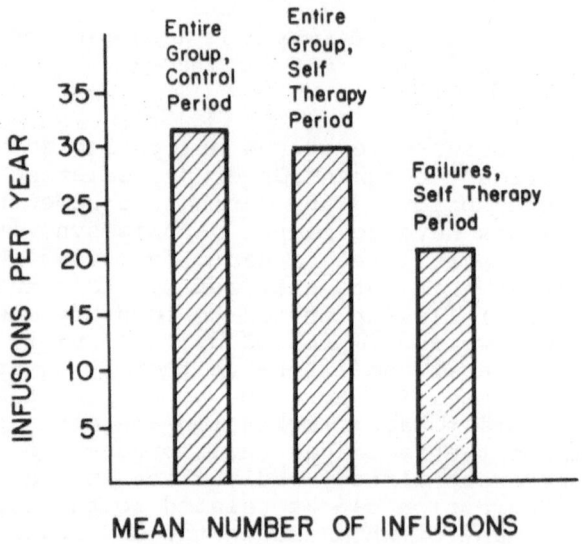

Fig. 4. Average number of infusion episodes per year of patients exhibiting new or progressive arthropathy while on home therapy (third column) as compared to study group as a whole.

CONCLUSIONS

Over the last fifteen years, we have evolved a system of care for hemophilia that is designed to meet both the medical and psychosocial needs of our patients. The central theme of the clinic has been a team approach involving a hematologist, an orthopedist, nurse, social worker, genetics associate, physical therapist, a dentist, and other consulting staff, as previously discussed. The mainstay of our therapeutic approach is a good solid education program designed to allow the patient, with the support of the center, to make most of the decisions relating to the therapy of their hemophilia. We then provide the patient with the technical expertise to implement this program. The result of this is the supervised self therapy program which we feel has revolutionized the care of hemophilia.

Over the fifteen years we have collected data that supports our hypothesis that the home infusion program improves the patient's life style and does it in a cost effective manner. The data also demonstrate that these concepts can be applied to a larger, more heterogenous population. Unfortunately we do not have the data that allows us to support our strong feeling that the psychosocial aspects of this chronic disease are also ameliorated by our program. We believe, however, that our program has resulted in a tremendous sense of well being by the normalcy which has been achieved in the lives of a majority of our patients and their families, and our patients and families agree with this opinion, with rare exceptions.

The short term results also demonstrate a significant effect of a Home Therapy program on the development of new or progressive joint disease. Long term studies will need to be done to define the limits of our ability to decrease the musculoskeletal morbidity that is associated with hemophilia.

We feel that the efficacy of home infusion programs is proven beyond a doubt. We continue to gather data that will allow us to look at unanswered issues facing patients with hemophilia today. Among these are:

1. The approach to patients with inhibitors to Factor VIII and IX;

2. The long term sequelae of liver dysfunction presumably caused by multiple transfusions;

3. The optimal factor regimen that will allow maximum benefit from treatment in the most cost effective manner and in a way that will allow for optimal use of the limited plasma resource.

REFERENCES

1. Bidwell, E., Dike, G.W.R., Snape, T.J.: Therapeutic materials. In: Human Blood Coagulation, Hemostasis and Thrombosis (2nd ed), editor R. Biggs. Blackwell Scientific Publications, Oxford, 1976, p. 262.
2. Feissly, R.: Etudes sur l'hémophilie. Mem. Soc. Med. Hosp. Paris 47:1778, 1923.
3. Graham, J.B., Buckwalter, J.A., Hartley, L.J. et al.: Canine Hemophilia. J. Exp. Med. 90:97, 1949.

4. Levine, P.H., Britten, A.F.H.: Supervised patient-management of hemophilia: A study of 45 patients with Hemophilia A and B. Ann. Int. Med. 78:195, 1973.
5. Poole, J.G., Hershgold, E.J., Pappenhagen, A.R.: High potency antihemophilic factor concentrate prepared from cryoglobulin in precipitate. Nature 203:312, 1964.
6. Tullis, J.L., Melin, M., Jurigian, P.: Clinical use of human prothrombin complexes. New Engl. J. Med. 273:667, 1965.

Discussion

Moderator: E.J.M. Sjamsoedin-Visser

C. Smit, Amsterdam:

Dr. Jones, when you were talking about the rest of the family with a hemophilic child, you were also talking about the involvement of the parents, brothers and sisters, and grandparents. Do you have a special program or project to get these people involved in the treatment of hemophilia in your center?

P. Jones, Newcastle-upon-Tyne:

We do have a special program. I think it is important to point out that when you are looking at the rest of the family, you work from the center. I mean the center of the family. So the first person is obviously the child with hemophilia. As he gets into his teen-age, when he is 10 or 11 years old, I see him in private. He is the only person in the room for at least part of the consultation of the sort of follow-up as is being described by dr. Cederbaum. Then the parents: I always speak to parents and patient together. After the parents, and with their permission, we go to grandparents and aunts, uncles and cousins. We worked out that for every index case we see, of whatever severity, at least five other people have to be tested in the laboratory and something like 10 other people have to be involved in some stage in consultation.

J.J. Van Loghem, Amsterdam:

I am very interested in the problem of making antibodies. The antibody you mentioned, dr. Cederbaum, occurs in about 20% of patients who have been treated with factor VIII concentrate. Is it possible to think about the idea that you may add anti-antibodies. If you make antibodies against the idiotype of the factor VIII antibody, the problem would be that you have to have a pure antibody of course. You could produce this either by monoclonal antibody techniques, or by other ways to purify it completely. Then you inject normal individuals with this antibody and you produce antibodies against the antibody. If you inject these antibodies into your hemophilia patients with antibodies, you suppress the formation of the antibodies and will solve the problem of antibody formation. What do you think about it?

A.I. Cederbaum, Worchester, USA:

I would start off by saying that if the 8th symposium in Groningen is on antibodies to factor VIII, I hope I am re-invited back. Antibodies are obviously a major problem in the treatment of factor VIII, and as your countrymen ele-gantly published very recently*, there are efforts of trea-ting. There are also major efforts being made to look at the immunology of the problem. In fact, I do not know if anyone is practising the concept of injecting antibodies to an antibody into the patient, but there are certainly test-systems now available of using monospecific anti-factor VIII antibody in a mechanism of being able to pu-rify plasma over a column. Presumably some day, much like the dialysis people do, we will be able to run blood through a column and remove antibody. Although clinically, I do not know if anyone has done this.
As far as injecting into the individual, I think that is obviously looked at in other forms of therapy and may in fact be applicable to the hemophiliac.

P. Jones, Newcastle-upon-Tyne:

It is a lovely idea. Unfortunately we are dealing with a heterogenous collection of what we call antibodies.
We are also dealing with the very, very few patients who have really high titer antibodies. The sort of testsystem which you referred to, like the measurement of CAG, as well as the measurement of the clotting activity of that specific part of the molecule, is relatively recent. It has not really yet come into the clinical forum. This sort of ideas is thrown around. It is the difficulty of finding the specific antibody and being able to develop it to the extent that we are able to use it for an anti-antibody.

J.G. Jolly, Chandigarh, India:

Could you enlighten us about the psychological problems of a young person? When a young one, about 15 or 16 years old, starts to realize what hemophilia is and what impact it is going to have on his life, on his intellectual abi-lity and performance as a student? Do you think that this sort of problem makes a difference when the young one is on home therapy?

---

* Sjamsoedin-Visser, E.J.M. et al., New Engl. J. Med. 1981, 305, 717.

A.I. Cederbaum, Worchester:

The patient who has been with us from the time of infancy
or childhood, in fact grows up with hemophilia and the
concept of the hemophilia being openly discussed with
that individual. In fact in almost every country adolescence - I am sure there are cultural differences - must
be a problem time.
Going through adolescence with hemophilia as an additional
problem is like any other chronic ailment. Our aim is that
by the time they become an adolescent a hemophiliac and
the treatment of hemophilia is as close to normal as is
reasonable to expect. These are children who, from the
time they went to school, have been with their peers.
There are children who have been encouraged to ride bi-
cycles, to go outside and play with their friends, to
engage in sports of the non-contact variety. We actually
have a number of our youngsters who play socker routinely
and organize leagues. We try to avoid hockey and football,
which are common in the area, but we talk them out of it.
So, hopefully, when they enter the adolescent period they
can deal with the problems of adolescence like most of
their peers. In fact the hemophilia has become a minor
issue to them, because they understand that they have the
way to correct it. A more difficult problem is the individual who comes to us during adolescence. At that point
they have to be educated, they may have already 1 or 2 de-
formed joints. More importantly, they may have been over-
protected and not allowed to develop with their peers.
This becomes a much more difficult team-effort. The social
and psychological aspects become much more difficult to
adjust to, than in fact infusion and getting the joints
taken care of.

P. Jones, Newcastle-upon-Tyne:

The only comment I can make is that the saddest thing a
doctor can see, is a patient who has not had comprehensive
care, either in adolescence or any stage into adult life.
Because as soon as they walk into the room, you can tell,
they are dependent people. It can not be measured, it has
to be anecdotal, but it is there. The difficulties in
helping them to overcome the next 5 or 6 years are immense.

I. Temperley, Dublin:

I would like to comment primarily on dr. Cederbaum's results when he compared the number of bleeding episodes
before and after the introduction of home therapy. The
criticism to the introduction of home therapy has been the
possibility that the treatment might go wild and that too
much treatment might be given. It is very encouraging to
see that your figures roughly speaking approximate before
and after the introduction of home therapy. I did an exer-

cise in our center, where I did not quite compare before
and after home therapy, because we have gradually introduced home therapy. I did compare the number of bleeding
episodes treated as it were with people who were coming
to the center versus those who are on home therapy. In
fact the results were approximate to yours. I think we had
about 29 or 30. So it is very encouraging, and I think it
should be broadcasted more to health authorities, that
home therapy does not necessarily increase the amount of
treatment given.

A.I. Cederbaum, Worchester:

It is encouraging to hear that someone gets similar data.
I think it is fair to say that the number of bleeding episodes for which the patient infuses will undoubtedly go
up. As a matter of fact, we encourage that. We encourage
the concept when you are in doubt, infuse. We consider
the total number of infusions not important, it is the
total health care costs that are important. When you keep
people out of the hospital, it is cheaper. A fact to the
matter.is, that there will be abuses, you just have to keep
them out by a good control system.

J. Stibbe, Rotterdam:

As I understood, dr. Cederbaum, you wanted to point out
the beneficial effects of home care. You gave several numbers which you all expressed in percentages. You said that
the change was minus 50 to 80%. Mathematically, 80 is plus;
so I want to make sure whether you wanted to say minus 50
to minus 80, or minus 50 to plus 80, which is different.

A.I. Cederbaum, Worchester:

I think what I wanted to say in my presentation was minus
50 to minus 80.

V. Hemophilia home care: Social and legal aspects

SOCIAL ASPECTS OF HEMOPHILIA

Th.P.B.M. Suurmeyer

QUANTITATIVE AND QUALITATIVE ASPECTS OF HEMOPHILIA: SOME PRELIMINARY REMARKS

According to Swaak (20), 7-10% of all children, aged 0-18, has a more or less severe chronic disease with a physical cause. If all kinds of chronic disorders (such as: mental retardation; hare-lip; speech, educational, or behavioral disturbances) are included *one in every four* children has one or more chronic disorders. Some of the chronic conditions with the highest prevalence are presented in Table I.

TABLE I. Some prevalence rates[*](children aged 0-18)

- Asthma	20 per 1,000
- Epilepsy	10 per 1,000
- Congenital heart disease	5 per 1,000
- Spasticity	5 per 1,000
- Diseases of bones/joints	5 per 1,000
- Diabetes	1 per 1,000

Adapted from: Swaak (20)

[*]These prevalence rates are estimates. However, complete agreement is missing as to these rates. Compare, for instance, the rates given by Swaak (20) and those given by the CBS (7). Hull and Johnston (13) mention a lower prevalence rate of hemophilia than the authors mentioned in the text. See also Suurmeijer (19) regarding some possible causes of the differences of prevalence rates (of epilepsy).

Hemophilia (A and B) occurs in approximately 8 in 100,000 population or in 1 in 6,000 males. This means that there are some 1,200 people with hemophilia in the Dutch population (11,21). Therefore, seen from this quantitative point of view hemophilia seems to be a relatively unimportant chronic condition.

Nevertheless in connection with a more qualitative point of view, the quantitative point of view should not be underestimated. As has been said there are only 1,200 hemophilia patients. Consequently, there will be one patient per five general practitioners (GP's). The unfamiliarity of GP's with hemophilia will probably affect the adequacy of the diagnosis, the information and social help given to

the patients and/or parents, especially when there is no
'family history' of hemophilia. Denial, delay of referral,
misinterpretation of symptoms, accusation of parental mis-
treating (or even abusing) their child might be a consequence. Maybe the same holds for specialists as well. And
this may considerably aggravate 'problems' of patients.
And so will those of their families. Because 'patients
have families', approximately 5,000 to 7,000 family members (parents, brothers and sisters; marriage partner,
children)   are or will be involved in, and affected by
the disease (apart from relatives, friends, peers, colleagues).

With 'problems' is not meant the medical aspect of hemophilia. What I have in view are the so-called psychosocial
problems possibly associated with hemophilia, e.g. behavioral restrictions and their consequences, family distur-
bance, problems in social relations, educational, vocational and occupational problems, feelings of inferiority,
guilt, shame, fear or stress (of patients and/or family
members). Many of these problems have to do with the way
'society' reacts to the label 'hemophilia'.

In the next sections I will discuss some of the psychosocial aspects of hemophilia. Where relevant, use will be
made of depth interviews, in October 1981 held with five
hemophilia patients and their partners or their parents.
It must be noted that these patients/parents, all members
of the Dutch Association of Hemophilia Patients, northern
region, probably were not all 'average patients or families'
In a social sense they were, speaking generally, the 'better' patients or families (in terms of social relationships,
marriage and employment). I learned a lot of these interviews on subjects such as: diagnosis; information and social help (not) given by doctors; (un-)desirability of
home-treatment; attitudes of GP's and specialists to this
treatment; expected improvements of family functioning because of this treatment; child socialization; the integra-
tive function of the coagulant laboratory of the Academic
Hospital of the State University of Groningen, the Netherlands, until some years ago; the disintegrative function
of the pediatric clinic of the same hospital; and last but
certainly not least, the important function of the Dutch
Association of Hemophilia Patients, northern region may perform (and already performs in many cases) for the patients
and their families in social, emotional as well as informa-
tional respects.

However, in this discussion I will confine myself mainly
to the more general judgments and prejudices in society and
some of their consequences. This is not because the other
subjects mentioned are not interesting or important, on
the contrary, but because (a) I have been asked to offer a
more general social view on hemophilia, because (b) the
amount of time available, and because (c) several of the
other topics will be dealt by some of the other speakers.

HEMOPHILIA AS A SOCIAL PHENOMENON

Although people with a chronic condition are lifelong in
need for medical help (e.g. drugs) this does not mean that
they are feeling themselves always chronically ill. No,
sometimes, they have, for instance, a seizure, attack or
a bleeding. But these impairing episodes aside they can
often function normally.

In his book 'The future of children', Hobbs (12) remarks: 'Categorization is necessary to open doors to opportunity: to get help ... to write legislation ... to appropriate funds ... even to communicate about the problems..'
However, classification and labeling may produce unexpected consequences. Children as well as adults '...catego-
rized and labeled as different may be permanently stigmatized, rejected by others ... and excluded from opportuni-
ties essential for their full and healthy development'.
Therefore, 'to take care' of different (or deviating)
people can and should be read with two meanings (8,12):
A. to give these people help, and B. to exclude them from
normal social interaction.

It is this exclusion or social segregation, providing
separate facilities and encouraging the disabled to interact primarily with their own minority group, that forms one
of the grim aspects of (some) chronic conditions. It is
being suggested that the justification of segregation as
'best' for the disabled, may be a rationalization of society's unease and guilt (1,2,15,17,19).

It has been assumed that the degree of feelings of unease and guilt and (consequently) the degree of segregation will vary according to the degree and attribute or
behavior is *defined* as 'different', 'abnormal' or 'undesirable'*. It is the *imputed meaning* to a set of physical
attributes that counts (whether or not a person actually
shows or has 'these attributes'). According to Freidson
(8,9) the degree of 'undesirability' can be explored along
three dimensions:

1. The *diagnosis*, or the imputed responsibility one has
for a deviant attribute or behavior;

2. The *prognosis*, or the degree a deviating phenomenon
is believed to be curable or improvable; and

3. The *stigma*, or the assigning of a negative label (often with a moral connotation) to certain deviating attributes or behaviors. In particular, those forms of organic
dysfunction or maldevelopment (for which, theoretically,
the sufferer is not held responsible) will be sigmatized
which evoke reactions of fear and disgust because of the
grim physical appearance and/or unpredictability of its manifestation (e.g. dwarfism; disfigurements; mental retardation; schizophrenia).

---

*What is called 'different', what is singled out as 'undesirable' or 'ab-
normal' or 'deviance' is not absolute. It is often historically and cul-
turally variable, defined by particular societies at particular times
for particular purposes (8,9,12).

It will be clear that whether or not an individual is believed to be responsible, incurable and (therefore) stigmatized, will have important consequences for his management (e.g. temporary versus permanent segregation), his treatment (e.g. permissivity versus punishment) and his self-concept (e.g. feelings of worth or worthlessness).

TABLE II. Types of deviance, by imputed responsibility, stigma, and prognosis (8)

Imputed prognosis	Responsibility		Not responsible	
	No stigma	stigma	Stigma	No stigma
Curable	parking violation	syphilis	leprosy	pneumonia
Improvable, not curable		burglary	crippling	hearing loss
Incurable and unimprovable		sex murder	dwarfism	cancer

In Table II some examples of kinds of deviances have been presented (8). It must be noticed that the examples presented refer to judgments of the 'man-in-the-street'. It is a *'lay diagnosis'* which probably will be at variance with the 'professional diagnosis'. This is not to say that they are (or may) not be related. Or, according to Freidson (8), '...so long as the agent or agency not publicly label or segregate individuals only a 'rate-producing-process' is involved....But if public labeling or visible segregation from which a labeling conclusion can be drawn occurs, the process may be said to be *deviance-producing* in that, by labeling the individual, it may organize the response of the community towards him as a stereotyped deviant. Whereas those around him might never have attained any consensus about his behavior before, each responding to him according to his individual relationship, public labeling establishes a common focus for uniform community response....'.

This means that once publicly labeled as, for instance, an 'epileptic', 'hemophiliac' or 'mental retardate' he may be regarded as an undifferentiated member of the category 'epileptics', 'hemophiliacs' or 'mental retardates' rather than an individual who happened, amongst all his other characteristics, to have a physical impairment. By what Safilios-Rothschild (17) calls the 'spread phenomenon' the disability trait overshadows and qualifies all other traits and abilities. The whole person becomes a 'dis-abled', he *is* the disability! (2,15).

This stereotyped, negative definition will seriously constrain and simplify the relationships between the disabled and the non-disabled. And this will have more or less

negative consequences for the feelings of worth and value
of the individuals concerned. For, as has been said in the
introduction, in hemophilia as in other disorders, the reactions of 'society' determine to a great extent the individual's feelings about who he is, what he can or may do,
and how he should behave. Thus, if the non-disabled, for
instance, parents, peers, teachers or employers, define
a person as 'different', they will treat him 'different'
and (may thereby) encourage him to become as he is percei-
ved. If they, for instance, believe him to be incompetent
(for normal social relations, education or employment)
they protect him from exposure to experiences (again: normal education etc.etc.) from which he might learn greater
competence (12,17).

Let us turn back to Table II. What could be the place
of hemophilia? Obviously, the answer to this question depends largely on who is doing the assigning, because mostly there will be no (complete) agreement in a society as
to 'responsibility', 'curability/improvability' and 'stigma'
Nevertheless, let us have a try: hemophilia is an incurable,
unimprovable, stigmatized, congenital physical impairment
for which, theoretically, one is not held responsible but
which '...in some way damage his identity because of the
halo of moral evaluations' (8) that in fact surrounds hemophilia.

HEMOPHILIA AND EXCLUSION

It must be emphasized that this description is supposed to
be a hypothetical lay diagnosis, made by the man-in-the-
street. Although, as one of the respondents interviewed
remarked:
- 'One sometimes wonders what doctors are talking about
  when they are talking about hemophilia. You may hear
  from them the same prejudices: 'untouchable', 'stanch-
  less bleedings' and 'bleeding to death'.'

This is definitely a wrong conception of hemophilia, certainly nowadays with the new developed (highly purified)
concentrates, (cryoprecipitate; PPSB) and, connected with
that, the ever increasing possibility of home-treatment.
Nevertheless, it is a conception coming from the near-by
past and induced by the most severe forms of hemophilia,
until the mid sixties often leading to more or less serious impairment of the joints and orthopedic disabilities.

From the interviews it turned out that this conception
still exists, sometimes leading to an involuntary restric-
tion or even denial of activities, particularly in the
areas of education and employment, but also in the area of
more general social activities and relationships. Let me
illustrate this point by some quotations.
- In first instance, people are staring on hearing it ...
   at the hemophilia. Friends and acquaintances also assume
   that I have to be spared and taken care of, because they

really think 'you surely can't do that'.
- The name 'bleeding disease' still frightens people
  (somewhat) ... being careful with you ... that image,
  you know, it's still maintained. I haven't had really
  negative reactions of friends and so. But sometimes
  their reactions are so stupid, for instance, when they
  slap you on your shoulder and then say: 'I can't do that
  with you, can I?! It hurts a little ... they are pushing
  me back on the hemophilia ... and that's annoying and
  frustrating. These are the adults who make the problems,
  such as 'what are you walking foolish ... in fact, you
  can't do anything, can you?! You like to join, to 'play
  up', and at that moment you are pressed hard upon the
  'facts': 'you can't do that .... you have hemophilia'.
  Things like that. It hurts.
- When my brother was attending a normal school, one time
  the teacher told him '...that he had to attend a special
  school ... because he had the bleeding disease'.
- Hemophilia is a 'reason' to be rejected as a civil ser-
  vant. That was the reason why I, in first instance, was
  not admitted to that school. But the former doctor of
  the coagulation laboratory in Groningen, whom I and many
  other patients owe a lot, said: 'are you crazy, we try
  to make you function as normal as possible and now society says: you are not normal. We don't take it!' The
  doctor who rejected me as medically unfit was an old
  one; young doctors do know more about hemophilia.
- When my employer heard that I had hemophilia, then he
  fired me at once ... While I always lost less days from
  work than my colleagues...!

What may be concluded from these events? Are they mere
incidents, many people may experience one day or another?
I don't think so for several reasons. Firstly, the restrictions of activities are always associated with the hemophilia. Insufficient knowledge of hemophilia and the modern
means of treatment as well as certain feelings of uneasi-
ness gives rise to stereotyped treatment of the patients.

Secondly, the respondents interviewed referred to other
hemophilia patients who have had the same kind of negative
experiences. Unemployment was no exception.

In the third place, from the investigations of the Dutch
Central Bureau for Statistics (CBS; 6,7), of Gorter and
Terpstra (10) and of Bos (3) it turned out that the handi-
capped are always more unemployed than other people. According to the trade unions this difference in (un-)employment
rate still increases in times of economic recession.

Fourthly, if the former head of the coagulation laboratory (of the Academic Hospital at Groningen, the Netherlands
had not actively intervened and assisted some of the respondents, probably they would not function quite as well as
they did and do now in an educational and/or occupational
sense. In this way, the events did not occur by accident.

There are more or less obvious indications that 'healthy'

people confronted with people with hemophilia feel unease
and tend to exclude them from normal activities and experiences. And that would be of course 'beneficial' for the
hemophilia patient.

HEMOPHILIA AND SELF-CONCEPT

But there is still more to be worried about. As has been
said before, in my opinion the experiences of the hemophilia patients quoted were no incidents. Nevertheless, they
may blame themselves sometimes. This 'blaming oneself' is
a very well-known phenomenon in disability. Mostly, it is
connected with feelings the patient has about himself. As
has been discussed before (Table II) the feelings a patient
with hemophilia may have about himself and his illness are
to a great extent determined by the reactions of his social
environment.
From the interviews it appeared that the male respondents have (had) feelings of inferiority. Seldom they are
aware that these feelings largely have been evoked by 'society'. Therefore, they may blame themselves when problems
arise*. These feelings of inferiority may be demonstrated
in various ways: from withdrawal from social relations to
over-compensation in terms of conspicious behavior and/or
over-ambition. Let the next quotations speak for themselves.
- I was strongly motivated to achieve better ... that's me.
  And I have still that strong ambition.
  Yes, (his wife said; T.S.) in those days you were also
  very, very serious, you would have been hurt very quickly .... you had really quite an inferiority complex ...
  but still you have that strong ambition ... not to be
  inferior ... to prove yourself.
- I think you are always proving yourself, your whole life
  long, that you are not inferior, not of less value than
  someone else. By 'kicking up a row' you try to keep in...
  to remain friends ... to belong to them ... really belong
  Perhaps someone else would have said: 'I don't do it or
  I don't dare it', but I did.
  On the other hand, because of the hemophilia I broke off
  relationships with the other sex in advance. That idea:
  'be inferior' ... perhaps it was only in my mind. But,
  you know, hemophilia is very central in your life!

These experiences of their own lives aside they had ample
examples of the same kind of feelings and experiences of
other hemophilia patients.

---

*This is not to say that a chronic illness cannot possibly be used
as a 'perfect alibi' for failures in social, educational or occupational respects, for which he no longer blames himself but blames the
disability. Disabled persons who react in this way are often referred
to as those who derive 'secondary gains' from their disability (17).

The manifold hospitalizations, particularly those during their youth, the many behavioral restrictions imposed (life-long), the fear to be excluded from normal interaction, to be 'pushed back on the hemophilia' and to be dependent on others (parents; peers; colleagues) during impairing episodes in their lives as well as other more or less poignant experiences (of themselves or of other patients) probably are responsible for these feelings of diminished worth and value. If consistent and strong enough these experiences, reinforcing one another and leading to a downward spiral of self-respect and self-confidence, may ultimately manifest itself in more overt ways, e.g. in severe emotional or behavioral maladjustments, for which, to be sure, they themselves will be blamed once again.

IMPLICATIONS AND CONCLUSIONS

From the interviews quoted it must not be derived that the patients and their families with whom I have spoken were in a bad way. From a social point of view they could be conceived of as the 'better patients and families' (as has been remarked in the introduction). Nevertheless, also from their experiences it can be inferred that there are still certain prejudices towards people with hemophilia, some-times coupled with exclusion from normal activities, re-lationships and experiences and allied to often deeply rooted and hidden worries, fears and feelings of diminished value and worth, manifesting themselves in feelings of an-noyance and frustration, uncertainty in social relation-ships and/or conspicious attitudes and behavior.

One can only guess about the situation of other hemo-philia patients but listening to the remarks of the res-pondents I am not over-optimistic. There may be at work a process called 'self-fulfilling prophecy' (16). For, the consequences of a physical impairment viz. hemophilia may be to place the patient in stigmatized categories, identi-fied with the uneducable, the unemployable, the poor or the dependent. Consequently the non-disabled may feel that it is justified to think of hemophilia as a stigmatized, uncurable and unimprovable physical impairment and that it is 'beneficial' for the hemophilia patients to prevent them from exposure to experiences from which they otherwise might have learned greater competence. Because they have not the abilities, have they! In this way the process of stigmati-zation may be self-reinforcing: negative reactions of other people continually provide new grounds for stigma. Rarely, a man manoeuvred into this position'... may find himself the resources to re-plan his life, to take definite posi-tive steps to break out of a vicious circle ... He is like-ly to feel trapped in an environment too powerful for him to overcome by his own efforts' (1). And eventually, this may lead to what I have called elsewhere *social inheritance* (19): a transfer of negative social conditions from one ge-neration to another (14).

Chronic illness
Child
Family
Environment

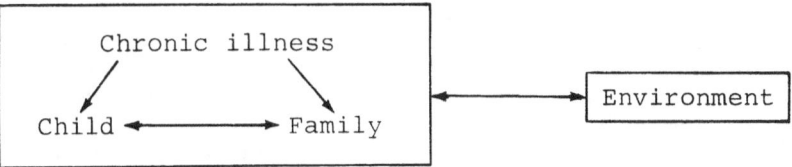

Fig. 1. Basic relations between hemophilia, child and family functioning, and environmental reactions.

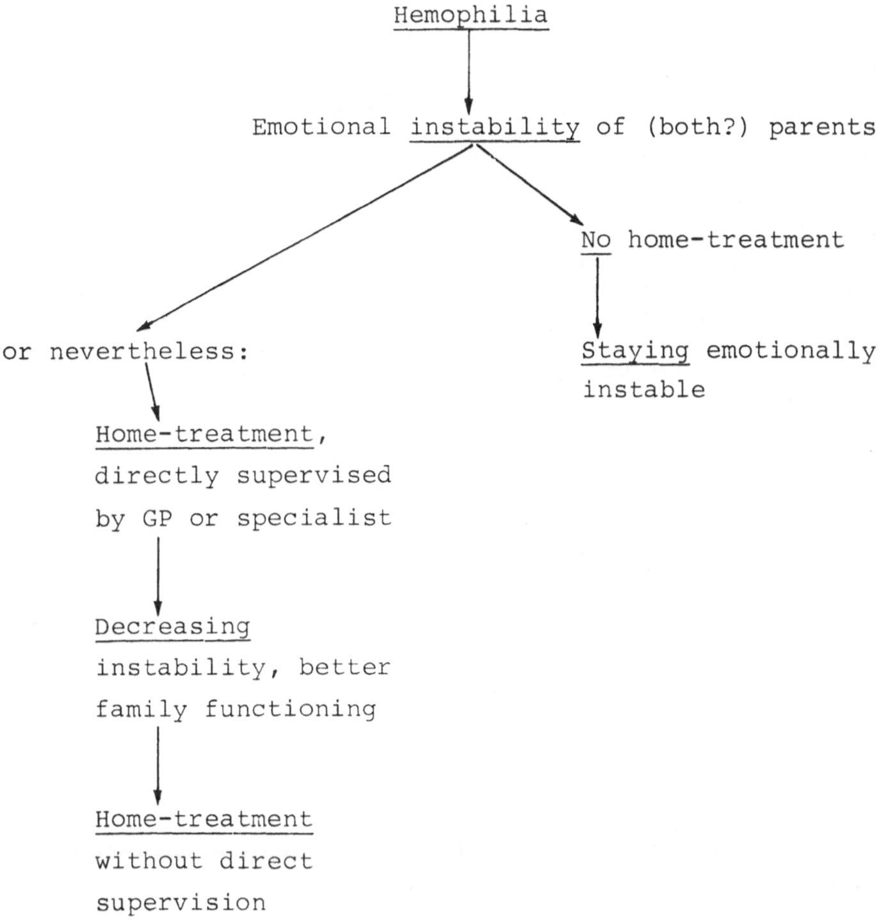

Hemophilia
Emotional instability of (both?) parents
No home-treatment
Staying emotionally instable
or nevertheless:
Home-treatment, directly supervised by GP or specialist
Decreasing instability, better family functioning
Home-treatment without direct supervision

Fig. 2. Some possible relations between hemophilia, emotional stability, and home-treatment.

As a very prejudiced person until now I have spoken of *the* hemophilia patient. Of course, there are several degrees of severity of hemophilia (although the 'average man' will not take this into account when speaking and judging over hemophilia).

But there is another very important line along which patients with hemophilia can be differentiated, namely the age of the patient. Compared to the 'older' patients children born in the mid sixties or later are born under much more favorable conditions of life (in a medical sense) because of the development of new methods and means of treatment. In particular I will point at the possibility of home-care, which has been made possible by the development of freeze-dried concentrates. I shall not say very much about this subject because other speakers have already done this or will do so. But something I would like to say because of the impressive influence this kind of treatment may have on the way not only the patient but also his family will function.

1. Firstly, this kind of treatment may, among others, prevent (serious) orthopedic impairments because 'the medication is always at home'. Delay of treatment will considerably decrease (5,18). Therefore, also home-treatment of children at an early age may be indicated. Pediatricians or pediatric clinics ought to be more benevolent and actively promoting in this respect. General practitioners, too, ought to be more sympathetic and ready to help.

2. It may cause not only a physical but also a mental and social liberation, i.e. a greater physical mobility and less behavioral restrictions as well as increasing self esteem and self-confidence, independency and social mobility (5,18).

3. It will increase the level of family functioning in instrumental as well as in emotional respect. Particularly, the emotional aspect seems to be important because it is often used as one of the criteria for (not) selection for a home-care program (4).

One must remember, however, that one of the causes, often underestimated, for personal and/or family stability is the chronic condition itself (19)! (see Fig. 1). In this way, not allowing home-care for emotional reasons may increase the emotional stress: another example of 'self-fulfilling prophecy'. In Figure 2 some possible relations between hemophilia, emotional stability, and home-treatment are presented.

4. Last but not least, the better way the patient functions in physical, social and mental respect because of this, home-treatment may be the best *example* that hemophilia is only an impairment and as such is only *one* of the characteristics a person may have. Possible changes in society's concept of hemophilia by the mass media aside, this 'exampling' may be the best remedy against social prejudices.

ACKNOWLEDGEMENTS

I am very grateful to the patients, their partners or their parents who were willing to grant me so much of their confidence and time.

REFERENCES

1. Blaxter, M.: The Meaning of Disability. Heinemann, London 1980.
2. Blommestijn, P.J.: Zorg voor lichamelijk en zintuigelijk gehandicapten. In: Organisatie van de gehandicaptenzorg, editors G.J. Kronjee et al. Van Gorcum, Assen, 1980, p. 97.
3. Bos, J.M.: Hard tegen hart. Een social-wetenschappelijk onderzoek onder jongeren die enkele jaren daarvoor werden geopereerd aan een aangeboren hartafwijking. Swets & Zeitlinger, Amsterdam, 1978.
4. Breederveld, C.: Home-therapy: risk factors and complications. In: Home-treatment for Haemophilia: Perspectives and Limitations. Proceedings of a workshop on haemophilia, editor C. Th. Smit Sibinga. Drukkerij Schut, Groningen, 1979, p. 47.
5. Britten, A.F.H.: A concept of home-treatment for haemophilia. In: Home-treatment for Haemophilia: Perspectives and Limitations, editor C.Th. Smit Sibinga. Drukkerij Schut, Groningen, 1979, p. 15.
6. CBS: Gehandicapten wel geteld, deel 5, Staatsuitgeverij, Den Haag, 1974.
7. CBS: Gehandicapten wel geteld; bijlage bij deel 3: tabellen. Staatsuitgeverij, Den Haag, 1976.
8. Freidson, E.: Disability as social deviance. In: Sociology and Rehabilitation, editor M.B. Sussman. American Sociological Association and Vocational Rehabilitation Administration, Washington, DC, 1965, p. 71.
9. Freidson, E.: Profession of medicine. Dodd, Mead & Company, New York, 1973, p. 205.
10. Gorter, K.A., Terpstra, J.B.: Zorgen door en voor lichamelijk gehandicapten. NIMAWO and ITS, Nijmegen, 1979.
11. Hemofilie in Nederland, Academisch Ziekenhuis, Leiden, 1979.
12. Hobbs, N.: The futures of children. Categories, labels, and their consequences. Jossey-Bass Publishers, London, 1975.
13. Hull, D., Johnston, D.I.: Essential paediatrics. Churchill Livingstone, London, 1981, p. 183
14. Jones, P.: Home-therapy: cost effectiveness and society aspects of home-treatment. In: Home-treatment for Haemophilia: Perspectives and Limitations. Proceedings of a workshop on haemophilia, editor: C.Th. Smit Sibinga. Drukkerij Schut, Groningen, 1979, p. 51.
15. Meiresonne, J.B.: Zorg voor geestelijk gehandicapten. In: Organisatie van de gehandicaptenzorg, editor: G.J. Kronjee et al. Van Gorcum, Assen, 1980, p. 31.
16. Merton, R.: Social theory and social structure. The Free Press, New York, 1967, p. 421.
17. Safilios-Rothschild, C.: The sociology and social psychology of disability and rehabilitation. Random House, New York, 1970.
18. Smit, C., Veltkamp, J.J., Willeumier, H.T.L., Van Dijck, H.: Home-treatment for haemophilia in the Netherlands 1972-1978. In: Home-treatment for Haemophilia: Perspectives and Limitations, editor:

C.Th. Smit Sibinga. Drukkerij Schut, Groningen, 1979, p. 27.

19. Suurmeijer, T.P.B.M.: Kinderen met epilepsie. Een onderzoek naar de invloed van een ziekte op kind en gezin. Veenstra Visser Offset, Groningen, 1980.

20. Swaak, A.F.: Ongeneeslijke ziekte heeft grote emotionele invloed op ontwikkeling van het kind. Maatschappelijke Gezondheidszorg, 5:20, 1977.

21. Veltkamp, J.J.: Prevalence and variety of picture in haemophilia in the Netherlands. In: Home-treatment for haemophilia: Perspectives and Limitations, editor: C. Th. Smit Sibinga. Drukkerij Schut, Groningen, 1979, p. 11.

HEMOPHILIA AND THE BORDERS OF LIFE

J.L. Prothero

The borders of any individual's life will be set by the circumstances into which he is born and which encompasses his childhood and the use that he and others may make of any chances that may occur for changing those borders and circumstances over the following years. Those chances may be dictated purely by fate, or they may be created by the person involved or those close to him. There will be some borders which are immovable and others which in some circumstances may seem so, but which in fact can be moved by a degree of extra consideration. For example, there is no way that a woman can become a firefighter, involved with putting out fires in houses and factories, because generally she is considered physically unsuited to the job and nothing will change that particular border in her life. In parts of the United Kingdom there is a minimum height level of 6 feet for men wishing to join the police force, and again, there is nothing that a shorter man can do to change that, no matter how desperate he may be to become a policeman in that area. However, he has the chance to change his life's borders radically by moving to a different area of the country where the minimum height level is less and where he may be accepted. Thus it is with hemophilia. If you are born with hemophilia, then that is one border of your life that you can never change and it is a factor affecting almost all of the other borders of life to a greater or lesser extent. It is an added complication to all the other factors that affect the life of a hemophiliac, as they do all people's lives and it results in a lessening in the chances of a hemophiliac altering some of these factors. It is no good a hemophiliac moving from one area to another where he will exceed the minimum height requirement needed to become a policeman, for his height is no longer the main factor and it is the fact of his hemophilia that will prevent him even being given the chance to try to become a policeman for his application would be immediately turned down without his height being considered.

In that particular instance, the attitude of the people concerned would be correct, but the attitude of many other people to hemophilia, which often has a very great effect on the borders of a hemophiliac's life and the chances that exist for alteration are based on misconceptions and wrong thinking.

The attitude of others is governed not by what hemophilia actually is and means today, but by how they perceive hemophilia. All to often their perception is based on an out-of-date picture usually remembered from some over-dramatic story or television program, or even a half-remembered legend of the sufferings of the most famous hemophiliac of all, the last Tsarevitch of Russia. Their ideas most certainly seldom bear any resemblance to the real lives of hemophiliacs. When I was 11 years old, my parents applied for my admission to a local grammar school as I had successfully completed the primary stage of my education. The headmaster was a charming man and after some discussion, agreed to accept me, but suggested I should carry a soft cushion with me from classroom to classroom, so that I need not sit on a hard wooden chair, for his idea of hemophilia was someone who bruised so easily that just sitting could bring out a large bruise! Fortunately, for my acceptance among my school mates, on an ordinary basis, he was subsequently persuaded that nature had provided me with a very serviceable built-in cushion which really needed no supplementing!

Even today it is seldom that anyone who is not actively concerned with a hemophiliac as a close relative or friend, or who is involved in their treatment and care, appreciates just what effects hemophilia has on the life of a hemophiliac and even fewer can comprehend what it means to live as a hemophiliac. The usual response of most people is still to expect the hemophiliac to bleed to death from a small cut in, say, a finger, as was the response of most people decades ago. There has obviously been a failure to convey to the general public the real meaning of hemophilia and the revolutionary effect on hemophiliacs' lives of the development of modern treatment materials, coupled with home care or self-therapy. People as a whole do not realize how the capabilities of hemophiliacs have been expanded in a way that would have been beyond dreams even 15 years ago when I was little more than a boy.

It must not be forgotten, however, that even with the recent developments in hemophilic care, living and coping with hemophilia still imposes a great strain on many people apart from the hemophiliac himself. From the point of view of the hemophiliac, there remains the uncertainty of his day to day life, his problems in planning the smooth running of such simple things as work schedules and holidays: the boredom of the extra and continuing arrangements he must make day in day out, month in month out, year after year, to cope with his need for treatment, ideally within minutes of identifying the onset of a bleeding episode. Let us not forget that even with the advent of self-therapy it is still impossible to treat all bleeding episodes in this way. Two of the worst bleeding episodes I have had in the six years I have been on self-therapy happened only a few months ago because I was unable to treat them soon af-

ter they commenced. The first, a very severe bleed in a
knee, started very soon after I started to interview someone at my office. As the interview concerned an alleged
crime, it was impossible to halt the interview as quickly
as would have been preferable, with the result that by the
time I was able to treat myself, about an hour had passed
and the knee had reached the stage where I was unable to
walk for several days. The second, in an elbow, started
when I was asleep and woke me eventually because of the
pain - by which time obviously the bleeding had been under
way for some time. Thus, a hemophiliac still must learn
to cope with considerable pain and discomfort. Older hemophiliacs must also try to accept the possibility of increasing degrees of crippling as joints damaged by bleeding
episodes in the past when there was no treatment, deteriorate further under the stresses imposed on them and also
by the normal effects of the ageing processes.

These effects are ones to which it is possible for a
hemophiliac to adjust, and one to which he has to adjust
if he is to hope to lead a normal life. It is however,
frequently more difficult for the hemophiliac to accept
and adjust to the effect his hemophilia has on others.
This starts from a young age when excuses have to be made
for such things as arriving late to collect a girlfriend
for a date, or even worse, not turning up to collect her
at all! The options then are either to explain all about
hemophilia, which to a young boy with his first or second
girlfriend is really an impossibility, or inventing some
other excuse. If it happens too frequently the girlfriend,
not unnaturally, will find a more reliable boyfriend! As
relationships grow however, the effect of a hemophiliac's
problems on others become less simply resolved. The adjustment by both parties to the shift in the traditional
roles between husband and wife needs a great effort. In
my household, normally it is my wife who carries the heavy
bags or climbs up and down stepladders to paint ceilings!
I hope our relationship is such to take such role rever-
sals without too many problems, but for many it is a cause
of great stress. Frequently, a hemophiliac is unable to
experience with his son the normal relationship between
father and son involving so frequently as it does, especially as the son gets bigger, so much physical effort,
as for example in the rough and tumble of things like
teaching him football, or just indulging in physical activities such as running in the course of normal play activities. The problem of explaining to a daughter that she
is a carrier of hemophilia and may give birth to a hemophilic son can cause great anguish to the hemophilic father and indeed to his wife, in addition to the problems
it presents to the daughter. The problems his hemophilia
causes to others therefore add to the stresses a hemophiliac suffers himself in just coping with his complaint
and trying to persuade outsiders to accept him on a normal
basis. Fortunately, as the treatment of hemophilia has im-

proved, these problems have lessened to some degree and as treatment continues to improve will, no doubt, be less of a burden in the future, but their effect on a hemophiliac's life must not be ignored.

The revolution in treatment has affected the life of a hemophiliac, but without this becoming apparent to the world at large. The fact that with modern treatment a hemophiliac is not restricted in anywhere near the same degree as in the past is just not comprehended by most people and the blame for this and the lack of correcting the image is one that must be shared by the hemophiliac, his family, his close friends, his doctors and all who he deals with at his hemophilia center. The increase in the capabilities of hemophiliacs today in comparison with even the recent past varies according to the age of the hemophiliac. Obviously a young hemophiliac who has had the advantage of modern treatment all his life will suffer few restrictions on his capabilities as a result of his hemophilia. An old hemophiliac who had no adequate treatment for perhaps the first 50 years or so of his life is unlikely to show much change as a result of new developments. The majority of today's hemophiliacs will lie in between these two extremes and it is perhaps on these that a large amount of the responsibility lies for communicating the up-to-date position to others. Not only is it essential to show to schools, prospective employers, insurers and all others involved in hemophiliacs' lives the capabilities the modern hemophiliac has with the latest care, but it is also essential to demonstrate to other hemophiliacs who do not avail themselves of the best treatment, or do not seek to find it, just what they could achieve, for if they fail in this respect, not only will they suffer personally, which would be most regrettable, but also they fail to present a picture of modern hemophilia to others and this will adversely affect not only themselves, but also other hemophiliacs. As an example, consider an employe who has a hemophiliac employee who does not avail himself of the benefits of modern care. Without doubt he will spend a considerable number of days away from work, or working at a level well below his best, which would lead his employer to be very reluctant to employ anyone else with hemophilia. With the proper use of home care programs many hemophiliacs have little extra time away from work for sick leave. For example, in the last 6 years I have a mean level of 9 days sick leave a year, which apart from absences due to bleeding episodes, also includes non-hemophilia illness such as influenza, upset stomachs and hangovers! In fact if I exclude the extra-ordinary sick leave attributable to a car crash I was in last year, that mean drops to 6 days a year. These sorts of levels are sufficiently low not to deter an employer from employing other hemophiliacs. The effect on other hemophiliacs, particularly younger sufferers and on the parents of young hemophiliacs especially where the disorder is newly diagnosed, of talking to those who have an outdated attitude to their own treatment, and therefore their own capabilities will only add to their problems and despondance, whereas seeing and talking to hemophiliacs who cope properly with their complaint, and work towards reducing it to the lowest possible nuisance value, can only encourage them and hopefully make them determined to do the same.

In talking about modern care of hemophilia involving, as it does, concentrates, home care, etc., we should not lose sight of the fact that this form of care is still not available to a majority of hemophiliacs around the world. Without such care, or care at a level approaching it, hemophiliacs are dependent on others to a large degree, and their ability to contribute to the society in which they live is substantially reduced, if not removed altogether. With the highest level of care, hemophiliacs live fulfilling lives and make a worthwhile contribution to their community. In economic terms, they will be contributing to, if not totally covering, the cost of their hemophilia care and this point is one which is important to convey whenever the care of hemophiliacs is discussed.

The keynote of modern care of hemophilia and perhaps the largest single change in the borders of the life of a hemophiliac, is summed up in the word 'independence'. Independence from relying on others for the administration of treatment, and indeed independence in managing his own care, as well as independence from the ties of having to be close to a hemophilia center or source of treatment, and independence of movement about his country or indeed the world. This independence is not always easily achieved as it requires a radical adjustment in the attitudes both of the hemophiliac, his doctors and the staff at his hemophilia center. The doctor and center staff are used to administering treatment to their patient, coping with his needs and seeing their care rewarded by an improvement in the hemophiliac's condition. The hemophiliac need take no active role and had only to get himself to his hemophilia center, explain where he was bleeding and then lie back and wait to be treated and made well. Now, however, this style of treatment is not encouraged, but the implementation of home care needs a great deal of understanding and thought on both sides to add this extra dimension to a hemophiliac's life. The doctor is basically relegated to the role of spectator in the day to day care of hemophilia. His role becomes, at most, an advisory one for his job of diagnosing the problem, deciding on the course of treatment necessary and overseeing its administration has been transferred to his patient. Probably now he is involved more in the treatment of complications that arise, such as those with inhibitors, or in the decisions as to how best to rectify damage done to joints, etc. before modern treatment was available. For him to have the confidence to allow his patient the freedom to get on with his own treatment requires a radical change in outlook, surpassed

only by that of the hemophiliacs themselves, many of whom
are very conservative by nature! Even if the training for
home care given to the hemophiliac is exhaustive and the
best available, the switch to doing your own treatment is
quite dramatic! Usually all goes well until the first tim
a small problem is encountered and then a mild state of
panic can set in! I would suggest that it takes some year
on a home care program before the hemophiliac is really
coping with his complaint to the best advantage. By this
I mean being able to do more than slavishly follow a set
of instructions for his treatment. He will have mastered
the technicalities and procedures of his care and be able
to overcome any problems with venepunctures, etc., but he
will also have the confidence and ability to vary the dosage and frequency of his treatment. He should also be
able and allowed to make decisions as to when he should
institute short periods of prophylaxis. To do this he
must have a very good relationship with the staff at his
hemophilia center, who should support him in such a program and they need to encourage him to develop his confidence in this way if he is to extract the maximum benefit
from home care programs and thus make the most of his capabilities.

By such a program of care both the hemophiliac, his
doctor, the staff at his hemophilia center, his own family, friends and all those with whom he is involved, wil
benefit and the hemophiliac will be able to demonstrate
he can cope efficiently, and without dramatic fuss, with
his disorder and that he can be placed in the same category as the great part of the population who have some
sort of physical problem to a greater or lesser extent.
He can show his self-sufficiency, self-reliance, and fore
sight can overcome to a large degree the problems with
which he has been afflicted.

The modern way of caring for hemophilia has meant that
the borders of life for hemophiliacs have been significantly extended in the past few years. It is confidently
expected that the next few years will see an even greater
expansion of these borders.

HEMOPHILIA IN PROFESSIONAL LIFE

C. Breederveld

In social life hemophiliacs meet many problems, caused by recurrent bleeding episodes. Postponement of appointments, irregular school attendance and absenteeism from the job are familiar to every severe hemophilia patient. However, prophylactic treatment and home therapy completely changed the picture of frequent hospital visits and absenteeism from almost any social event.

Everybody recognizes the importance of a happy family life. However, a steady and pleasant job is at least as important as that. It gives the opportunity for a meaningful life, without being an exception in all aspects of society. For this reason there is no need for finding jobs without real responsibility, for this will only confirm the feeling of being of no use for society.

The importance of developing a clear policy of appreciation of a hemophiliac's professional life is illustrated by the results as obtained in a survey by Prof. Veltkamp and his coworkers (1). This survey concerns 435 hemophiliacs, of whom over 60% was younger than 20 years of age at that time. Six years later a clear shift of age groups was noted in the same population (2). This means that in the past years more hemophiliacs finished school education and are now looking for jobs.

Concerning the education of hemophilia patients, figures presented in Table I, were revealed by the survey.

TABLE I. Education level of hemophiliacs according to age

Age (years)	Level	Hemophiliacs (%) (n=160)	Male population (%)
10-19	Secondary or high school	52.6	32.6
15-19	Trade school	9.6	38.8
15-19	Higher trade school	15.1	12.7
20-24	Technical college	14.2	12.6
20-24	University	18.6	16.8

J.J. Veltkamp et al., 1979

Comparing the population of hemophiliacs with the male dutch population it is clearly shown that far less hemophiliacs are trained for jobs demanding physical strength, like carpenters or building constructors, etc. Heavy jobs must be considered as not advisable to severe and moderately severe hemophiliacs.

However, the possibility of exceptions is always there. In every big treatment center, there are a few people who show this by being a farmer or so.

Delay in education was experienced by many respondents. However, in 1978 a slight improvement was seen compared to the situation in 1972. A delay of over one year was noted in 28% of the cases while in 1972 35% experienced this delay. The number of interruptions of education showed an even better improvement. In 1978 only 21 hemophiliacs had to interrupt their education, while 58 cases were noted in 1972. There is no doubt that home care and prophylactic treatment is one of the main reasons for this improvement.

In contrast to the educational level of the younger hemophiliacs the older working population shows an equal distribution over all jobs available, compared to the normal male population. For the future one may expect a shift to higher income levels because of a better or at least different educational level. The joy of a pleasant job is partly determined by the appreciation by direct colleagues This appreciation might easily be disturbed by frequent ab senteeism.

The average absenteeism of the working severe hemophili was 38 days in 1978. A slight improvement compared to the situation in 1972 was noted. However, absenteeism is still very high. Less affected hemophiliacs like the mild and sub-groups show an average absenteeism which is equal to the dutch male population. A striking result is seen when from the group of severe hemophiliacs those are excluded who show an absenteeism of over 60 days. In that case aver age absenteeism is only 13 days per year, which must be considered as very low. This should be an encouragement to employers.

Satisfaction with the job seems to increase in the hemo philic population. Almost 80% of the respondents to the second survey described their job as suitable for their situation, an increase of almost 10% compared to 1972.

In conclusion: Concerning the hemophiliacs professional life and education an improvement was noted in the course of 6 years. This improvement was concurrent with better treatment facilities, development of home care programs an the availability of sufficient amounts of factor VIII for prophylactic regimens. However, the situation should be improved further by good cooperation of the Dutch Society for Hemophiliacs, treatment centers and employers.

ACKNOWLEDGEMENTS

We are indebted to Prof. Dr. J.J. Veltkamp for providing us with the results of the survey and his approval for using these results for this review.

REFERENCES

1. Veltkamp, J.J. et al.: Hemofilie in Nederland I. Werkgroep Hemofilie Onderzoek Leiden, 1973.
2. Veltkamp, J.J. et al.: Hemofilie in Nederland II. Werkgroep Hemofilie Onderzoek Leiden, 1979.

THE LEGAL ASPECTS OF HEMOPHILIA. WHAT IS POSSIBLE IN THE NETHERLANDS AND WHAT ARE THE CONDITIONS?

P.W.J. De Graaf

Most people, and especially my fellow countrymen with enough self-knowledge know that the average Dutchman likes to do the things he has to do, as good as possible, but without much red tape and formal organization via laws, regulations and so on. This applies to home-treatment, too. Nevertheless, some of us, both among patients and among physicians, felt from time to time that we were walking on a knife's edge with regard to the legal aspects of home-treatment. The only question so to speak was, who would be the first to cut himself, thus undermining the whole framework of the home-treatment system that seemingly functions in such a nice informal way at the moment in our country.

Only two months ago, C. Breederveld in a statement added to his thesis (1) formulated it as 'with regard to the legal position, home-treatment of hemophilia is absolutely unsatisfactorily organized in the Netherlands'. Actually he did not say 'and inefficiently', but I think he will defend that just as well as I would. Quite a bad situation as it seemed to him and many others at that moment.

It was thus decided that within the framework of this symposium, somebody had to start some action to improve the legal framework in question. The organizing committee looked for a long time for a well-informed speaker on this subject, but did not succeed in finding one, and finally asked the Dutch Hemophilia Society to do some desk research.

Our findings were as follows:

First of all, we found that nothing is wrong with the legal framework. Home-treatment is possible, but mind you, only provided certain conditions are properly defined and adhered to. The question is of course: what are these conditions?

First of all, it is necessary that physicians involved in hemophilia treatment must have a uniform policy regarding home-treatment. This uniform policy does not exist at the moment. Thus, both the patient and the physician needlessly expose themselves to judicial claims, by not having this uniform policy.

Let us first consider some of the framework and conditions mentioned above necessary to let the system work from a legal point of view, and then come back to the destined

uniform policy in general. These conditions can be found
in an excellent recent book on the relation between law
and the medical profession by Dr. Leenen (2), undoubtedly
known to all my countrymen.

He bases his statements on a verdict of the Dutch Supreme Court, somewhere in the sixties, and on some additional verdicts from a lower court, and concludes on the
following points:

1. The physician has to decide as to diagnosis and indications. These decisions can not be delegated. Within the
framework of these decisions for which the physician is
responsible, however, certain procedures can be delegated
to others. Although not explicitly mentioned, home-treatment is most certainly among the procedures that can be
delegated. One could consider the patient, the home-treater
as a kind of long-distance instrument in the hands of the
physician. Not an every day instrument, because:

2. The patient can refuse home-treatment. A situation
that will not too often arise, but still it happens. So
home-treatment is among the procedures that can be delegated. How is this delegation formally organized?

3. Delegation must be accompanied by clear instructions
concerning the performance of medical and related procedures, possible complications and their treatment.

4. This delegation only can take place when the capability to perform the necessary medical procedures is achieved by the patient. A kind of examination one could say.
Not only to know how to make the venepuncture, but especially as to when, where, how much and questions like that

It looks thus as if we did allright, at least from a
legal point of view. No, not completely because:

5. This delegation must be in writing and signed by the
physician and the patient. When delegating, clear instructions must be given as to the execution of the procedure,
possible complications and what to do when these arise. In
other words: the physician has to sign a written delegation
just as well as the patient has to. As far as we know, no
physician in the Netherlands signs a home-treatment delegation document in the above-mentioned way.

Suppose we organize everything in a legally perfect way
Even then, the home-treatment system we have, is far from
being perfect. So we, the physicians, the Hemophilia Society, and other people involved in hemophilia treatment
propose to start and organize some real work, without red
tape, but nevertheless firmly organized. First of all, we
have to be able to implement the desired uniform policy.
It is necessary that home-treatment is organized through a
limited number of regional hemophilia centers, may be by
a mother center and satellites. Organization of such centers is a joint task of the government, physicians and the
hemophilia society.

These regional hemophilia centers must conform to certain qualitative criteria. It will take us quite some time

to decide what these criteria are, but in the early morning sessions some good and reliable statements were made on that subject. Only under conditions of quality assurance, an optimal approach to hemophilia treatment will be possible. We must do it real good this time.

Finally, both from a medical and legal point of view, an adequate report and registration system should be institutionalized in these regional hemophilia centers.

Concluding: legally speaking home-treatment is possible. All points taken together, both the strictly legal aspects, the circumstantial and organizational aspects on which I commented, form the conditions under which home-treatment is theoretically possible.

The signing and countersigning of the relevant documents is not quite optimal at the moment, but that is the easiest thing to improve. Once that is arranged, a lot of work can still be done to improve the practical system. I hope we can start this work together.

ACKNOWLEDGEMENT

The author wishes to thank Mr. H. van Dijck. Legal opinions mentioned in this lecture are based on his research and interpretations.

REFERENCES

1. Breederveld, C.: Factor V and hemostasis, clinical and experimental studies. Thesis, Amsterdam, 1981.
2. Leenen, H.J.J.: Gezondheidszorg en recht; een gezondheidsrechtelijke studie. Alphen a/d Rijn etc., 1981, p. 331.

Discussion

Moderator: H. Van Dijck

J. Stibbe, Rotterdam:

Ik zou van deze gelegenheid gebruik willen maken en in
het Nederlands overgaan. Ik vermoed dat de heer de Graaf
niet bekend is met het feit dat in 1974 een discussienota
is gemaakt over de thuisbehandeling, waarin alle aspecten
van thuisbehandeling, o.a. de juridische, behandeld zijn*.
Daarin is in grote lijnen behandeld hetgeen U hier naar
voren hebt gebracht. De discussienota is besproken door de
hemophilie-behandelaren. Sinsdien is, in elk geval in mijn
centrum en zover ik weet, in een groot aantal andere cen-
tra, aan iedere patient die overgaat op thuisbehandeling,
een document voorgelegd, waarin staat dat hij de instructie schriftelijk gekregen heeft en dat hij die heeft be-
grepen; verder dat de arts de instructie gegeven heeft en
de indruk heeft dat de patient de behandeling wil en kan
doen. Dan tekenen beiden dit stuk.

P.W.J. De Graaf, Voorburg:

There is a document in use in the Netherlands and this
'legal' document is quite uniform. That is true. Let me
first point out that my comment was not only to construct
a legal framework. My conclusion was that with a correct
legal framework, still a lot of work has to be done to get
a uniform policy into practice. That is the main point.
Then there is a document. I know that document, my wife
signed it. The point which is lacking is, that the factual
saying that the physician in question delegates the right
and responsibilities for home treatment to the patient is
not in the document. The home treater and transfuser signs
that he has learned all the technical tricks. However, the
doctor does not sign.
To say it quite simple: the doctor in question can get in
trouble by not countersigning this document.

* Stibbe, J. Thuisbehandeling van Hemofilie, Rotterdam 1974.

J. Stibbe, Rotterdam:

De discussienota is indertijd door mij opgesteld. Omdat
ik geen jurist ben, heb ik dus contact hierover opgenomen
met prof. Rang en met mr. Langemeier. Prof. Rang heeft
dit document gezien en heeft daarmee ingestemd. Dat is
het enige wat ik erover kan zeggen. In hoeverre dit juri-
disch wel of niet juist is, wil ik verder niet beoordelen.

P.W.J. De Graaf, Voorburg:

Of course it is difficult when doctors in law say different things. Dr. Leenen is just as well a coryphaen as
prof. Rang is. Perhaps we can rediscuss this issue with
these two experts.
We cannot finish this discussion by some simple statements
of course, I agree, but the intention is, to restart the
discussion for the 1980's.

E.J.M. Sjamsoedin-Visser, Bilthoven:

I am confirming the statement dr. Stibbe made about the
document. We are always signing a document for all the
patients who go on home treatment.

C.Th. Smit Sibinga, Groningen:

Of course, we are all well aware of the 1974 note and the
document, but times have changed and the legal points of
view are changing as well. Home therapy is now well accepted all over the world.
There is a parallel situation, home dialysis, which has
even more impact on the health care situation in the home
outside the immediate control of the medical profession.
The question is in the 5th point of the conditions for a
legal system of home treatment which dr. de Graaf has
shown about the informed consent. It is not the consent
part of the informed consent, it is the informed part of
the consent, which has to be signed.
You need to inform optimally and properly. Not only the
physician who is in charge of the home therapy, you need
to inform the patient and his family as well, to get a
good understanding of what is really going on, what the
legal impacts of home therapy are. It is the informed
part of the consent which is the crucial part.

C. Smit, Amsterdam:

I have a question to dr. Breederveld and a remark on the
figures he presented about the grade of disability among
the people in the age-group of 15-29 years. The increase
in number of disabled persons in that group is due to a
change in the social security system in Holland in 1976.
There was a new social law introduced and because of that

fact, it was no longer possible for a number of students to receive a grant from the government. They were transferred to a social law system which enabled them to follow university courses. There was also a relation that most of the group were also on home-treatment. My question to you, as chairman of the Hemophilia Treaters Meeting in Holland, goes back to the uniform policy on registration and control of home-treatment in the Netherlands. Do you think that there are some special reasons why the uniform policy has not developed in the last 5 years in spite of the fact that there is a national hemophilia plan, made 5 years ago?
There are some reports from our society, asking all people involved in hemophilia treatment to develop guidelines which can be used nationally. I also would like to extent this question to the people who are not on home treatment, because also for those hemophiliacs it is important that there is a good registration and control system.

C. Breederveld, Amsterdam:

Concerning your remark about the percentage disability: that might be so because of the different social law. Nevertheless, in view of the presentation of dr. Suurmeijer, this is an unfavorable law, because it causes stigmatization. I do not think it makes any sense putting a hemophiliac, going to university, in the disablement class, because he is not disabled at all.
Concerning your question about the uniform policy on home treatment, I think there is a uniform policy. We have regular meetings of hemophilia treaters, 3 to 4 times a year.
Like in any other country, everybody was very enthusiastic when home therapy was institutionalized. The regional orientation of centers in countries like England and the United States made it possible to have a uniform policy for a large area, because there was only one hemophilia center, and all the people, even 100 miles from the center, were in this region. In Holland we have quite a lot of doctors, quite a lot of small hemophilia centers. They all want to be important and think about hemophilia. The more doctors there are, the more ideas there are about home therapy. Part of the local home therapy regimen is being developed at the center itself. That makes it difficult to develop a rule for the whole country.
I think there should be a uniform policy in the way dr. de Graaf mentioned, but not a uniform policy in the way how you teach your patient.
You have to have a doctor who has well balanced ideas about home therapy. In Holland the health care system is good enough to arrange that.

J.G. Jolly, Chandigarh, India:

It is very important that this legal question is sorted
out. Is there a profile or a specimen acceptable to the
legal profession in a particular country as well as to
the profession, which could be utilized as a guideline
for those countries where this security does not exist
for the profession. It does become very important that
we have a document available.

P.W.J. De Graaf, Voorburg:

The laws on this point differ from country to country in
fairly large degrees. For the Netherlands there is no
simple profile within the law; as I said we had to go to
the Supreme Court to get a verdict which gave a kind of
solution to this whole problem.
Every country must devise his own system, both from a
legal point of view and then from a practical point of
view.

C.Th. Smit Sibinga, Groningen:

May I just add a remark to what dr. de Graaf said. There
is one country, Italy, where there is a type of regulation, and home therapy has been profiled in a law. Prof.
Manucci is not here, but he could comment on that better
than I can. This profile was reported last year at the
1980 Bonn meeting[*].

L.H. Siegenbeek Van Heukelom, Alkmaar:

Can you tell me whether it is possible that a hemophilia
patient controls his home care by measuring his own clotting time?

C. Breederveld, Amsterdam:

This is an interesting question. I never have thought
about that system. I think there are some technical problems. I don't think there is a good relationship between
the shortening of the clotting time, the factor VIII level
after transfusion, and the clinical improvement. I think
that is the most important thing. Measuring glucose gives
you direct information about the effect of therapy, but
measuring the APTT or KCT or cephalin time does not say
anything about the curing of a bleed. I do not think there
is any good correlation between those two.

---

[*] Marchello, M. National Status Report Italy, Haemostasis 1981, 10
(suppl.1), 150.

P. Jones, Newcastle-upon-Tyne:

Can I just make some general comments on the legal position? Dr. Suurmeijer said that there was no reason for
not starting home therapy for emotional reasons as he
showed in his figures. I just like to go back to that all
the way. I think it is the right of every single hemophiliac who bleeds sufficiently and who wants on home therapy,
to go on home therapy. I do not think that any emotional,
psychological, physical or any other sort of hang-up
should prevent that. Having said that and stated that
very firmly, I think that you could turn the argument
that you had about the legal position completely the
other way round, and state that it would be possible to
bring legal constraints on a doctor for not starting
home therapy. I do not believe that if you have a doctor today who has not got his patient on home therapy,
that he is treating his patient properly.

The question of a uniform policy was raised. Doctors
have uniform policies on absolutely nothing except for
payment and perhaps retirement. But the system of bringing hemophilia center directors together once a year,
as we do in England, or once every 3 months as you do
in the Netherlands, is obviously a good policy. If you
have doctors who do not come to those meetings and will
not advance modern medicine to their patients, then surely the patient can go to a doctor who will implement
correct treatment. To deny home therapy to a severely
affected hemophiliac is exactly the same as denying insulin to a diabetic, or denying home dialysis in the way
that one mentioned earlier on.
I get worried about legality. I know that this had to
happen in Italy. I do not think, certainly not in the
British system that any doctor could be sued for something that went wrong with home therapy, provided that
he had prescribed it into good faith. That is the level
in which we would interprete the law. If you try to go
beyond that, you are putting up barriers and making it
difficult and you are playing into the hands of those
people who may be ultra-conservative.

P.W.J. De Graaf, Voorburg:

As to the closing remark you made, I quite agree with
that. As to your first remark the right of every hemophiliac for home treatment, I certainly would not advise
to bring that into the law. It would come close to the
situation as dr. Britten described.
We do not like to be a pressure group. What we like to do
is to come to discussions with physicians and other people
involved in hemophilia treatment, to organize a home-care
system in such a way that everybody who wants to have it,
can have it.

Th.P.B.M. Suurmeijer, Groningen:

I mentioned emotional stability especially because you
can read in the proceedings of the 1979 Workshop on He-
mophilia* that it was one of the criteria for not putting
someone on a home program. In my opinion, deciding whether or not a family or a person is emotionally stable,
is not a medical act, it is a social act.

A.F.H. Britten, Albany, USA:

I have a question regarding the frequency of home treatment availability in the Netherlands. We heard from dr.
Cederbaum that approximately 80% of the patients at the
Worchester center are on home treatment and it is my understanding that there are about 600 hemophiliacs in the
Netherlands. How many of these patients are utilizing
home treatment?
I am also interested in the technology here. I saw a picture in the presentation of Breederveld of home treatment
by infusion. I wonder if the opportunity for infusion
by syringe is available in the Netherlands?

C. Breederveld, Amsterdam:

Concerning the percentage of hemophiliacs who are on home
treatment, I think in the last survey the number of 120
was mentioned, which is about 1/3 of all severe hemophiliacs. This is different from the situation in England,
because there distances play an important role. I know
quite a lot of hemophiliacs who think it is still quite
comfortable to go to the center and arrive there when the
factor VIII has already been dissolved, get the injection
and just leave without the problems of selftreatment. But
I think there will be an extension of the number of hemophilia patients on home treatment.
I presented the first slide on purpose. This was really
cryoprecipitate which was in the bottle, and given by an
infusion system. It was merely the expression of the fact
that in Holland there is still discussion about whether
one can use cryoprecipitate for home care or not.
There are some in favor, some are against. We did not
finish that discussion, but I think the biggest group
is using the syringe, and therefore concentrates.

---

* Home-treatment for hemophilia: perspectives and limitations. Smit
  Sibinga, C.Th., ed. Groningen 1980.

VI. Hemophilia home care for the future

A. Factor VIII

FACTOR VIII SUPPLY: THE SWORD OF DAMOCLES IN A NATIONAL SELF-SUFFICIENT PLASMA PROCUREMENT PROGRAM

C. Vermijlen

The Belgian Red Cross blood- and plasmapheresis program provides yearly 12,000 - 13,000 liters of plasma per 10^6 inhabitants. This amount allows to cover all the national needs of plasma derivatives.

Our program allows adequate hemophilia A treatment, even on a prophylactic basis and (or) on home-treatment. Up to 50,000 units per patient are available as the yearly mean under the form of lyophilized cryoprecipitate.

By refusing this aid and requiring only highly purified concentrate the availability drops to a mean of 15,000 units per patient per year, which is insufficient.

The hemophilia A patients and their physicians must be aware of the fact that permanent national self-sufficiency of the life-saving drug is their best guarantee for a normal life. The abuse of highly purified factor VIII concentrates dislocates even the best national self-sufficient plasma procurement programs.

Note: abstract only, manuscript not available. (eds)

NATIONAL RESOURCES AND THE USE OF FACTOR VIII

I. Temperley

The report 'Preparation and Use of Coagulation Factors VIII
and IX for Transfusion' in 1980 was prepared by Drs. R. Masure, G. Myllyla, I. Temperley and K. Stampfli for the European Public Health Committee, Council of Europe. All member
countries including Finland were circulated for information
and most were visited by the above. The report contained the
best information which could be extracted from the various
national health authorities. No information was provided
by Austria and little from Sweden where production is in
the hands of semi-state bodies. There was no co-operation
from commercial producers.

Non-commercial producers used a total of 432,000 l plasma for F VIII concentrate production in 1977. This was split
in the following manner: frozen cryoprecipitate 117,000 l,
freeze dried cryoprecipitate 163,000 l and more purified
products 152,000 l. It is likely that many smaller producers of frozen cryoprecipitate were not included in the returns.

It was calculated from the above that the total production of F VIII concentrate in Council of Europe countries

TABLE I. Factor VIII concentrate production (i.u.) in Council of Europe
countries per million population

	Frozen cryo. $(\times 10^6)$	Lyophilized cryo. $(\times 10^6)$	Purified con- centrate $\times (10^6)$	Total $(\times 10^6)$
Belgium	0.19	1.16	–	1.35
Denmark	0.02	0.26	0.42	0.70
Finland	–	1.61	0.09	1.70
France	0.07	0.37	0.05	0.49
Germany	–	0.05	0.03	0.08
Ireland	0.75	–	–	0.75
Netherlands	1.00	0.59	–	1.60
Norway	0.39	0.26	–	0.65
Spain	0.10	0.03	–	0.13
Switzerland	–	0.52	0.39	0.90
UK	0.34	–	0.27	0.61

was about 130,000,000 i.u. The quantity and type of concentrate produced per million population in each country is shown in Table I. Other countries' returns revealed only insignificant production.

The number of all hemophiliacs both A + B, all hemophilia A subjects and severe hemophilia A subjects per million population in Council of Europe countries except Cyprus, Iceland, Luxemburg and Malta is shown in Table II. The incidence of subjects with hemophilia A varies from 34 to 70 with a mean of 48 per million population and of those with severe hemophilia A from 20 to 32 with a mean of 23.

TABLE II. Hemophilia in Council of Europe countries per million population

	Hemophilia A + B	All hemophilia A	Severe hemophilia A
Austria	81	70	–
Belgium	55	49	–
Denmark	58	51	29
Finland	42	34	21
France	57	48	–
Germany	69	56	–
Greece	67	61	–
Ireland	74	55	32
Italy	45	38	–
Netherlands	48	41	–
Norway	78	59	27
Portugal	56	48	–
Spain	45	38	22
Sweden	68	53	23
Switzerland	61	53	20
Turkey	11	9	–
UK	78	67	24
Mean	55	48	23

Most countries face difficulties in collection of fresh frozen plasma. These will be alluded to later. Once collected two factors affect the adequacy or apparent adequacy of F VIII concentrate production. First, the yield of the method of manufacture is of importance. Frozen cryo. yields a mean of 425 i.u./liter plasma, lyophilized cryo. a mean of 350 i.u./kg plasma and purified F VIII concentrate a mean of 175 i.u./kg plasma according to figures made available to the Council of Europe's study (Table III). The results used to obtain a mean for frozen cryo. yield was based on the assumption that five donations are equivalent to one liter plasma. Obviously a country relying heavily on purified F VIII has to obtain much more plasma than that producing mainly freeze dried cryo.

TABLE III. Final yield in vitro (for clinical use) i.u./kg plasma

	Lyophilized cryo.	Purified F VIII
Belgium	450 (mean)	
Finland	400	300
France (Paris)	400	145 (mean)
Germany (Frankfurt)	300	100 (Baden-Baden)
(Ulm)		
Netherlands	260	
Switzerland	320	120
UK (Elstree)		220
Mean	350	175

The second factor is the number of hemophiliacs requiring treatment. A figure commonly quoted for the incidence of hemophilia is seven per 100,000. Assuming a national production of one million units per million population then approximately 14,000 i.u. F VIII would be available for each hemophiliac (Table IV). The incidence of hemophilia A based on the figures available to the Study was 55 per million. This means 13,000 units per hemophiliac. However, from information available to the National Hemophilia Treatment Center, Dublin, Ireland, only 6% of treatment is utilized by mild and moderate hemophiliacs. If this is the case generally and the incidence of severe hemophilia A is only 23 per million (Table IV), then one million units production per million population will supply about 40,000 units per severe hemophiliac.

TABLE IV. F VIII concentrate availability and incidence of hemophilia A

Hemophilia A per 10^6 population	Information source	F VIII production 10^6 units/10^6 pop/annum
		Units/Hemophilia A/annum
70 (all)		14,300
55 (all)	C. of Europe	18,200
23 (severe)	C. of Europe	43,500

Another communication which deals with availability of F VIII concentrates is 'A study of Commercial and non-Commercial Plasma Procurement and Plasma Fractionation 1980' (IFPMA). From information available in this communication a further assessment of the utilization of hemophilia concentrates can be made (Table V). There is evidence from the IFPMA publication that non-commercial production supplies about 136 million units F VIII, a figure close to that estimated by the Study Group of the Council of Europe. Assuming that production of one million units F VIII per million population is minimum adequate treatment for hemophiliacs then hemophiliacs in Council of Europe countries are dependent upon commercial companies for 66% of their therapy.

TABLE V. F VIII concentrate utilization in Western Europe

Country	10^6 units utilized per million population
Austria	0.8
Belgium	2.6
Finland	0.7
France	0.3
Germany	2.1
Italy	0.5
Netherlands	2.5
Sweden	0.9
Switzerland	0.8
Spain	1.0
UK	1.1

From the information made available to the Study Group and that provided by the IFPMA communication it would appear that of the countries whose national resources appear inadequate to meet minimum adequate needs as defined above Germany, Spain and the United Kingdom are heavily dependent upon commercial (non-national) products to meet the level required. Austria and Sweden present a somewhat different situation in that they reach close to the minimum required by use of commercial national products.

It is clear that the basic structure of the blood transfusion service in some countries is grossly inadequate to initiate a F VIII concentrate program to meet the needs of indigenous hemophiliacs. In some countries the basic structure of the blood transfusion service is adequate but organization of a satisfactory program is hampered by lack of co-operation between local blood banks and fractionation centers. A hint of this may be noted in Table VI. This information would suggest that local blood banks take more care of their local frozen cryoprecipitate production than they do of the plasma sent to fractionation laboratories. There

TABLE VI. Time between donation and separation of plasma

	Number of replies					
	for frozen cryoprecipitate			for Factor VIII concentrate		
Hours	< 6	6–18	> 18	< 6	6–18	> 18
	35	10	2	3	14	4

is no doubt that assuming a red cell concentrate utilization all countries except the Netherlands could double
fresh plasma production. To meet the needs in some countries
from national resources it may be necessary to introduce
a plasmapheresis program along the lines of that now in
operation in the Red Cross Blood Transfusion Center, Brus-
sels, Belgium.

REFERENCES

1. Preparation and use of coagulation factors VIII and IX for transfusion. European Public Health Committee, Strasbourg, 1980.
2. International Federation of Pharmaceutical Manufacturers Associations.
   A study of commercial and noncommercial plasma procurement and
   plasma fractionation. Zürich:IFPMA, 1980.

NEW DEVELOPMENTS IN F VIII PURIFICATION, AN OVERVIEW

F. Feldman

The preparation of antihemophilic Factor (AHF) for replacement therapy in hemophilia A has evolved through several phases over the last 15 years (Table I).

1. Up to the mid 1960's fresh or fresh frozen plasma was the predominant source of AHF available for infusion. The low plasma AHF concentration, the high non-AHF protein concentration, and the decay of AHF activity on long term storage were major factors limiting its use.

2. The development of concentrated forms of AHF suitable for infusion and for allowing rapid build-up of AHF activity in vivo followed two major alternative fractionation routes.

In one, Fraction I was utilized as a source material by the Blombäcks (1956) in Sweden and they developed a series of potential AHF concentrates suitable for replacement therapy. One of these, Fraction I-O is still available for use today.

In the other route, the discovery of the cold precipitation of AHF in a cryoglobulin by Pool and co-workers in 1964-65 led to the widespread use of cryo concentrate as a replacement product initially as a fresh frozen product, and later adapted commercially as a pooled, sterile-filtered, freeze-dried product.

Concentrates represented a major therapeutic advance by allowing the infusion of AHF in a concentrated form of about 10 units per ml rather than the 1 unit per ml or less previously available from plasma. These early concentrates, however, still suffered from a high protein concentration (low purity) and poor solubility and many allergic reactions have been reported in their use. Their high fibrinogen content further limited their use in many surgical procedures.

3. In the third phase, concentrate technology was further refined by pharmaceutical manufacturing. Intermediate purity concentrates became generally available in the 1970's with most existing fractionation schemes relying upon cryo-precipitation as a starting point and incorporating aluminum hydroxide adsorption to remove traces of the vitamin K dependent factors. Several variations in fractionation technique have further been utilized to gain additional purification - such as precipitation with polyethylene

glycol (PEG) detergents or high concentrations of glycine or subtle adjustments of pH and temperature. These concentrates have now been available worldwide and with a purity of 0.5 to about 1 IU per mg of total protein now constitute the intermediate purity AHF concentrate therapeutic.

TABLE I. Evolution of replacement therapy for AHF

Product	Source materials	
	Potency	Purity
1. Plasma	1 unit/ml or less	0.016 unit/ml
2. Fraction I-0 cryo	5 unit/ml	0.2 unit/mg
3. Intermediate purity concentrates	10-25 unit/ml	0.5-1 unit/mg
4. High potency, high purity concentrates	25-40 IU/ml	2-4 IU/mg

Over the past few years, Armour Pharmaceutical Company developed a new high purity AHF concentrate as an improvement over cryo and the types of concentrates discussed above. This was adapted to a large commercial scale as an addition to our usual intermediate purity AHF products. We felt that a high purity material would be useful in long-term treatment, as well as in inhibitor therapy or in surgery where large amounts of products may be used and where the potential for complications or sensitization may be a concern.

Today we would like to present a comparison of this concentrate to others available on the world market. The concentrates we examined are the generally recognized intermediate purity materials produced by the other major U.S. and European companies as well as one high purity fibrinogen free product available outside the U.S.

In speaking of high purity, we use a different definition than that in use in many current publications where high purity is defined as being only more pure than cryo.

We use the definition suggested by Allain (1) where there are three categories:
1. Cryo
2. Intermediate purity (specific activity of about 1 unit per mg), and
3. High purity (specific activity much above 1 unit per mg).

Table II shows a comparison of manufacturer A with Armour's high purity AHF preparation (FACTORATE, Generation II). As can be seen, manufacturer A offers several potency ranges (low and high) but the high potency is not high purity. The 1,000 unit vial of manufacturer A has three times the protein content of the Armour Generation II FACTORATE which is both <u>high potency</u> and <u>high purity</u>.

TABLE II. Biochemical parameters: Manufacturer A vs. Armour

Manu-facturer	MI Diluent	AHF U/ml	AHF U/vial	Protein mg/ml	Protein mg/vial	Fibrinogen mg/ml	Fibrinogen mg/vial	Specific activity U/mg protein	Specific activity U/mg fibrinogen
A	10	21.4	214	24.1	241	6.5	65	0.9	3.3
	10	23.2	232	21.6	216	7.0	70	1.1	3.3
	10	27.1	271	21.3	213	7.0	70	1.3	3.9
	30	24.4	732	20.5	615	7.7	231	1.2	3.2
	30	33.3	1000	33.3	1000	10.0	300	1.0	3.3
Armour high purity factorate	30	37.1	1113	11.7	351	8.2	246	3.2	4.5

Vials were reconstituted according to manufacturer instructions. Potency was measured in units per ml using a modified activated partial thromboplastin time (APTT) against a freeze-dried plasma standard. Protein was measured on a reconstituted aliquot by the Biuret assay; fibrinogen was measured using the Dade DATA-FI clotting assay.

A comparison of manufacturer B to Armour Generation II shows the same comparison (Table III).

TABLE III. Biochemical parameters: Manufacturer B vs. Armour

Manu-facturer	MI Diluent	AHF U/ml	AHF U/vial	Protein mg/ml	Protein mg/vial	Fibrinogen mg/ml	Fibrinogen mg/vial	Specific activity U/mg protein	Specific activity U/mg fibrinogen
B	10	22.0	220	23.0	230	6.7	67	1.0	3.3
	10	35.0	350	24.6	246	6.8	68	1.4	5.1
	10	24.5	245	19.2	192	5.5	55	1.3	4.5
	40	24.5	980	17.8	712	6.0	240	1.4	4.1
	40	24.5	980	20.5	820	7.8	312	1.2	3.1
Armour	30	37.1	1113	11.7	351	8.2	246	3.2	4.5

For Legends see Table II.

Table IV shows that manufacturer C also offers low potency and high potency AHF but all of a lower intermediate purify form. Armour's preparation is up to 5-6 times more pure than this product. In instances where product is required for surgery or inhibitor patients, the same effective treatment can be given with Armour product with only 1/5th to 1/6th the total infusion of unnecessary non AHF protein.

FACTORATE Generation II further differs from these preparations in being totally clear and colorless compared to

the others being hazy and yellow. Armour's product also
has very low levels of cold insoluble globulin and excellent solution solubility with a low content of insoluble
protein or floaters after reconstitution in marked contrast
to some of the other preparations. In addition, the Armour
preparation was very low in glycine content, contained no
residual PEG and was approximately isotonic, in contrast
to some of the preparations which had high concentrations
of glycine, substantial residuals of PEG, and were up to
three times hypertonic.

TABLE IV. Biochemical parameters: Manufacturer C vs. Armour

Manu-facturer	MI Di-luent	AHF U/ ml	U/ vial	Protein mg/ ml	mg/ vial	Fibrinogen mg/ ml	mg/ vial	Specific activity U/mg protein	U/mg fi-brinogen
C	10	29.5	295	45.1	451	15.8	158	0.6	1.9
	20	28.4	568	40.9	818	12.1	242	0.7	2.3
	40	25.0	1000	50.0	2000	17.0	680	0.5	1.5
Armour	30	37.1	1113	11.7	351	8.2	246	3.2	4.5

For Legends see Table II.

Table V shows another high purity product sold in parts
of Europe. It was about 1/2 - 2/3 the purity of the Armour
preparation but differed in having no fibrinogen at all.
Data that we will show indicate this to be a less stable
preparation than all the others seen (manufacturers A, B,
and C).

TABLE V. Biochemical parameters: Manufacturer D vs. Armour

Manu-facturer	MI Di-luent	AHF U/ ml	U/ vial	Protein mg/ ml	mg/ vial	Fibrinogen mg/ ml	mg/ vial	Specific activity U/mg protein	U/mg fi-brinogen
D	10	25.0	250	11.0	110	0.6	LT 6	2.3	42
	20	28.6	572	14.1	282	-	-	2.0	-
Armour High purity factorate	30	37.1	1113	11.7	351	8.2	246	3.2	4.5

For Legends see Table II.

Table VI shows the reproducibility of the Armour Generation II process. Consistent product in the 1,000 unit
range with a high purity of 3.0 - 3.7 units per mg is
routinely and reproducibly produced.

TABLE VI. Reproducibility: Armour high purity factorate

Lot No.	MI water	AHF U/ml	AHF U/vial	Protein mg/ ml	Protein mg/ vial	Fibrinogen mg/ ml	Fibrinogen mg/ vial	Specific activity U/mg protein	Specific activity U/mg fibrinogen
318	30	36.1	1083	11.9	357	8.6	258	3.0	4.2
360	30	33.7	1011	10.4	312	6.4	192	3.2	5.3
368	30	37.7	1131	12.6	390	8.6	267	3.0	4.4
696	30	37.3	1120	10.7	321	7.5	226	3.5	5.0
726	30	38.7	1160	10.9	327	6.8	203	3.5	5.7
849	30	42.5	1275	11.4	342	7.2	216	3.7	5.9

For Legends see Table II, but potency was measured using a Thrombo-plastin Generation Test; clotting was measured on a Bioquest Fibro-meter. Potency was assigned as a weighted mean assayed to 95% statis-tical confidence.

Table VII shows another major difference between the products studied. The higher the product purity, the lower the contaminating immunoglobulins. Armour's preparation had the lowest content of contaminating IgG (about 1/9th that found in preparation C). There has been speculation by Allain, Verroust and Soulier (1) that high levels of IgG and IgM contaminants may induce the formation of anti-immunoglobulin antibodies.

TABLE VII. Radial immunodiffusion (Mancini)

Manufacturer	IgG (mg/100 ml)	IgA (mg/100 ml)	IgM (mg/100 ml)
Armour	42	17	28
D	70	17	18
B	127	40	30
A	146	18	31
C	380	80	55

IgG, IgA, and IgM were assayed using commercially available antisera and agar plates and measuring radial immunodiffusion with BEHRING PARTIGEN PLATES.

Table VIII shows data obtained and recently published by Nilsson et al. (8) indicating a 1:1 ratio of Factor VIII coagulant antigen to clotting activity. All other concentrates examined by that group showed a higher level of Factor VIII antigenic material with less activity and indicates the Factor VIII CAg is less denatured during processing in the Armour fractionation. This observation has now been confirmed in at least two other major labo-ratories.

In the last five years, considerable doubt was raised in the literature whether a higher purity AHF product

TABLE VIII. Comparison of antigen and procoagulant ratios factorate (high purity) and hemophil

	F VIII C-Ag / F VIII C	F VIII R-Ag / VIII C		VIII RCF
		EI	IRMA	
Factorate	0.9	2.2	0.8	25
Hemophil	1.6	3.8	2.1	32

F VIII C: One-stage assay
F VIII C-Ag: IRMA using 2 spontaneous inhibitors
F VIII R Ag: EI-Laurell assay
              IRMA - Immunoradiometric assay (Nilsson)

Personal communication, I.M. Nilsson

could be manufactured without modifying the Factor VIII coagulant protein structure and sacrificing solution stability and clinical half life. The data which follow show Armour Generation II FACTORATE to have the best solution stability of all products analyzed as well as excellent clinical in vivo half life.

Figure 1 shows the half life of the Armour preparation in solution in vitro to be about 88 days at room temperature. This is in marked contrast to literature reports of the instability of the AHF molecule in solution and is due to the gentle fractionation and high quality of the fresh frozen plasma.

Figures 2 and 3 show manufacturer's B and A AHF preparations to have substantial lower in vitro half lives, implying their preparations to have undergone more alteration than the Armour preparation.

Figure 4 is of particular interest because it shows the other high purity preparation (the one with no fibrinogen) to have the worst in vitro half life, implying the most alteration of its structure during fractionation.

It is interesting to compare these data with the stability of the AHF from manufacturer C (Fig. 5) the crudest preparation studied.

That preparation is closest in its stability properties to Armour's Generation II process. Using accelerated degradation solution stability studies is a classic biochemical approach to investigating alterations in structure caused by fractionation or differences between isozymes or apparently similar enzymes. The excellent solution stability was exploited by Levin and co-workers (6) (Johns Hopkins University) who recently published results on use of this product by continuous infusion therapy; they concluded that with continuous infusion that they were able to achieve a steady state potency level in vivo. In addition to the clinical benefit derived, the authors concluded that this technique was also more cost effective than administering a single bolus of an intermediate purity concentrate during

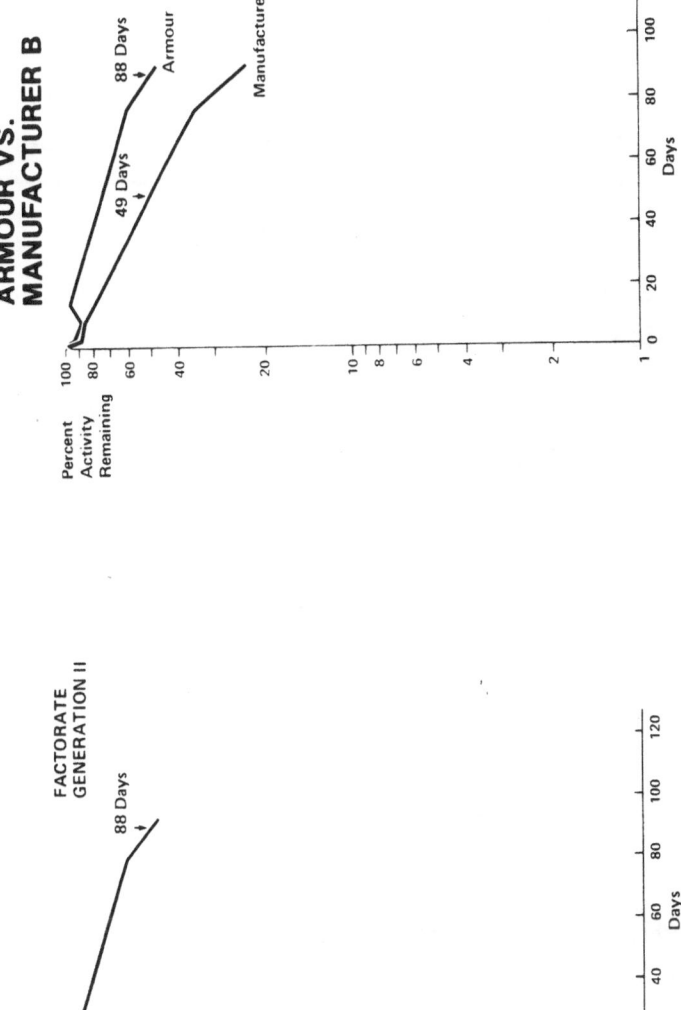

Fig. 1 and 2. Vials were reconstituted under laminar flow using sterile handling conditions and following manufacturer recommendations. Reconstituted vials were stored at room temperature, sampled periodically using aseptic technique and assayed for AHF activity using the APTT assay.

256

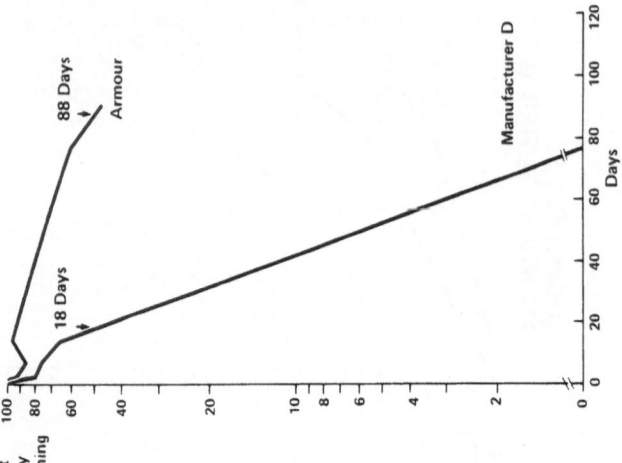

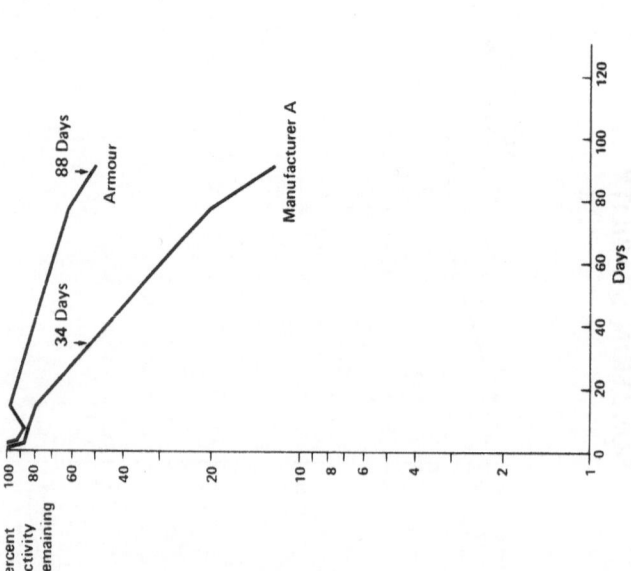

Fig. 3 and 4. For Legends see Figs. 1 and 2.

ROOM TEMPERATURE
SOLUTION STABILITY

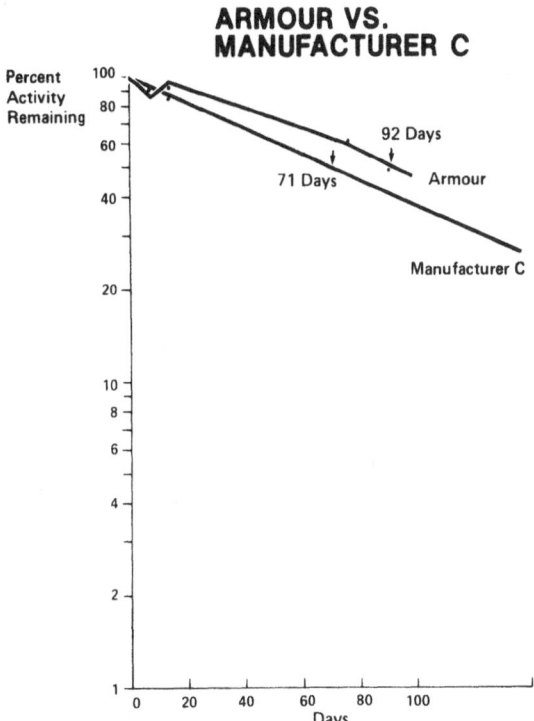

Fig. 5. For Legends see Figs. 1 and 2.

intermittent therapy. Despite their excellent results, we do not recommend holding the product beyond 3 hours as a concern for maintaining product sterility.

The FACTORATE - Generation II process has been evaluated in a number of leading laboratories around the world. The most comprehensive data obtained to date was obtained by the Bonn Center for experimental hematology and some of their clinical data are shown below.

Table IX summarizes data in 13 patients and shows a recovery of 1.6 - 1.7% increase per unit per kg administered and an average in vivo half life of 14 hours by the one stage assay and 18.5 hours by the two stage. The next three figures (Figs. 6, 7, 8) show the half life data in three patients and show the excellent results obtained.

In this study, AHF was administered at about 50 units per kg patient and initial response monitored for recovery at 5 minutes, 15, 30, 45 and 60 minutes. This was essential since the peak of recovery varies from patient to patient (as shown in several publications by Margarita Blomback); in some investigators hands (J.P. Allain), the peak of recovery is never seen until 1 hour. Unless the precise peak

TABLE IX. Bonn clinical study – Summary

Patient	Recovery	1st stage		Recovery	2nd stage	
		Half life t½	Half disappearance time		Half life t½	Half disappearance time
1	1.7	14.5	5	1.77	15.5	5.5
2	1.53	8.5	3.5	2.14	11.5	3
3	2.0	13	4.3	2.0	18	5
4	1.4	10	3.7	1.7	12.5	3
5	1.7	12.5	3.7	1.67	15	5.5
6	2.0	16	2.3	2.0	22.5	7.5
7	1.8	22.5	4	1.9	25	6
8	1.2	14	7.7	1.4	28	6
9	1.0	17.5	5.5	1.1	21.5	5.5
10	2.6	20	3	2.3	21	6
11	0.8	11.5	4	0.8	14	5
12	1.4	12	3.5	1.8	17.5	4
13	1.9	11	5	1.7	18	5
x̄	1.62	14	4.25	1.71	18.46	5.15
σ	.48	4	1.35	.41	4.93	1.25

Personal communication – H. Egli.
Armour Factorate Generation II, Lot 29212 was reconstituted according to manufacturer directions and infused at a dosage of approximately 50 units per kg body weight. Recovery and kinetics of AHF decay in vivo were measured by both the APTT and TGT methods. Half disappearance time was recorded as the time for activity to decay from its peak initial value to 50% of that value; half life was measured as the 50% decay of the second phase of the disappearance curve.

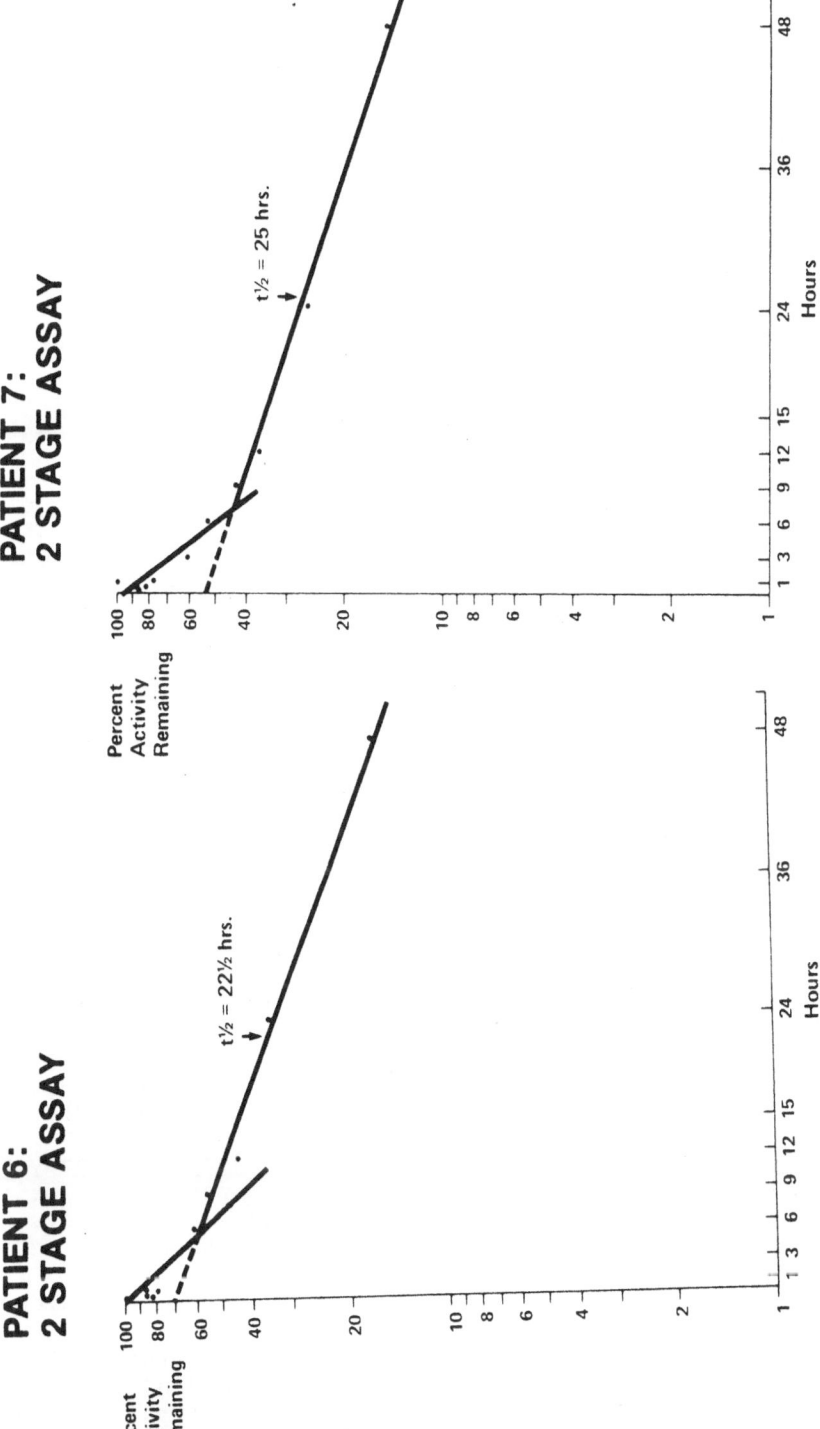

Fig. 6 and 7. For Legends see Table IX.

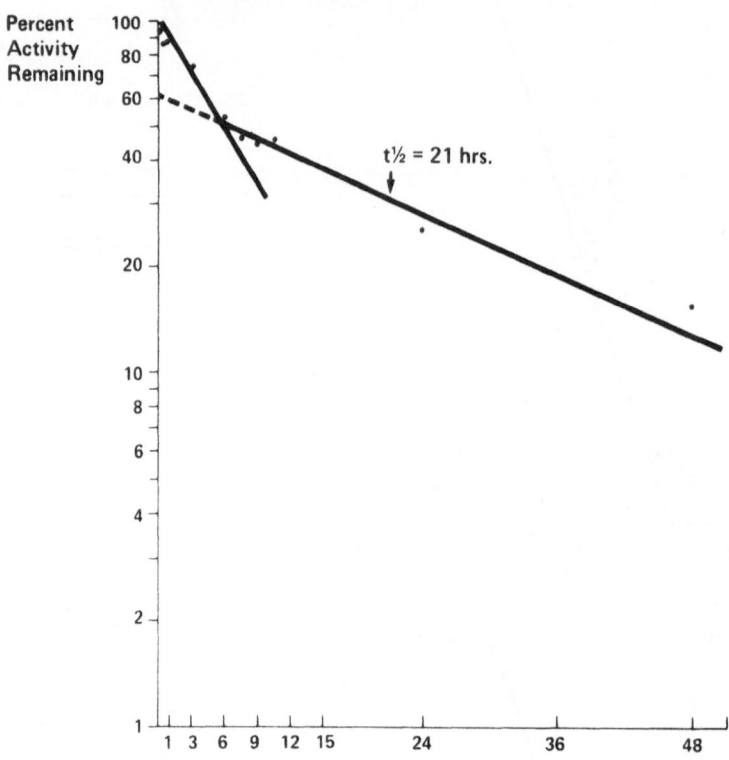

PATIENT 10:
2 STAGE ASSAY

Fig. 8. For Legends see Table IX.

of recovery is determined, estimates of percent recovery, half disappearance time, and half life for the Factor VIII will all be in error. Although this may be of little intere during routine clinical treatment, it is critical if one is characterizing a new preparation or studying the kinetics of Factor VIII decay. To precisely characterize the Factor VIII decay, this study examined many time points and carried the study out to 48 hours. This is essential to obtain enough points during the secondary AHF decay to accurately characterize the half disappearance time of the molecule. Both 1 stage (APTT) and 2 stage (TGT) assays were used to monitor patient performance. As documented by Kirkwood and Barrowcliffe (5), higher AHF activity is seen when using the 2 stage assay and assaying a concentrate against a calibrated plasma standard.

Our study has demonstrated the Armour Generation II process and the high plasma quality to yield a high purity AHF concentrate with better solution stability than seen by other products and with excellent clinical parameters.

In the course of our study, we found the preparation with no fibrinogen to have the worst solution stability and suggest that the presence of some fibrinogen stabilizes the AHF molecule in solution during fractionation.

The increasing availability of Factor VIII concentrates has resulted not only in increased patient survival but improvement in the quality of life of the hemophiliac. However, as the hemophiliac's life span has improved, new problems have surfaced and have been discussed at this meeting as well as in a number of recent reviews of Drs. Aledort, Hilgartner, Levine, White and others.

In a recent publication by Egberg and Blombäck (2), patients on long term therapy with intermediate Factor VIII concentrates showed subnormal haptoglobin values and the authors speculated that alloantibodies (either anti A or anti B or other irregular antibodies) caused intermittent episodes of hemolysis leading to a consumption of haptoglobin. Besides being available in higher purity, FACTORATE Generation II is also available manufactured from group specific plasma (A, AB or B) and may be useful in avoiding hemolysis complications, especially in circumstances where high doses are necessary.

In addition to reports of hemolysis and liver disease, there are reports of an increased incidence of hypertension as well as an increase in renal complications such as hematuria. Antibodies to a wide variety of proteins (such as the blood group substances, beta lipoprotein, IgG and IgA) have been demonstrated in multiply transfused hemophiliacs and there has been some speculation that immune injury may be involved in some hematuria problems. In addition, there has been a recent report by Helmer et al. (4) (University of Texas and Mayo Clinic) in Clinical Research documenting adverse immunologic reactions (including severe anaphylaxis) to some component(s) in intermediate purity concentrates in one of their patients. Myers et al. (7) (University of Conn. Health Center) also reported a patient with hemophilia A who experienced five episodes of something resembling acute hepatitis within 7-16 days following five separate infusions of other AHF intermediate purity concentrates. Neither hepatitis A nor B were implicated and the authors indicated the episodes were not suggestive of non-A non-B hepatitis patterns. These authors instead proposed a mechanism of immune sensitization to some protein contaminants in the intermediate purity concentrates.

There have also been reports from European laboratories (such as those by Sutor in Freiburg (9) or Gadner in Berlin (3)) documenting complications such as paradoxical bleeding in using lower purity concentrates even when the Factor VIII activity achieved in vivo was in the normal range.

These reported incidences indicate the importance of further clinical experience with higher purity concentrates and may in fact prove to be justification for their use in preference, to other materials.

Several other approaches have been reported in the past

for fractionating more purified AHF, but these have invariably resulted in preparations showing physical or biological stability, as discussed above. Other approaches are now being tested clinically. As other fractionation methods become available for concentrates, retention of a stable relatively undegraded coagulant structure may be important in preventing modifications which could be deleterious.

Results obtained with the Armour Generation II FACTORATE so far have demonstrated:

1. An improved concentrate with much lower levels of contaminating non AHF protein and lower levels of immunoglobulins than previously available commercial preparations

2. A product with better solution stability than other concentrates studied.

3. The only concentrate to have a 1:1 ratio of coagulant antigen and procoagulant activity, indicating retention of native properties.

4. Excellent clinical parameters.

ACKNOWLEDGEMENT

The author acknowledges the excellent technical assistance of Mr. Robert Kling.

REFERENCES

1. Allain, J.P., Verroust, F., Soulier, J.P.: In vitro and in vivo characterization of Factor VIII preparations. Vox. Sang. 38:68, 1980.
2. Egberg, N., Blombäck, M.: High frequency of low plasma haptoglobin values found in hemophilia A patients on prophylactic treatment with factor VIII concentrates - a sign of hemolysis? Thrombos. Haemostas. (Stuttgart) 46:554, 1981.
3. Gadner, H., Odenwald, E., Jarofke, R., Reihm, H.: Alteration of platelet function during intensive replacement therapy in hemophilia A. Klin. Wschr. 55:1165, 1977.
4. Helmer, R.E., Alperin, J.B., Yunginger, J.W., Grant, J.A.: Anaphylactic reactions to Factor VIII in a hemophiliac. Clin. Res. 28:348 1980.
5. Kirkwood, T.B.L., Barrowcliffe, T.W.: Discrepancy between one-stage and two-stage assay of Factor VIII:C. Brit. J. Haematol. 40:333, 1978.
6. Levin, J., Ness, P.M., Bell, W.R.: Continuous infusion of Factor VIII concentrate for therapy of hemophilia A. Blood 58:220, suppl. 1, 1981.
7. Myers, T.J., Tembrevilla-Zubiri, C.L., Klatsky, A.U., Rickles, F.R.: Recurrent acute hepatitis following the use of Factor VIII concentrates. Blood 55:748, 1980.
8. Nilsson, I.M., Holmberg, L., Stinberg, P., Henriksson, P.: Characteristics of the Factor VIII protein and Factor XIII in various Factor VIII concentrates. Scand. J. Hematol. 24:340, 1980.
9. Sutor, A.H., Jesdinsky-Buscher, C.: Bleeding in hemophilia during massive treatment with AHG. Dtsch. Med. Wschr. 100:1183, 1975.

10. Sutor, A.H., Jesdinsky-Buscher, C.: Bleeding times in hemophilia patients treated with lyophilized antihemophilic globulin (AHG). Dtsch. Med. Wschr. 101:1715, 1976.
11. White, G.C., Blait, P.M., Campbell, W.M., Webster, W.P., Lesesne, H.R., Roberts, H.R.: Medical complications of hemophilia. Southern Medical Journal 73:155, 1980.

PURIFIED FACTOR VIII: A HIGH YIELD PRODUCTION METHOD FOR ROUTINE BLOOD BANKS

H. Welbergen, P.C. Das and C.Th. Smit Sibinga

The demand for factor VIII as a therapeutic material for hemophilia appears to be the main driving force in donor plasma procurement. Because of the ease of handling and the high yield cryoprecipitate is still widely produced by blood transfusion services for hemophilia treatment.

However, it has to compete more and more with mostly commercially freeze dried and purified preparations.

The convenience of the latter for hemophilia home therapy is no longer a matter of debate, but the current fractionation procedures imply about 80-85% loss of plasma factor VIII during the production of purified preparations.

This therefore demands a large pool approach resulting in enormous logistic problems, high cost price and considerable hepatitis risk. Over the past couple of years attempts have been made to increase the yields and purity of factor VIII products applying thaw-siphon principle (1, 3,6) or plasma heparinization (8,9) for cryoprecipitation at blood bank level.

These attempts so far have not led to a widespread introduction at routine level, because of lack of practicability.

Instead of harvesting cryoprecipitate by this approach we envisage production of purified and freeze dried Factor VIII in blood banks without elaborate fractionation facilities (11).

Our results confirm those reported by Rock and others from Ottawa at the 1980 Washington AABB meeting (9).

METHODS

Thaw syphoning principle as previously described (1,2,3) was the starting point for development and production of a factor VIII concentrate. Our main aim in developing the method was not to interfere with routine blood bank procedures and techniques.

For the experimental production of our concentrate a small pool of 12 donations was used.

Donor blood was collected in heparin-CPD triple bags (Fenwal) with in the main bag 1500 IU of heparin in a 20 ml volume and in the first satellite bag 63 ml of CPD, while the second satellite bag was empty.

The fresh heparinized plasma was separated from the red cells by centrifugation and harvested in satellite bag nr. 2. Out of the first bag 25 ml of CPD was added to the red cells which makes a 70% hematocrit and allows a normal shelf life of the red cells. The red cells are available for clinical use.

The plasma was cryoprecipitated using the standard technique at $-55^{\circ}C$ in an alcohol dry ice bath.

The frozen packs were allowed to thaw in a rocking water bath, while a constant temperature of $4^{\circ}C$ was maintained during the thawing process. Complete thawing is reached within 75-90 min. The cryoprecipitate was harvested by centrifugation and the clear supernatant plasma was expressed in satellite bag nr. 1, which still contained 48 ml of CPD.

This plasma is made available for clinical use as a plasma volume expander.

The bag containing the cryoprecipitate was sealed off, the precipitate redissolved at $37^{\circ}C$ and the precipitates of 12 bags pooled, using a 0.9% sodium chloride solution containing one IU of heparin per ml.

The satellite bag with the pooled precipitates was placed in a $0^{\circ}C$ ice bath. After about 15 minutes floculation of cloudy cold insoluble material was observed and after 2 hours the cold insoluble fraction was harvested by centrifugation.

The supernatant fluid was decanted and the cold insoluble precipitate was redissolved in a saline, citrate, glycine, dextrose buffer, pH 6.5.

This solution was filtered through a 170 micron filter to remove insoluble polymers. Aliquots of 10 ml were collected in 25 ml freeze drying bottles. The bottles were quick frozen and freeze dried. During the freeze drying process no heat was applied, the final product being a white powder.

The different production steps were assayed for factor VIII:C and factor VIII:RAg, total protein, albumin, fibrinogen and immunoglobulins.

The final product was also assayed for heparin using a chromogenic substrate technique.

Independent assays were done on the final product by the Research Laboratory of the Scottish National Blood Transfusion Service and the Edinburgh and South East Scotland Blood Transfusion Service at Edinburgh.

RESULTS

Frequent in vitro assays of this two step cold precipitation method indicate increasing potencies of the product to about 27 IU of factor VIII/ml.

The total protein content is significantly reduced especially during the second step of the process, where the total protein concentration is 26 mg/ml (Table I).

Table II represents the yield of factor VIII clotting

TABLE I. High yield purified factor VIII production method. Mean
values of small pool preparation

	Total volume (ml)	Factor VIII:C (IU/ml)	Total protein (g/l)
Original plasma	2818	1.2	66.6
Step 1 cryoprecipitate	89	28.1	52.7
Step 2 final product	78	27.4	26.0

TABLE II. High yield purified factor VIII production method. Mean
values of small pool preparation

	Factor VIII:C (total IU)	Yield (%)
Original plasma	3382	100
Step 1 cryoprecipitate	2499	73.8
Step 2 final product	2143	63.4

activity after each of the two steps, varying between
44-70% with an average of 63.4%.

The results of the use of heparin is already clearly
visible after the first precipitation step since a yield
of 73.8% is obtained which is remarkably higher than the
average 40% yield obtained with the normal cryoprecipitate
procedure where CPD anticoagulant is used.

After step 2 still 63% of the original factor VIII activity is retained which is remarkably high for a freeze
dried concentrate of this potency and purity.

When compared with international standards available
in our laboratory, the specific factor VIII activity as
shown in Table III almost doubles during the last step
to a value of about 1 IU of factor VIII per mg total protein, varying between 0.68 to 1.27. The same values for
the various commercially dried factor VIII products available presently on the market range between 0.3-2.7, while
that of the national fractionation product is 0.6.

We followed the enzymatic degradation of factor VIII by
measuring the factor VIII related antigen concentration.
The factor VIII:RAg / factor VIII:C ratio shows very little
factor VIII activity loss because of enzymatic degradation
(Table IV).

The factor VIII:CAg assays as done at the Research Laboratory of the Scottish National BLood Transfusion Service result in a factor VIII:CAg, factor VIII:C ratio of
1.05 (Table V).

The total protein was reduced to 1.08% and averaged
26.0 g/l in the reconstituted final product.

Protein analysis showed a considerable reduction

TABLE III. High yield purified factor VIII production method. Mean
values of small pool preparation

	Factor VIII:C (IU/ml)	Total protein (g/l)	Specific activity
Original plasma	1.2	66.6	0.02
Step 1 cryoprecipitate	28.1	52.7	0.53
Step 2 final product	27.4	26.0	1.06

TABLE IV. High yield purified factor VIII production method. Mean
values of small pool preparation

	Factor VIII:C (IU/ml)	Factor VIII:RAg (IU/ml)	Factor VIII:RAg/C ratio
Original plasma	1.2	1.3	1.08
Step 1 cryoprecipitate	28.1	32.2	1.15
Step 2 final product	27.4	30.4	1.11

TABLE V. High yield purified factor VIII production method. Mean
values of small pool preparation

VARIOUS FACTOR VIII ASSAYS (freeze-dried final product)	Groningen	NBTS Edinburgh[*]
Factor VIII:C	27.4	21.9
Factor VIII:RAg	30.4	32.2
Factor VIII:CAg	-	20.9
Factor VIII:RAg/C	1.11	1.47
Factor VIII:CAg/C	-	1.05

[*]assays of batch nr. 10.

TABLE VI. High yield purified factor VIII production method. Mean
values of small pool preparation

	Total protein (g/l)	Total albumin (g/l)	Total Ig (g/l)	Total fibrinogen (g/l)
Original plasma	66.6	39.9	12.3	2.6
Step 1 cryoprecipitate	52.7	26.1	7.2	19.4
Step 2 final product	26.0	5.0	1.9	11.3

in total albumin, immunoglobulins and fibrinogen content to 0.34, 0.8 and 11.8% respectively as compared to the starting plasma pool (Table VI).

Further differentiation of the immunoglobulin fractions showed a substantial reduction of IgG, IgM and IgA (Table VII).

TABLE VII. High yield purified factor VIII production method. Mean values of small pool preparation

	Total IgG (g/l)	Total IgM (g/l)	Total IgA (g/l)
Original plasma	10.4	0.4	1.5
Step 1 cryoprecipitate	5.9	0.3	0.9
Step 2 final product	1.5	< 0.1	0.3

TABLE VIII. High yield purified factor VIII production method. Mean values of small pool preparation

HEPARIN CONCENTRATION			
Collection	1500	IU	vol. 500 ml
r.c.c.	0.8	IU/ml	vol. 350 ml
cryosupernatant plasma	2.5	IU/ml	vol. 234 ml
final product (12 donations pool)	9	IU/ml	vol. 10 ml

Analysis of the heparin concentration showed that the red cell concentrate contained 0.8 IU/ml, the cryosupernatant plasma 2.5 IU/ml, while the final pooled freeze dried and reconstituted product contained a heparin concentration of 9 IU/ml (Table VIII).

This means that on the average 250 IU of factor VIII in a 10 ml volume contains 90 IU of heparin.

The final pH varied between 7.2-7.4, while osmolarity was found to be between 310 and 335 mosm/kg.

The test results from the Research Laboratory of the Scottish National Blood Transfusion Service and the Edinburgh South East Scotland Blood Transfusion Service in Edinburgh, as done randomly on one of the batches confirm the validity of the method (Table V).

The product showed complete reconstitution within 5 minutes. No signs of precipitation, clotting or fibrin strands were noticed within 6 hours following reconstitution.

DISCUSSION

Since in 1964 Pool and Shannon (5) introduced the cryo-precipitation technique for harvesting factor VIII, much work has been done to optimalize the isolation and puri-fication of factor VIII, while preserving its clotting ac-tivity.

Freezing and thawing of plasma is known to cause consi-derable loss of factor VIII procoagulant activity mainly believed to be related to the volume of plasma (4).

However, Rock and others (7,9) have clearly demonstra-ted that heparin as an anticoagulant dramatically impro-ves the yield of factor VIII when precipitating plasma in the cold.

A second cold precipitation step then allows separation of different cold insoluble globulin fractions, purifying factor VIII (8,9).

By maintaining a physiological calcium concentration and a slightly alkaline pH, heparin seems to stabilize the factor VIII molecule (10), preventing it from enzyma-tic degradation, as demonstrated by the good factor VIII: RAg/factor VIII:C ratios.

Starting from small pools, allowing the red cells and supernatant plasma to be preserved for clinical use, the high yield good purity final product provides blood banks a possibility for safe and balanced solution of plasma procurement logistics for hemophilia care.

For the production of 1 million IU of this factor VIII concentrate only 8000 donations will be needed. In contrast, 22,500 donations would be needed for the equivalent amount of factor VIII as yielded by the average commercial or na-tional fractionation center using a high purity fractio-nation method with a minimum of 80% loss of activity during fractionation.

The use of standard triple packs commercially prefilled with heparin in the main bag and CPD in a satellite bag may improve and facilitate the method in routine practice.

Although the product is still in the developmental stage, it filfills already most of the World Health Organization Requirements (12).

If, in the future, this small pool product meets all the pharmacopoeial criteria on which works are progressing satisfactorily here, then a purified and dry factor VIII preparation without an elaborate fractionation procedure is within the reach of most blood banks who would supply this product for hemophilia therapy both at home and in hospital.

ACKNOWLEDGEMENT

Our thanks are due to Dr. D.S. Pepper, Brenda Griffin and Dr. C. Prowse of the Scottish National Blood Transfusion Service, Edinburgh.

REFERENCES

1. Das, P.C., Smit Sibinga, C.Th.: Thaw siphon technique for factor VIII cryoprecipitate. Lancet ii:273, 1978.
2. Das, P.C., Smit Sibinga, C.Th.: In: Proceedings workshop home-treatment for haemophilia. Drukkerij Schut, Groningen, 1980, p. 57.
3. Mason, E.C.: The thaw siphoning technique for production of cryo-precipitate concentrate of factor VIII. Lancet ii/15, 1978.
4. Pool, J.G.: Preparation of testing of antihaemophilic globulin (factor VIII) sources for the transfusion therapy in haemophilia. Description of a new sterile concentrate process for blood banks. Scand. J. Clin. Lab. Invest. 17(suppl.84):70, 1965.
5. Pool, J.G., Shannon, A.E.: Production of high-potency concentra-tes of antihaemophilic globulin in a closed-bag system. N. Engl. J. Med. 273:1443, 1965.
6. Prowse, C.V., McGill, A.: Evaluation of the 'Mason' (continuous thaw siphon) method of cryoprecipitate production. Vox Sang. 37: 235, 1979.
7. Rock, G.A., Cruickshank, W.M., Thackaberry, E.S., Palmer, D.S.: Improved yields of factor VIII from heparinized plasma. Vox Sang. 36:294, 1979.
8. Rock, G.A., Palmer, D.S.: Intermediate purity factor VIII produc-tion utilizing a cold insoluble globulin technique. Thromb. Res. 18:551, 1980.
9. Rock, G.A., Palmer, D.S.: Intermediate purity factor VIII produc-tion utilizing a cold insoluble globulin technique. Transfusion 20:651, 1980.
10. Rock, G.A., Palmer, D.S.: The role of calcium, thrombin and other proteolytic enzymes in factor VIII degradation. Transfusion 20:652 1980.
11. Smit Sibinga, C.Th., Welbergen, H., Das, P.C., Griffin, B.: High-yield method of production of freeze-dried purified factor VIII by blood banks. Lancet ii:449, 1981.
12. World Health Organization Technical Report Series 626. Geneva 1978.

THE EFFECTS OF HEPARIN ON FACTOR VIII RECOVERIES: MARKEDLY IMPROVED YIELDS

G.A. Rock

HEPARIN AS PRIMARY ANTICOAGULANT

Recent investigations in our laboratory have shown that when blood is collected into heparin rather than the standard citrate-containing anticoagulant solutions the level of factor VIII in the plasma is greatly increased (1) (Table I). Collection of blood from the same individuals into heparin, CPD, or CPD plus heparin permits a direct comparison between values obtained in these different anticoagulants and shows a significantly higher level of factor VIII in heparin collected plasma.

TABLE I. Comparison of factor VIII activity in plasma and cryoprecipitate from blood collected into different anticoagulant solutions

Anticoagulant	Plasma		Cryoprecipitate		Cryosupernatant	
	total units	% recovery	total units	% recovery	total units	% recovery
Heparin	235±21	100	184±16*	78	46±8	20
CPD	175±4	100	88±11	50	38±5	22
CPD + heparin	189±6	100	117±12	62	43±3	23

Results are the average of 3 pools, each of which contained 3 subjects. Plasma volumes were 220-255 ml and were not significantly different for any anticoagulant.
*Significantly different (p<0.005) from standard CPD values.

The mixture of citrate and heparin was used to elucidate the specific role of the anti-thrombin action of heparin versus the calcium sparing effect in this phenomenon. The results show the importance of the calcium ion (1) in protecting against the loss of factor VIII. Further evidence of the essential role for calcium in preserving factor VIII activity was shown by an experiment in which blood from a single normal healthy individual was collected into varying concentrations of citrate. As shown in Table II, as the citrate level increased the level of factor VIII activity decreased.

TABLE II. The effect of various concentrations of CPD on the distribution of factor VIII procoagulant activity

Anticoagulant	Initial % of factor VIII per ml in plasma	% Distribution after chromatography*	
		V_O (HMW)	2.3 V_O (VLMW)
CPD + Heparin	110%/ml	77%	23%
1/5 CPD + Heparin	110%/ml	79%	21%
1/10 CPD + Heparin	110%/ml	80%	20%
1/20 CPD + Heparin	140%/ml	71%	29%
1/40 CPD + Heparin	159%/ml	63%	37%
1/80 CPD + Heparin	168%/ml	62%	38%
Heparin alone	168%/ml	63%	37%

*Blood from a single donor was collected into 7 test tubes, each containing a different mixture of anticoagulant solutions, and the plasmas were then immediately chromatographed on Sepharose CL-6B. All samples were assayed for procoagulant activity.

TABLE III. Stability of factor VIII at room temperature

Anticoagulant	Factor VIII activity		
	0 hours (%/ml)	24 hours (%/ml)	% of original activity remaining at 24 hours
CPD	92 ± 22	59 ± 10	64
CPD + Heparin	124 ± 25	101 ± 16	81*
Heparin	176 ± 22	174 ± 38	99*

*Significantly different, $p < 0.005$.

Heparin also has a beneficial effect of stabilizing factor VIII in plasma (Table III). This may be of profound advantage in permitting blood collection at areas far removed from processing centers while still permitting the production of factor VIII for transfusion.

A further advantage of the heparin system is that cryoprecipitates prepared from this plasma contain as much as 80% of the starting factor VIII level with the remaining 20% found in the cryosupernatant (Table I). This is significantly increased from the 40-50% recovery commonly seen in citrated plasma. Further, while the percent recovery is high, the actual number of units of factor VIII is also considerably increased over that found in blood collected from the same individuals into either citrate or citrate heparin anticoagulants.

CONCENTRATES PREPARED BY LARGE SCALE FRACTIONATION

1. PEG

The cryoprecipitate obtained from heparin collected blood

can be further purified using any of the standard batch fractionation processes. These include ethanol extraction, glycine or polyethylene glycol (PEG) precipitation. Data obtained using the 4 to 11% PEG precipitation technique of Wickerhauser (2) are shown in Table IV. Using this method it is possible to obtain a high purity factor VIII preparation with a final yield of 530 units per liter of starting plasma (1).

TABLE IV. Comparative recoveries of factor VIII units in the PEG precipitates

Anticoagulant	Plasma			Cryoprecipitate		
	Starting factor VIII units	PEG pre-cipitate	% Re-covery	Starting factor VIII units	PEG pre-cipitate	% Re-covery
Heparin	235±21	232±26*	99±2	184±16	128±12*	70±3
CPD	174±4	118±5	67±4	88±11	54±7	62±1
CPD + Heparin	189±6	147±9	78±4	117±12	70 ** (62,77)	61 ** (60,62)

Three pools each containing 3 donors were collected.
*Significantly different from CPD values (p < 0.005).
**Only two sets of data available.

2. Application of a cold insoluble globulin precipitation step to cryoprecipitate

In 1938 Morrison et al. (3) reported the precipitation, in the cold, of a globulin fraction of a patient's plasma. Since that time, extensive investigations have revealed that this protein, cold insoluble globulin, now called fibronectin, will precipitate in heparinized plasma of even normal individuals when that plasma is exposed to the cold.

TABLE V. Recovery of factor VIII:C from heparinized plasma using a cold precipitation technique

Fraction	Total units of F.VIII:C	Total protein	Specific activity	Purity over plasma	Recovery per liter plasma
Plasma pool*	2246 U (100%)	135,479 mg (100%)	0.0166 (U/mg)	1x	1500 units per liter
Cryoprecipitate pool**	1814 U (81%)	5,409 mg (4%)	0.3354 (U/mg)	20.2x	1211 units per liter
Cold-insuluble cryoprecipitate	1193 U (53%)	1,208 mg (0.9%)	0.99 (U/mg)	60x	797 units per liter

*Plasma from 6 units of blood.
**Resolubilized as required in heparin-saline diluent (heparin at 1 unit/ml, 0.9% NaCl, pH 7.2).

We have incorporated this principle into the production
of factor VIII by introducing a cold insoluble globulin
precipitation step to the heparin-collected cryoprecipitate. Specifically, cryoprecipitate is resolubilized in a
heparin buffer, then incubated at 0-4°C for 1 hour. This
produces another precipitate containing a high purity factor VIII preparation (4). As shown in Table V the precipitate obtained from these cryos contains most of the factor
VIII activity but relatively few of the other contaminating
proteins. Thus, by introducing one simple cold incubation
step to heparinized cryoprecipitate, it is possible to obtain a high purity factor VIII preparation without the necessity of using any of the usual salting out agents.

Utilization of the cold insoluble precipitation step
can also be done on a small scale in a Blood Bank. Cryoprecipitates from 6 to 20 bags of heparin-collected blood
are pooled and the cold incubation step carried out in the
presence of appropriate buffers to produce a precipitate
which is greatly enriched in factor VIII but which contains
relatively few other plasma proteins. This technique, which
requires few additional steps other than those usually used
to pool cryoprecipitate prior to administration to a patient
permits the generation of a high purity factor VIII preparation which, when filtered and lyophilized could allow
even an isolated service to provide high purity factor VIII
concentrates, of a known volume and potency, without access
to fractionation facilities.

APPLICATION OF HEPARIN TECHNIQUES TO BLOOD COLLECTED INTO
CITRATE SYSTEMS

In some areas it may be desirable to use the standard anticoagulant and to collect blood directly into citrate rather than into heparin. Under these circumstances, it is
still possible to produce some of the benefits of the
straight heparin collection system. Specifically, if heparin is added to the fresh plasma immediately after separation of red cells from plasma and prior to freezing of
the plasma there is again a marked increase in the amount
of factor VIII which will precipitate in the cryoprecipitate. We have reported the recovery of 80% of the starting
level of factor VIII in cryoprecipitate made from citrated
heparin plasma to which heparin was added prior to freezing
(5). This material can then be fractionated using large
scale chemical extraction procedures or alternatively it
is possible to apply the small batch preparations outlined
above for heparin plasma. When applied to citrated plasma
this procedure produces a product of intermediate purity
with a yield in excess of 600 U/liter of plasma (5).

SUMMARY

These studies extend the original discovery of Poole et al.
in 1965 that factor VIII can be concentrated by cold pre-

cipitation. However, the high yield product produced by maintaining physiological levels of calcium and/or altering the cold precipitation environment results in a much greater recovery than for citrated cryoprecipitates and also provide a higher purity product. The technique has the added advantage in that it can be easily carried out on a small scale in a blood bank. Alternatively large scale fractionation procedures are also possible.

REFERENCES

1. Rock, G.A., Cruickshank, W.H., Tackabery, E.S., Palmer, D.S.: Improved yields of factor VIII from heparinized plasma. Vox Sang. 36:294, 1979.
2. Wickerhauser, M.: Preparation of antihemophilic factor from in-dated plasma. Transfusion 16:345, 1976.
3. Morrison, P.R., Edsall, J.T., Miller, S.G.: Preparation and properties of serum and plasma proteins. XVIII. The separation of purified fibrinogen from fraction I of human plasma. J. Amer. Chem. Soc. 70:9, 3103, 1948.
4. Rock, G.A., Palmer, D.S.: Factor VIII concentrates: a high yield product prepared in the blood bank. New Engl. J. Med. in press.
5. Rock, G.A., Palmer, D.S.: Intermediate purity factor VIII production utilizing a cold-insoluble globulin technique. Thromb. Res. 18:551, 1980.

USE OF DDAVP IN BLOOD DONORS

B. Gullbring

A preliminary trial using DDAVP given to blood donors
started in 1978 in Sweden under the guidance of Professor
Inga Marie Nilsson, Department of Coagulation Disorders,
Allmänna Sjukhuset, Malmö, in collaboration with the Stock-
holm County Council Blood Transfusion Service, Kabi AB and
Ferring AB.

DDAVP (1-desamino-8-d-arginin-vasopressin) is clinically
used in patients with diabetes insipidus and has been used
by us in blood donors in i.v. doses of 0.1-0.4 µg/kg and
intranasally in doses of 0.25 ml (1,300 µg/ml).

DDAVP stimulates not only the release of factor VIII,
but also of plasminogen activator.

Fraction I-O obtained from donors who had been given
DDAVP 0.2 µg/kg and an inhibitor of fibrinolysis (tranexamic acid, 0.01 g/kg) contained about twice as much factor
VIII:C and factor VIIIR:Ag. It was given to two hemophiliacs and the survival time of factor VIII:C was the same
as for ordinary prepared fraction I-O.

Dose studies showed a significant correlation between
factor VIII and the increase in plasminogen activator.

To avoid the degradation of factor VIII the dose had to
be studied and also tested if it was necessary to give an
inhibitor of fibrinolysis.

Our studies showed that it was not necessary to give
tranexamic acid to the blood donors. It was sufficient to
add tranexamic acid in a dose of 50 mg to the transfer bag
for plasma.

The next stage was to try the intranasal administration.
The results showed that factor VIII:C rose to reach a maximum level of about 300% within 1 hour. By 6 hours it had
returned to its original level. Factor VIIIR:Ag rose to a
highest level of 180%. Also this level was normal again by
6 hours. Another parameter that changed was, of course,
the fibrinolytic activity.

The activity of the resuspended euglobulin precipitate
measured on fibrin plates rose from an average value of
135 to 231 mm^2 within 1 hour. It recovered its normal level within 6 hours. The APT time was slightly shortened
during the first few hours after administration of the
DDAVP. The platelet count, bleeding time, factors XI, XII,
IX, P&P and factor V were unchanged. No increase was seen

in platelet factor 3.

The ethanol gelation test was negative. No FDP appeared. Fibrinogen and factor XIII, determined by two methods, remained unchanged. It is also important to point out that no change occurred in the content of AT III determined immunochemically as well as with the substrate method or in the α_2-antiplasmin content. No change was found in the osmolarity of the serum. Apart from an increase in factor VIII and the fibrinolytic activity, then, no change suggesting any activation of the coagulation process was demonstrable.

After physical exertion, such as a quick running for 10 minutes around a park, exactly the same changes were seen.

No adverse effects were noted in about 300 blood donors, who had DDAVP administered intranasally.

Discussion

Moderator: W.G. Van Aken

C. Breederveld, Amsterdam:

I would like to ask a question to dr. Vermijlen. He is
in favor of treating hemophilia patients with cryoprecipitate. In that respect, how many patients in Belgium
are on home care and what is the incidence of allergic
reactions in these patients? By allergic reactions I mean
from the mildest to the most severe ones.

C. Vermijlen, Leuven:

In the group of hemophiliacs on home treatment in Belgium,
we had just to drop out 4 patients because of allergic
reactions. I know that a lot of allergic reactions can
occur, and a lot of side effects are described due to
cryoprecipitate, but it seems to me that these side effects described need to be analyzed very carefully because a great deal of them are due to the administration
of wet frozen cryoprecipitate.

C. Breederveld, Amsterdam:

In my experience, we see quite a lot of mild allergic
reactions using the lyophilized cryoprecipitate, like
urticaria for instance.
This is quite frequent. For that reason I am still afraid
of giving a patient on home care cryoprecipitate.
Can I ask another question? How does one measure reliably
factor VIII in heparin plasma?

H. Welbergen, Groningen:

That is a difficulty. The method we use is adding protamin and measuring the shortest clotting time.
To see whether our test results are reliable we therefore
did send samples to Scotland as well, to do duplicate
tests. We found not very great differences in both test
results.

C. Breederveld, Amsterdam:

Protamin on its own influences the clotting time of normal plasma, without heparin. That is well-known. So you compare your standard as well as using protamin in it.

H. Welbergen, Groningen:

Yes, we make first a dilution, add protamin and measure the shortest clotting time. The shortest clotting time we find, is correlated to the amount of factor VIII in the standard and the sample.

W.G. Van Aken, Amsterdam:

May I ask dr. Rock a question concerning heparin and factor VIII? You have been doing this for quite a number of years. Is this procedure yet introduced in your bloodbank? Do you have any in vivo experience with the preparation?

G. Rock, Ottawa, Canada:

We have been doing the technique for 4 years now. We are not using it routinely in our bloodbank, because of our national policy, which is that our plasma is send out for fractionation.
We have limited experience with the technique, in fact only in the last few years. What we did is develop it and then say 'fine'. If it is going on any further on the fractionation side, we have to ship heparinized plasma outside the country. Now, of course, there are a lot of difficulties in shipping heparinized plasma across the borders, reason why we had not had it fractionated except for experimental purposes. Very recently, however, we have been talking to Hyland, who is involved in taking a look at this procedure and I would tell you that this week some of the material is going to be infused into dogs in Albany.

W.G. Van Aken, Amsterdam:

So your recommendation to use it in a bloodbank is not followed as yet? Is it already tried in blood banks in the United States or Canada?

G. Rock, Ottawa:

No, not yet, and that is why I am so delighted to come over here and see that other people are in fact interested and have gone ahead of us and done something about it, particularly here in Groningen.

C.Th. Smit Sibinga, Groningen:

The state of the art here, in our center is now such that
we have come to a final experimental stage which will be
undertaken for the next 6 to 8 months: putting the procedure into routine practice and setting all the criteria
which are needed for final experiments in the clinic. We
expect to be that far by the end of spring 1982.

W.G. Van Aken, Amsterdam:

How do you think about the administration of heparin at
more or less regular intervals?
Because you will infuse each time about 90 units of heparin and although I do not believe that you are going
to disturb the hemostasis, still you are giving it very
regularly. We know that heparin can cause osteoporosis and
thrombocytopenia, what do you think when this product is
going to be used over a longer period of time?

C.Th. Smit Sibinga, Groningen:

It is well known that heparin is present in II, VII, IX,
X concentrates and some purified factor VIII concentrates,
and many of us have been using them for quite a number of
years. I am not aware of any of the rare side effects you
mentioned in using these concentrates. Talking about side
effects, aspirin - every man's medicine - is known to
cause pancytopenia. That is like the side effect you mentioned for heparin: a very, very rare incidence. Still
the drug is used widely.
The amount of heparin is very low. We have to find out
what will come out of that. Another point is, that of
course the other products, the red cell concentrates and
the supernatant plasma still contain heparin. We have
done already experiments in our center with the red cells.
We showed a completely normal shelf-life, there was nothing which appears to be different from any other units
collected into CDP or CPDA-1. Units of red cells have
been transfused into our patients and we could not trace
any heparin back. The supernatant plasma can be used for
either clinical purposes as a replacement fluid for e.g.
therapeutic exchanges or for fractionation. We have to
find out what the effect of the amount of heparin is on
e.g. albumin fractionation and II, VII, IX, X concentrate.
That is still under investigation.

J.J. Van Loghem, Amsterdam:

I am very much impressed by the communications of dr.
Welbergen, and of course dr. Rock, the inventor of the
whole system. Can dr. Rock tell us about the effect of
heparin on the stability of this factor VIII preparation.
It is of course a biologically very labile product. Do

you expect that e.g. some enzymes are neutralized which normally attack factor VIII?

G. Rock, Ottawa:

I could go on about this for an hour. It is really a very interesting problem you brought up. What we find in fact is that if you collect blood in heparin, and leave it on the desk for 24 hours, you have a 100% stabilisation of factor VIII, even at 22°. Now, if you take citrate plus heparin in the same blood, you don't have a 100% stability. That indicates, that in fact it is not thrombin which is contributing to the degradation. If you then take citrate, heparin and add calcium back, you will have stability. So it looks like calcium is very essential for the stabilisation of the factor VIII. We reported those results last year[*].
I would like to make one comment about the heparin content. The Hyland factor VIII concentrate does contain heparin in the final product.
Heparin is added to the cryoprecipitate because it stabilises the cryoprecipitate. Heparin is not added one step earlier on, but heparin is present during the purification procedure after the cryoprecipitate is reconstituted. That is the preparation people are using now for years.
There is one firm in the northern United States that has been plasmapheresing in heparin for diagnostic reagents collection for 20 years. They collect 20.000 liters per year. So this is one of the things we just found out, which is helping us to convince people in the United States that the heparin collection system, at least by plasmapheresis, may be feasible.

P.C. Das, Groningen:

I have the feeling that the commercial houses and the national fractionation centers play a cat and mouse game. In view of dr. Temperley's presentation, would dr. Temperley agree that one should complement each other?

I. Temperley, Dublin:

It would be fair to say that the fault of the lack of cooperation in the survey was not all together due to the commercial firms; they had a point in not cooperating perhaps. I think there is a lot of unnecessary tension between these two groups. Certainly I think a greater cooperation could go on, because I personally do not see very easily the various countries in the Council of Europe ever catching up on 66%. It is going to take a very long time and during that time the hemophiliacs are going to be dependent on

[*] Rock, G. and Palmer, D. Transfusion 1980, 20, 652.

the commercial firms for their treatment. It seems to me
only reasonable that these two groups should in some way
get together to find some way of cooperation, one way or
another.

A.F.H. Britten, Albany, USA:

I would like to congratulate dr. Das on his question. I
think the time is overdue for effective collaboration
amongst all of us who are involved in the provision of
plasma products. I look forward to implementation of that.
Could dr. Feldman tell us the production yield of your
factor VIII high purity product?

F. Feldman, Kankakee, USA:

In our production process we start with plasmapheresed
plasma. The plasma is collected and frozen within 1 hour
after collection. We then construct the pool after the
plasma is transported to the plant. In the pooling process,
the plasma goes to the cryoprecipitate stage as other
fractionators do. It is impossible to take a starting
alliquot there, because of the heterogeneity of the pool.
We do not measure the total number of input units into a
pool, so I cannot give you a precise recovery.

W.G. Van Aken, Amsterdam:

But can you tell us anything about the method you use to
make this preparation?

F. Feldman, Kankakee:

We have applied for a patent in Europe. The patent will be
granted in the near future. We can then disclose the method in a publication.

W.G. Van Aken, Amsterdam:

Is there any stabilisor added?

F. Feldman, Kankakee:

No, there are no stabilisors added at all. We tribute the
high stability of our product to be due to two attributes:
(1) We add no harsh materials to the product during fractionation, and (2) probably the primary factor: we use only
fresh frozen plasma, even though it is more expensive, and
freeze the plasma within 1 hour after collection. Some of
you have visited our plant and our collection centers, and
have seen the care with which we handle the plasma. With
other plasma, the same type of product is not obtained.
The yield drops and the quality drops as well.

B. Hepatitis

HEPATITIS B VIRUS VACCINE

F. Deinhardt

INTRODUCTION

It is appropriate to start this article by looking back briefly at the recent development of our knowledge of hepatitis viruses, of hepatitis as a disease, and of its natural history because this process is the background to the specific immune prophylaxis of hepatitis.

In the recent history of viral hepatitis, two events in the 1960s broke a log-jam in the progress of understanding hepatitis. The first event was the independent identification by Prince and Blumberg of an antigen associated with serum hepatitis, the SH-antigen (19) or the Australia antigen (1). During subsequent years, it was realized that some patients, both with or without clinically apparent chronic liver disease, were chronic carriers of this antigen, and that the antigen was almost always present in serum during the acute phase of what is now known as hepatitis B. In both the sera of acute phase patients and carriers, antigen could be seen as individual, small particles of about 22 nm diameter or as aggregates of tubular structures. The antigen was shown later to be an envelope component of the hepatitis B virus (HBV), the 45 nM Dane particle, and was named hepatitis B surface antigen (HBsAg). Antibodies to HBsAg (anti-HBs) develop rather late after the disease (3-13 months) but they persist for many years and perhaps lifelong. The ability to identify HBsAg and anti-HBs led to the first serological tests for hepatitis B, and it was the key to the further identification of HBV and its pathogenicity (for a summary of the background and references to these developments see references 5 and 28).

The second event was the transmission of hepatitis to laboratory primates. Human viral hepatitis was transmitted and passaged serially first in marmoset monkeys, and later also in chimpanzees. Later studies established that marmosets were susceptible to hepatitis A, and chimpanzees to both hepatitis A and B. In hepatitis A studies, both marmosets and chimpanzees may be infected orally or parentally, the disease is usually mild, and virus multiplication, excretion and antibody development follow the same general course seen in man. The subsequent identification of virus particles in acute phase human and marmoset stools and marmoset liver, agglutination of the virus particles, and fluorescent antibody staining by convalescent but not acute phase sera (for detailed reference see 7) provided the first identification of hepatitis A virus (HAV) particles, and formed the basis for detailed biochemical and biological characterization of HAV (20), and for developing diagnostic tests and defining the epidemiology and pathogenesis of hepatitis A.

The ability to recognize the antigens of HAV and HBV led indirectly to the identification of a third form (or forms) of hepatitis, the non-A, non-B hepatitides. Use of the diagnostic tests for HAV and HBV showed that many cases of post-transfusion hepatitis (PTH) were caused by a third form of hepatitis; in order to diagnose a non-A, non-B infection, hepatitis A as a possible cause must be excluded by testing for antibodies to HAV of the IgM class, and HBV must be excluded by testing for the various HBV markers (see 10 for further references). In addition, those forms of hepatitis which occur in association with herpes virus infection, particularly Epstein-Barr virus (infectious mononucleosis) but also cytomegalovirus (CMV) and herpes zoster, must also be excluded. Exclusion of other infections which cause liver disease, such as malaria, yellow fever, other hemorrhagic fevers and common viral infections such as mumps or coxsackie virus, is generally not difficult. Toxic liver damage must also be excluded, especially in cases of hepatitis with a very short incubation period after transfusion, surgery or injections.

PROPHYLAXIS OF HEPATITIS

For the immune prophylaxis of hepatitis A, normal immune serum globulin (NIG) can be used. All currently available NIG preparations contain sufficient antibodies to HAV (anti-HAV) to protect against disease (5), if the NIG is given before infection or early in the incubation period. Active immunization against HAV can already be foreseen: HAV has been grown in various cell cultures (for references see 9), and the first attenuated live virus vaccines are already in the first stages of evaluation (Hilleman, personal communication). In addition, HAV can now be cloned in plasmids and amplified in bacteria, thus enabling the future production of larger amounts of antigen for developing a non-infectious vaccine (25).

Despite the almost complete elimination of hepatitis B (HB) as a cause of PTH by the testing and selection of blood donors, HB remains a major public health problem. Two hundred million chronic carriers of HBsAg exist in the world, 50-100,000 deaths can be attributed to acute fulminant HB per year, and the number of deaths due to HBsAg-positive liver cirrhosis or liver cell carcinoma exceeds 1,000,000 per year. The HBsAg-carrier rate in central European countries is 0.3-0.5%, and it is higher in most tro-

pical countries. HB remains a frequent nosocomial infection, particularly in dialysis patients and personnel, and
its spread through sexual and other close bodily contact,
as well as through perinatal infection from HBsAg- and particularly HBsAg- and HBeAg-positive mothers to their newborns, guarantees that this problem will remain with us
for years to come.

Passive immune protection against HB with NIG is ineffective because NIG does not usually contain sufficient
amounts of neutralizing antibodies against HBV (anti-HBs).
Special immune globulin preparations with high anti-HBs titers (HBIG) protect but only if administered before infection occurs or within hours of infection. No hard rule can
be given for the timing of effective protection after infection but ideally HBIG should be given within the first
six hours after accidental inoculation because the efficacy
of the protection through HBIG declines constantly. In addition, passive immune prophylaxis with HBIG lasts only
for eight to maximally 12 weeks and is expensive, so that
its general, large-scale use for eliminating HB is not possible.   '

Active immunization against HB began with the observation by Krugman and his co-workers (13,14) that the inoculation of boiled human plasma containing HBsAg induced anti-HBs and subsequent resistance to challenge with live
HBV. This observation led ultimately to the development
of safe, effective non-living vaccines against HB. These
vaccines consist of purified HBsAg, extracted from the
plasma of HBsAg carriers and subsequently highly purified,
so that almost no residual protein other than HBsAg can
be detected in the vaccine. These vaccines contain no complete HBV or HBV DNA but even so the vaccines are 'inactivated' with formalin as an additional precaution (for detailed references see 11,17,18,27). In efficacy trials, no
side-reactions were observed in more than 10,000 vaccinees,
and 95-98% developed anti-HBs. It has been shown that persons developing anti-HBs as a result of vaccination were
protected against infections with HBV (2,4,12,23,27). In
these studies, three inoculations over three to six months
were given, and preliminary observations suggest that immunity lasts for at least three to five years.

Immunity against hepatitis B can also be established
by a passive-active schedule of vaccination (6,17,22,26).
Active immunity is stimulated with the HBsAg vaccine mentioned above, while passive protection is provided simultaneously by HBIG, and this approach is recommended after
accidental inoculation or exposure to blood (products),
for anti-HBs-negative persons in close contact with an
HBsAg- or HBsAG- and HBeAg-positive person (e.g. members
of a family into which a convalescent patient still positive for HBsAg or HBsAg and HBeAg will be reintroduced),
for people at particular risk of infection (personnel or
patients in dialysis units), and for newborns of HBsAg- or
HBsAg- and HBeAg-positive mothers (16). Passive-active im-

munization achieves an immediate immunity through the HBIG
inoculation, and during this phase the longer-lasting active immunity is simultaneously stimulated by the hepatitis B vaccine. In our own studies (4,6,26), we determined
the clinical and immunological responses to active and passive-active immunization with a vaccine containing highly
purified HBsAg prepared by Dr. Hilleman's group at Merck
Sharp & Dohme (11). This vaccine was produced in accordance
with WHO recommendations, it was free of blood group substances, and contained no trace of contaminants, i.e. the
protein content corresponded closely to the mass of HBsAg.
For passive-active immunization the vaccine was combined
with HBIG with high anti-HBs titers (1:380,000, as measured by radioimmunoassay and corresponding to 600 IU of
anti-HBs). Medical students, students of medical technology, and university staff members volunteered for this
study, and were assigned randomly to three groups. Group
I received three doses of vaccine (20 µg of HBsAg per dose)
initially, and after one and six months; group II received,
in addition to the first dose of vaccine, 3 ml of HBIG intramuscularly, and group III received HBIG along with the
first and second doses of vaccine. Results are given in
Table I. Only minor local or systemic reactions were observed in approximately 10% of vaccinated subjects. No reactions persisted for longer than 24 hours, nor did they
inhibit any of the subjects in their normal activities.
Anti-HBs developed in 40% and 98% of the subjects after
the first and second doses of vaccine respectively, and a
marked booster effect occurred after the third vaccination.
Although antibody development was slightly lower in group
II, titers obtained just before administration of the third
dose were comparable in all three groups, as was the response to the third vaccination and the persistence of anti-HBs titers over a total period of 18 months. None of
the subjects developed any clinical or serological signs
of an infection with hepatitis B virus during the entire
observation period. In a further study (group IV, Table I),
individuals were vaccinated with 10 µg instead of 20 µg of
HBsAg, and no difference in immune responses was seen, indicating that smaller doses of vaccine may be equally effective, at least in healthy young adults. In contrast,
immune responses are less good in immunocompromised patients
such as hemodialysis patients. Preliminary results of a
multicenter study in collaboration with Drs. Arnold (Mainz),
Grob (Zürich), Meyer zum Büschenfelde (Mainz) and Müller
(Hannover) indicate that only about 60% of dialysis patients
vaccinated thrice with 40 µg of HBsAg developed anti-HBs,
a result which is comparable to those of other groups. Different vaccination schedules with more frequent inoculations
may overcome this problem (3, 21). Nevertheless, our studies
further endorse the safety and efficacy (however limited in
immunosuppressed individuals) of the HB vaccine, and establish the feasibility of passive-active immunization for protecting a vaccinated subject against HBV infection within

TABLE I. Results of active and passive-active immunization against hepatitis B

		Months after vaccination										
		0	1	2	3	4	5	6	7	9	12	18
Group I* 20 µg	%**	0	38	82	90	91	90	91	94	94	94	94****
	mIU***	< 1	33	194	309	389	444	453	9782	5200	2972	1168
Group II 20 µg 1 x HBIG	%	0	100	100	100	100	98	96	95	95	95	95****
	mIU	< 1	43	77	122	221	301	237	7841	2978	1320	784
Group III 20 µg 2 x HBIG	%	0	100	100	100	100	100	100	98	98	98	98****
	mIU	< 1	28	400	342	533	517	530	8982	6870	3312	887
Group IV 10 µg	%	0	41	85	92	91	92	92	98	96*****		
	mIU	< 1	128	256	284	455	501	502	11488	NT		

*All four groups were vaccinated with 20 or 10 µg HBsAg at times 0 and 1 and 6 months later. Group II received 3 ml HBIG (600 IU anti-HBs/ml together with the first dose of vaccine intramuscularly at a contralateral site, and group III received HBIG at the time of the first and second vaccination.

**% of vaccinees positive for anti-HBs.

***Mean titer of anti-HBs in milli international units (12) of anti-HBs-positive individuals.

****No individuals which had seroconversion after vaccination became negative during the entire observation. The lower percentage is due to a loss of some of the responders for further observation whereas all non-responders were followed to the end of the observation period.

*****Preliminary data, sera not titrated as yet for anti-HBs.

hours of the first vaccination.

Vaccination with HB vaccine will become a generally routine protective measure for individuals at high risk; in general, health care workers (medical, dental, laboratory, blood bank and ancillary groups), patients and staff of institutions for the mentally retarded, hemodialysis patients and staff, recipients of certain blood products, household contact of HBV carriers, sexually promiscuous persons, frequent drug users, newborns of HBsAg-positive mothers, and patients before major elective surgery.

Vaccines are already licensed in several countries, e.g. USA, France, The Netherlands, Austria and Switzerland, and other countries are expected to follow in short order, but vaccine supply is and will continue to be limited. It is, therefore, particularly important that the HBV genome has been cloned in plasmids and amplified and expressed in prokaryotic and eukaryotic cells (for reference see 24); this advance provides an alternate means of producing HBsAg for future vaccines. Beyond the production of antigens, molecular cloning has enabled the entire HBV genome to be sequenced, and similar sequencing is now under way for HAV. This in turn will allow the determination of the sequence of aminoacids in the various viral antigens, thus opening the door for producing vaccines synthetically (8, 15). Such ideal vaccines should cost only a fraction of the current preparations, they would be free of any possible contaminant, and as they could be produced in any quantity, it would be possible to use them universally.

REFERENCES

1. Blumberg, B.S., Gerstley, B.J.S., Hungerford, D.A., London, W.T., Sutnick, A.I.: A serum antigen (Australia antigen) in Down's Syndrome, leukemia and hepatitis. Ann. Int. Med. 66:924, 1967.
2. Crosnier, J., Jungers, P., Couroucé, A.M., Laplanche, A., Benhamou, E., Degos, F., Lacour, B., Prunet, P., Cerisier, Y., Guesry, P.: Randomised placebo-controlled trial of hepatitis B surface antigen vaccine in French haemodialysis units: I. Medical staff. Lancet i:455, 1981.
3. Crosnier, J., Jungers, P., Couroucé, A.M., Laplanche, A., Benhamou, E., Degos, F., Lacour, B., Prunet, P., Cerisier, Y., Guesry, P.: Randomised placebo-controlled trial of hepatitis B surface antigen vaccine in French haemodialysis units: II. Haemodialysis patients. Lancet i:797, 1981.
4. Deinhardt, F.: Immune prophylaxis of viral hepatitis. Behring Institute Mitteilungen 69:36, 1981.
5. Deinhardt, F.: Serum markers of hepatitis in natural disease and after vaccination. In: Progress in Liver Disease, volume VII. Editors: H. Popper and F. Schaffner. Grune and Stratton, New York, in press.
6. Deinhardt, F., Zachoval, R., Schmidt, M., Frösner, H., Frösner, G. G.: Active and passive-active immunization against hepatitis virus infection. In: Hepatitis B Vaccine. Editors: P. Maupas and P. Guesl

Elsevier, Amsterdam, 1981, p. 167.

7. Dienstag, J.L.: The pathobiology of hepatitis A virus. International Rev. Exp. Pathol. 20:1, 1979.
8. Dreesman, G.R., Sanchez, Y., Ionescu-Matiu, I., Sparrow, J.T., Six,
   H.R., Peterson, D.L., Hollinger, F.B., Meinick, J.L.: Antibody to
   hepatitis B surface antigen after a single inoculation of uncoupled
   synthetic HBsAg peptides. Nature 295:158, 1982.
9. Gauss-Müller, V., Frösner, G.G., Deinhardt, F.: Propagation of hepatitis A virus in human fibroblasts. J. Virol. Meth. 7:233, 1981.
10. Gerety, R.J.(editor): Non-A, Non-B Hepatitis. Academic Press, New
    York, 1981, p. 1-301.
11. Hilleman, M.R., Buynak, E.B., McAleer, J., MacLean, A.A., Provost,
    P.J., Tytell, A.A.: Newer developments with human hepatitis vac-
    cines. In: Perspectives in Virology IX. Editor: M. Pollard. Allan
    R. Liss, New York, 1981, p. 219.
12. Hollinger, F.B., Adam, E., Heiberg, D., Melnick, J.L.: Response to
    hepatitis B vaccine in a young adult population. In: Viral Hepati-
    tis: 1981 International Symposium. Editors: W. Szmuness, J.W. May-
    nard and H.J. Alter. The Franklin Institute Press, Philadelphia,
    PA, 1982, p. 451.
13. Krugman, S., Giles, J.P., Hammond, J.: Hepatitis virus: effect of
    heat on the infectivity and antigenicity of the MS-1 and MS-2
    strains. J. Infect. Dis. 122:432, 1970.
14. Krugman, S., Giles, J.P., Hammond, J.: Viral hepatitis, type B
    (MS-2 strain): studies on active immunization. J. Amer. Med. Ass.
    217:41, 1971.
15. Lerner, R.A., Green, N., Alexander, H., Liu, F.-T., Sutcliffe, J.
    G., Shinnick, T.M.: Chemically synthesized peptides predicted from
    the nucleotide sequence of the hepatitis B virus genome elicit an-
    tibodies reactive with the native envelope protein of Dane partic-
    les. Proceedings of the National Academy of Sciences, USA 78:3403,
    1981.
16. Maupas, P., Barin, F., Chiron, J.P., Coursaget, P., Goudeau, A.,
    Perrin, F., Denis, F., Diop, Mar. I.: Efficacy of hepatitis B
    vaccine in prevention of early HBsAg carrier state in children.
    Controlled trial in an endemic area (Senegal). Lancet i:289, 1981.
17. Maupas, P., Guesry, P. (editors): Hepatitis B Vaccine (INSERM sym-
    posium 18). Elsevier, Amsterdam, 1981, p. 1-318.
18. McAuliffe, V.J., Purcell, R.H., Gerin, J.L.: Type B hepatitis: a
    review of current prospects for a safe and effective vaccine. Rev.
    Infect. Dis. 2:470, 1980.
19. Prince, A.M., Fuji, H., Gershon, R.K.: Immunohistochemical studies
    on the etiology of anicteric hepatitis in Korea. Amer. J. Hyg. 79:
    365, 1964.
20. Siegl, G., Frösner, G.G., Gauss-Müller, V., Tratschin, J.D., Dein-
    hardt, F.: The physicochemical properties of infectious hepatitis
    A virions. J. Gen. Virol. 57:331, 1981.
21. Stevens, C.E., Szmuness, W., Goodman, A.I., Weseley, S.A., Fotino,
    M.: Hepatitis B vaccine: immune responses in haemodialysis patients.
    Lancet ii:1211, 1980.
22. Szmuness, W., Oleszko, W.R., Stevens, C.E., Goodman, A.: Passive-
    active immunization against hepatitis B: immunogenicity studies
    in adult Americans. Lancet i:575, 1981.
23. Szmuness, W., Stevens, C.E., Zang, E.A., Harley, E.J., Kellner, A.:

A controlled clinical trial of the efficacy of the hepatitis B vaccine (Heptavax B): a final report. Hepatology 1:377, 1981.

24. Tiollais, P., Charnay, P., Vyas, G.N.: Biology of hepatitis B virus. Science 213:406, 1981.

25. Von der Helm, K., Winnacker, E.L., Deinhardt, F., Frösner, G.G., Gauss-Müller, V., Bayerl, B., Scheid, R., Siegl, G.: Cloning of hepatitis A virus genome. J. Virol. Meth. 3:37, 1981.

26. Zachoval, R., Frösner, G.G., Deinhardt, F.: Impfung gegen Hepatitis B. Münch. Med. Wschr. 40:1506, 1981.

27. Zuckerman, A.J.: Hepatitis B: its prevention by vaccine. J. Infect. Dis. 143:301, 1981.

28. Zuckerman, A.J., Howard, C.: Hepatitis viruses in man. Academic Press, New York, 1979, p. 1-269.

β-PROPIOLACTONE/ULTRAVIOLET TREATMENT: QUANTITATIVE STUDIES ON EFFECTIVENESS FOR INACTIVATION OF HEPATITIS B VIRUS IN HUMAN PLASMA

W. Stephan and A.M. Prince

For the isolation of biologically intact, non-infectious, protein-fractions from human plasma an alternative method to Cohn's alcohol fractionation was elaborated by Biotest in recent years (Fig. 1).

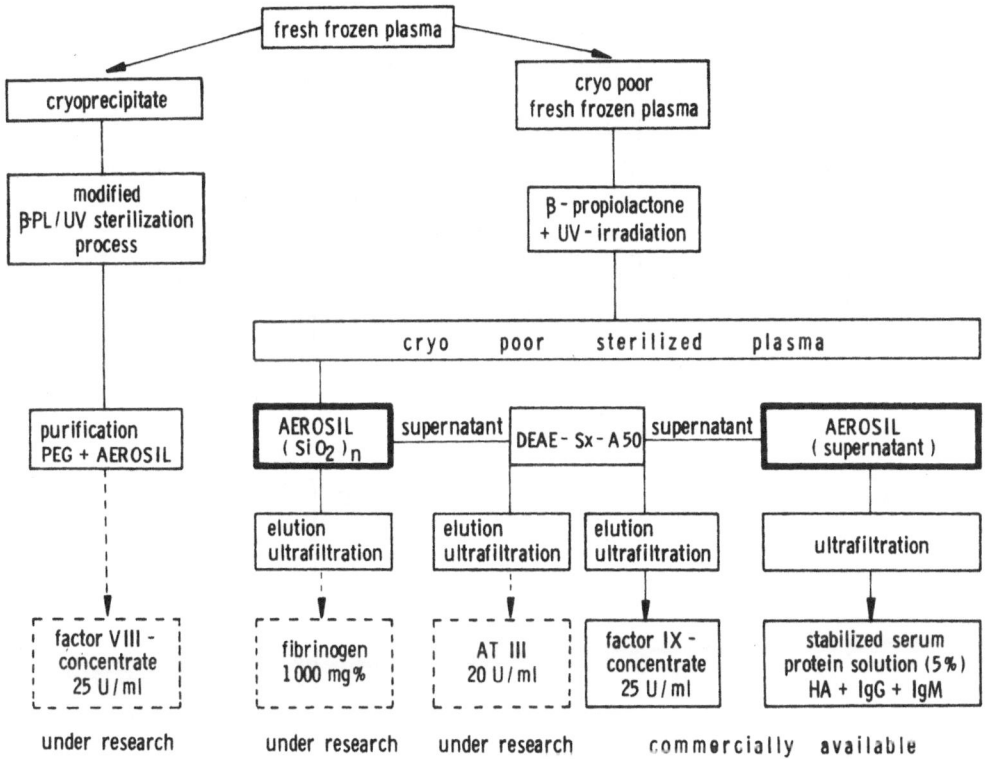

Fig. 1. Plasma protein fractions from β-propiolactone/UV-treated human plasma.

The most important steps of this method are:

1. The treatment of the plasma with 0.25% β-propiolactone (β-PL) and irradiation with UV-light (2 mW per cm^2 · min; 254 nm) (2).

2. The adsorption of the β-PL/UV treated plasma with AEROSIL[R], a special form of silicic acid with high specific

surface area $(380 \text{ m}^2/\text{g})$ (6).

Employing this procedure, the following products have been made commercially available by Biotest: factor IX concentrate (5) and the serum preparation BISEKO[R], which contains, in addition to albumin, trace proteins and the immunoglobulins IgG, IgA and IgM (4). Factor VIII concentrate and fibrinogen are meanwhile under clinical investigation.

The present study demonstrates the inactivating effect of β-PL/UV/AEROSIL[R] on hepatitis B virus in human plasma. The investigation was carried out at The Liberian Institute for Biomedical Research, Robertsfield, Liberia, West Africa, using seronegative, two- to four-year-old chimpanzees. During an observation period of six months, blood was withdrawn at weekly intervals and tested for hepatitis B serological markers and for transaminases. Liver biopsies were performed at intervals of 14 days.

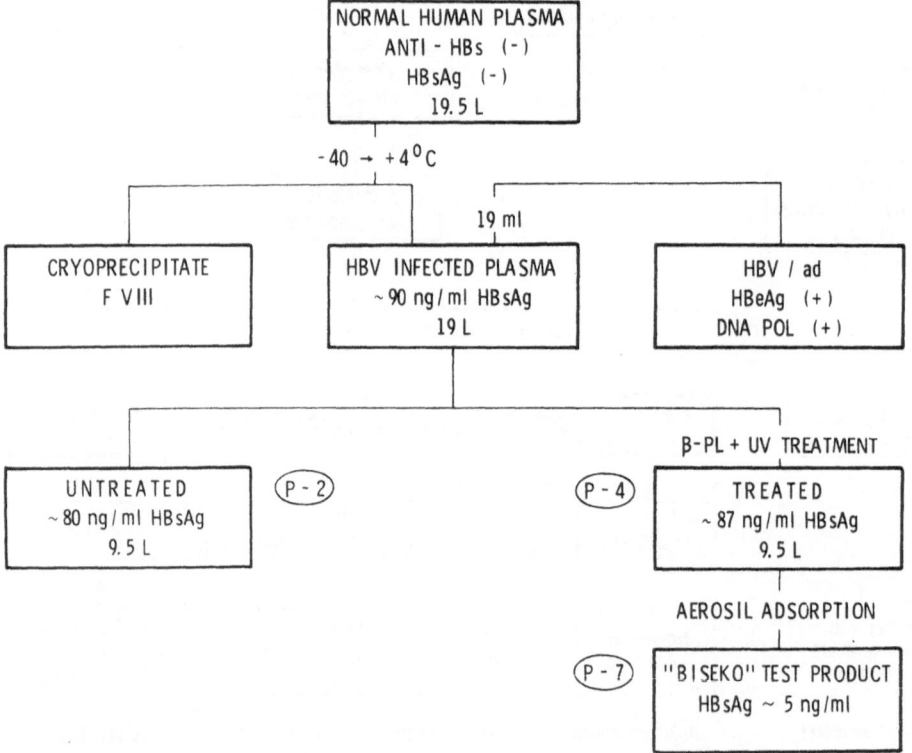

Fig. 2. Design of experiments described in this report.

Figure 2 shows the production of the test products derived from hepatitis B virus infectious human plasma. 19 ml of the New York Blood Center hepatitis-B-standard (HBsA 80 µg/ml, positive for Dane particles and DNA polymerase) were added to 19 l of cryopoor human plasma which was negative for HBsAg and anti-HBs. The contaminated plasma, P-2

(Fig. 2), was treated with β-PL and UV under production conditions at Biotest. From P-4 (Fig. 2) the test product, P-7, was derived by AEROSIL[R] adsorption. Each of the samples, P-2, P-4, P-7 (Fig. 2), was inoculated into two chimpanzees at a dosage of 10 ml per animal.

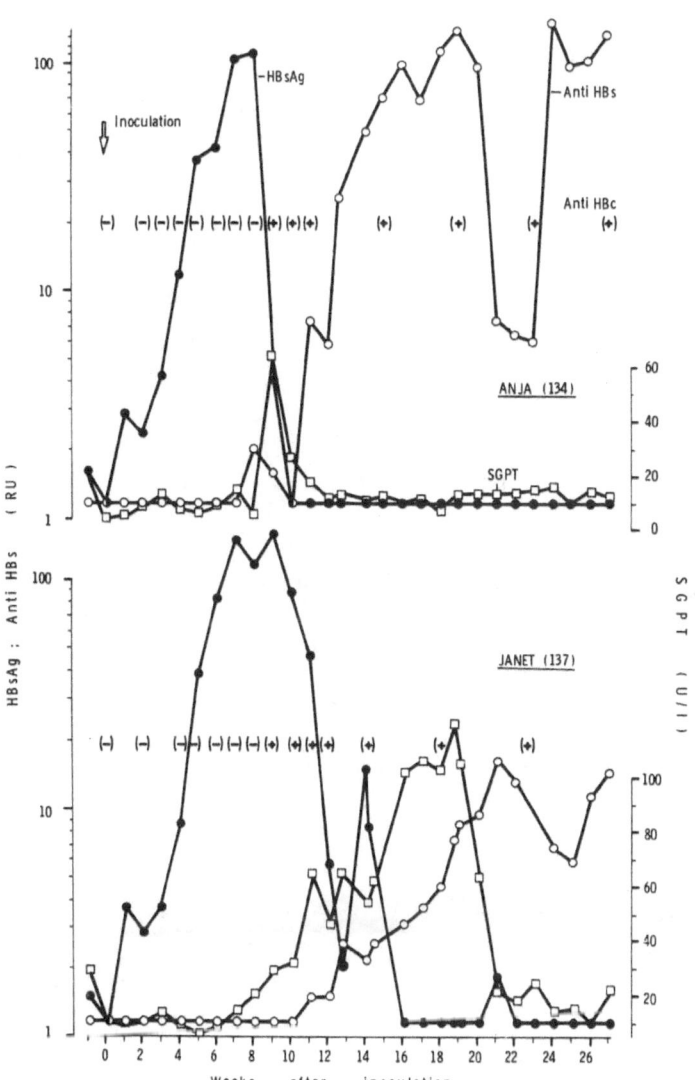

Fig. 3. Results of follow-up of chimpanzees Nos. 134 and 137 after inoculation with untreated HBV infective plasma (P-2). Closed circles: HBsAg. Open circles: anti-HBs. Squares: SGPT (ALT).

Figure 3 demonstrates the results of the testing of P-2.

The two inoculated chimpanzees developed clear cut hepatitis B, positive for HBsAg (incubation period four weeks), anti-HBc, anti-HBs and with elevated SGPT. Following the application of P-4 (Fig. 4), only one out of the two chimpanzees showed hepatitis B infection with an incubation time (appearance of HBsAg) of 20 weeks, an incubation time which is characteristic for borderline infectivity. The inoculation of P-7 (Fig. 5) showed no hepatitis in the two inoculated chimpanzees. To obtain quantitative values for the efficacy of the β-PL/UV treatment from these results, it is necessary to know the relationship between CID_{50} (50% chimpanzee infectious dose) and incubation period of hepatitis B infection (appearance of HBsAg).

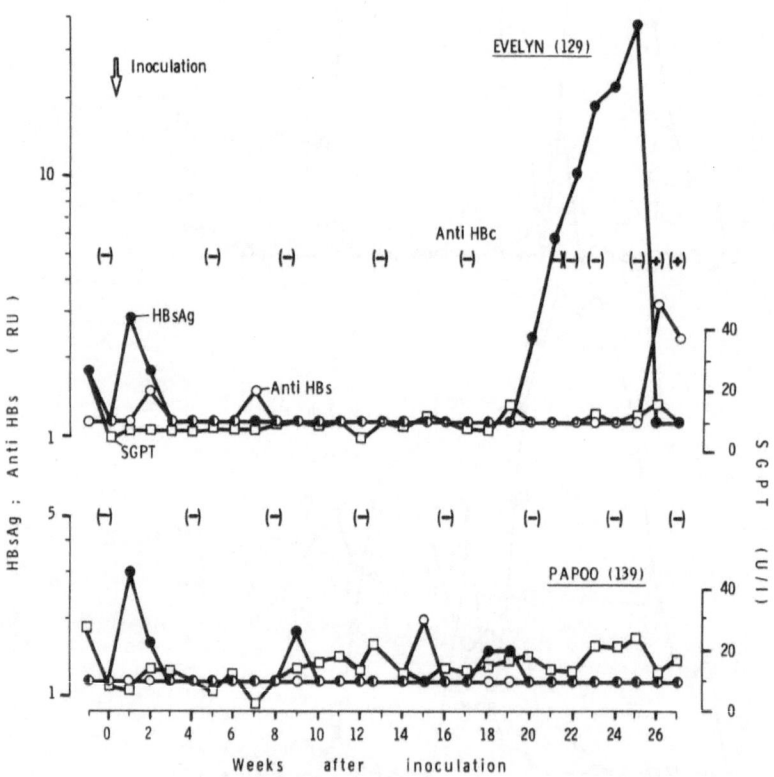

Fig. 4. Results of follow-up of chimpanzees Nos. 129 and 139 after inoculation with β-PL/UV-treated plasma (P-4). (See legend for Fig. 3).

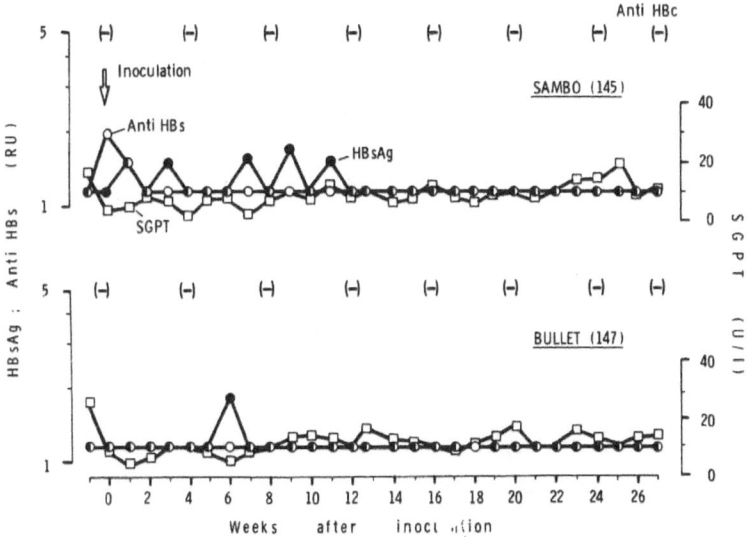

Fig. 5. Results of follow-up of chimpanzees Nos. 145 and 147 after
inoculation of β-PL/UV-treated AEROSIL^R-adsorbed serum test product
(P-7). (See legend for Fig. 3).

Figure 6 shows the reverse linear relationship between
the $\log_{10}$ of the CID_{50} and the appearance of HBsAg. This
curve was derived from the data published by Barker (1)
and our own chimpanzee infectivity experiments (Prince,
1978-1981). From this curve, P-2 was calculated to have
10^7 CID_{50} per inoculum. P-4, the β-PL/UV-treated plasma,
infected only one out of two chimpanzees (1 CID_{50} per inoculum). From this result, it is calculated that β-PL/UV
reduces hepatitis B infectivity ~ 10^7 fold. The test product, P-7, which was adsorbed on AEROSIL^R in addition to
β-PL/UV, showed no hepatitis in two chimps. If AEROSIL^R
adsorbs hepatitis B virus to the same extent as HBsAg (95%)
the whole process, β-PL/UV/AEROSIL^R, inactivates approximately 10^8 CID_{50}/ml of hepatitis B virus infectivity. Our
results are summarized in Table I: β-PL/UV-treatment is
10^3 times more effective than pasteurization (heating for
10 h at 60°C). The combination of β-PL/UV/AEROSIL^R is 10^4
times more effective than pasteurization, a process which
has been used for the production of hepatitis-safe, human
albumin for 30 years.

This study examined the effectiveness of the β-PL/UV-
procedure in the inactivation of hepatitis B virus. Two
recent observations suggest that this procedure also inactivates non-A, non-B viruses: in one study, aliquots of a

300

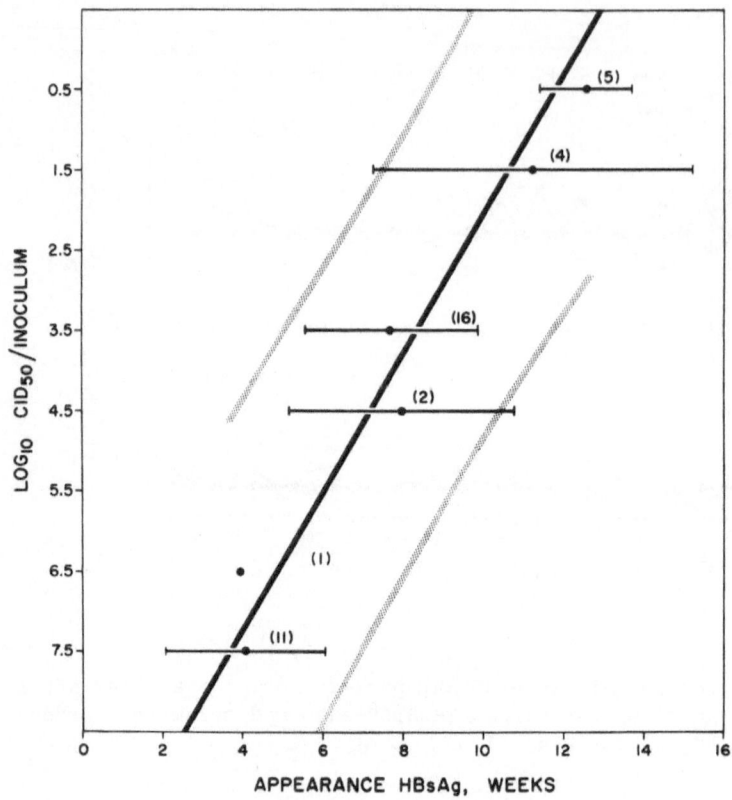

Fig. 6. Relationship between dose of HBV and incubation period to appearance of HBsAg based on results obtained with 39 chimpanzees. Point represent geometric means ± 1 S.D. Stippled line indicates the 95% confidence interval of the estimates when 2 animals are used.

TABLE I. Comparison of B-PL + UV cold sterilization with pasteurization (60°C, 10 hours)

Sterilization method		Process efficacy
Pasteurization (3)	:	$\sim 10^4$ fold inactivation
B-PL + UV	:	$\sim 10^7$ fold inactivation
B-PL + UV + AEROSIL^R	:	$\sim 10^8$ fold inactivation

starting plasma pool (~ 20,000 donors), used for production of BISEKO^R, and the final β-PL/UV/AEROSIL^R-treated product were each inoculated into two chimpanzees. Hepatitis non-A, non-B developed in both animals inoculated with the starting pool but not in either of the animals receiving the treated product (Prince, A.M., Stephan, W., Brotman, B., unpublished data).

In a second study, starting material for a pooled factor VIII preparation similarly induced hepatitis non-A, non-B in each of two inoculated chimpanzees, whereas two animals receiving a β-PL/UV treated experimental factor VIII preparation derived from this starting material remained uninfected (Prince, A.M., Stephan, W., Brotman, B., unpublished data). Further studies are needed, however, to evaluate quantitatively the process efficacy of these sterilization procedures on materials intentionally contaminated with hepatitis non-A, non-B viruses of known titer.

REFERENCES

1. Barker, L.F., Maynard, J.E., Purcell, R.H., Hoofnagle, J.H., Berquist, K.R., London, W.T., Gerety, R.J., Krushak, D.H.: Hepatitis B virus infection in chimpanzees: titration of subtypes. J. Infect. Dis. 132:451, 1975.
2. LoGrippo, G.A.: Status of betaprone for cold sterilization of biological products. Vox Sang. 17:52, 1969.
3. Shikata, T., Karasawa, T., Abe, K., Takahashi, T., Mayumi, M., Oda, T.: Incomplete inactivation of hepatitis B virus after heat treatment of 60°C for 10 hours. J. Infect. Dis. 138:242, 1978.
4. Stephan, W.: Hepatitis-free and stable human serum for intravenous therapy. Vox Sang. 20:442, 1971.
5. Stephan, W., Kotitschke, R., Prince, A.M., Brotman, B.: Long term tolerance and recovery of beta-propiolactone/ultraviolet (β-PL/UV) treated PPSB in chimpanzees. Thrombos. Haemostas. 46:511, 1981.
6. Wagner, E., Brünner, H.: Aerosil[R], Herstellung, Eigenschaften und Verhalten in organischen Flüssigkeiten. Angew. Chem. 72:744, 1960.

REPORT ON A DUTCH HB-VACCINE

W.G. Van Aken

In connection with the presentation of prof. Deinhardt, I
should like to comment very briefly on another vaccine
which is now produced in Holland by the Central Laboratory
of the Netherlands Red Cross Blood Transfusion Service
(CLB) in Amsterdam. This is a heat inactivated vaccine,
which after having been extensively tested in chimpanzees
and in a limited number of human volunteers during the
past 6 years, is now in the stage of extensive clinical
trials. Presently I only want to dwell on those studies
which are aimed at the demonstration of the safety, immunogenicity and efficacy of this vaccine in human volunteers.
In the first place it has appeared that the immunogenicity
of this CLB-vaccine is similar to the immunogenicity of
the vaccine mentioned by Prof. Deinhardt: 95-99% of normal
healthy volunteers (n = ca 300) have developed anti-HBs
antibodies already after 2 injections of 3 µg HB vaccine
(CLB). Secondly a study is in progress to investigate the
immunogenicity of the HB-vaccine in patients treated with
hemodialysis in centers in the Netherlands, where only
HBsAg negative patients are dialyzed. 225 patients have
been vaccinated in a randomized sequence either with 3 injections of 3 µg HB-vaccin or with 3 injections of 27 µg
HB-vaccine. It appeared that the number of patients who
formed anti-HBs after 2 injections of 3 µg, was less than
in the normal group (60%), but the number of persons forming anti-HBs after 2 injections of 27 µg was similar to
the percentage of normal persons forming anti-HBs after
3 µg. Other studies which are presently performed are first
of all a placebo controlled randomized double blind study
in 815 male homosexuals in Amsterdam and Rotterdam to test
the efficacy of this vaccine (supervisor Dr. R.A. Continho).
Secondly we are performing a double-blind randomized placebo controlled study in collaboration with prof. Desmyter
in Leuven (Belgium) in 330 hemodialysis patients of hemodialysis units, where HBsAg positive as well as HBsAg negative patients are treated, to demonstrate the efficacy
of the vaccine in a population which is known to have an
impaired immune response. We expect that the codes of these
placebo controlled trials can be opened by mid-1982 and
that we shall present the data shortly afterwards. Simultaneously, we are performing a placebo controlled random-

ized double blind trial in newborns of HBsAg-positive mothers in Hong-Kong, in collaboration with Dr. V. Wong and
in Surinam, in collaboration with Dr. E.A. Brunings. In
these latter clinical trials several regimens of vaccination alone or of vaccination in combination with the administration of one or more doses of anti hepatitis B immunoglobulin are tested.

Finally, we are in the process of performing a pilot
study in chronic HBsAg positive carriers to investigate
whether combined treatment with HB-vaccine, plasmapheresis
and anti-viral drug therapy will produce sero-conversion
from HBsAg-positive to HBsAg-negative.

Discussion

Moderator: P.C. Das

F. Feldman, Kankakee, USA:

I have a question for dr. Stephan. You showed that with pasteurization you get a 10^4 fold inactivation of virus and that with chemical sterilization you estimated approximate 10^7 fold inactivation. Concluding roughly a 1000 fold improvement by chemical sterilization versus pasteurization. Yet since albumin has been pasteurized, hundreds of thousands of units of the product have been used with practically no hepatitis reported at all. Yet in all the studies that have been reported over the last two years, out of 4 chimps one comes down with hepatitis.
Can you really conclude that cold sterilization is 1000 times more effective than pasteurization?

W. Stephan, Frankfurt:

We have compared our data with the data of Shikata. The number of animals are comparable and therefore the results are comparable.

H. Olthuis, Leeuwarden:

I want to know what the proportion is between the active and passive components in the vaccin? Is there any information about the possibility that patients getting blood-transfusion of donors who are anti-HBs positive get actively immunized?

F. Deinhardt, Munich:

As far as the first question is concerned, what we see during the initial stage of active passive immunization of course is passively administered antibody, if these antibodies decline. The active part of course is the rise again, without having given more antibodies.
From this curve you can exactly show what is passive and active. The second question I did not completely understand. Do you mean what happens if you vaccinate somebody who has already antibodies?

H. Olthuis, Leeuwarden:

Yes, I understood that in the combination of active and
passive vaccination, you give both the inactivated antigen and the antibody together. Is that true? I suppose they
combine.

F. Deinhardt, Munich, FRG:

No they are not combined, you administer the vaccin, and
the hyperimmune globulin at separate places. They are not
combined in the testtube and then given.
Can I ask dr. Van Aken a question? In your interesting approach to the vaccination of chronic carriers, could you
explain why you use plasmapheresis?

W.G. Van Aken, Amsterdam:

Well, you know better than I do that there are a number of
approaches to treat carriers, e.g. with corticosteroids,
with immunosuppressives and also, according to some preliminary reports, with plasmapheresis.
What we in fact are aiming for is a sort of pilot study
to see what happens when you combine all these types of
treatment, so if you can indeed convert patients from positive to negative. Because if you start to build it up
gradually, you have to wait quite a long time. So we try
to combine almost everything and then see if it indeed is
possible to convert.

F. Deinhardt, Munich:

So in fact you use in addition, treatment with corticosteroids just before vaccination and then stop abruptly?

W.G. Van Aken, Amsterdam:

The patients we select, have been on corticosteroids before the treatment is started, but the dosage of treatment
with corticosteroids should not be that high that stopping
might cause problems. So we select patients on the dosage
of corticosteroids.

E.E. Reerink-Brongers, Amsterdam:

Of course we all hope and expect in the very near future,
that a hepatitis-B vaccin will be available, but for the
time being that is not the case. The only way in which you
can prevent a chronic carriership in new-born infants, is
as you told, the treatment with anti-hepatitis B immunoglobulin. In that respect, I should like to recommend
strongly to give the anti-hepatitis B immunoglobulin not
3 times, but 6 times. Six injections at monthly intervals,

because it was shown in a publication by Reesink and others[*] from Amsterdam, that if you give so many injections then the effect is even better than after 3 injections as given by Palmer Beasley[**].

F. Deinhardt, Munich:

I know the publication by Reesink. I know the extensive discussion: once, 3 times, 6 times, may be 12 times.
However, in none of these studies, with the exception of Palmer Beasley's study[**], do we have enough cases. I agree on 6 times being better, but if this is absolutely necessary, I do not know.
I would say that in the future the passive-active immunisation will be much better than 6 times immunoglobulins administered.

E.E. Reerink-Brongers, Amsterdam:

I quite agree with you. I hope that the studies which are now ongoing in Hongkong will be presented in the near future.

P.C. Das, Groningen:

May I take the opportunity to ask a question, which we have not touched, about non-A, non-B hepatitis and the relationship with a donor who has got an increased level of transaminases. May I ask dr. Mitchell from Scotland to summarize his view?

R. Mitchell, Lanarkshire:

I was privileged to attend the Chicago 34th AABB meeting some weeks ago. A group looked at this problem of elevated ALT in blooddonors[***]. Their view is that there is no test for non-A, non-B hepatitis. One of the great difficulties which I would face as a regional bloodtransfusion director is the problem which is entailed on the donors.
Dr. Suurmeijer gave an excellent presentation on the dreadful anxiety which many people experience who have this kind of social problems.
The major difficulty in donors, who have elevated liver function tests, is that we do not know how long it might persist and what it really means.
I know that in certain times of the year this would persist perhaps for a week. So if I had to exclude donors on

---

[*] Reesink, H.W. et al., Lancet 1979, ii, 436.
[**] Palmer Beasley, R. et al., Lancet 1981, ii, 388.
[***] Alter, H.J. In: Hepatitis, a technical workshop. L.J. Keating and A.J. Silvergleid, eds, AABB 1981, Washington, DC.

this criterium, I have nothing to offer them but a liver
biopsy. I feel very strongly that, unless I have something
to offer the donor, I really cannot give him the anxiety
and trauma of exclusion, for the simple reason that these
people are volunteers. They volunteered as unpaid members
of society to give for others who are in worse state than
themselves. It seems to me that only 5% of the population
are blood donors. What does this really mean?
If there is carrier rate for non-A, non-B hepatitis then
it means that a very large number of people are walking
around with the carrier state and are not being picked
out. Just as we have with the hepatitis B. It is said
that there are 2.000.000 carriers in this world. I do not
think that hepatitis non-A, non-B is that kind of problem,
certainly not in the U.K.

A.F.H. Britten, Albany, USA:

I think that dr. Mitchell has brought up a very significant problem that would be encountered if one were to exclude donors whose transaminase level was found elevated
at the time of presentation to donation. As was pointed
out, this subject is under intensive review in the United
States at the moment. You are probably all familiar with
recent publications on the subject. If I can summarize the
attitude within the USA at the moment: although there is
not a clear consensus on this, the feeling is that there
is not sufficient information on the significance of non-
A, non-B infection on the cost of implementing a major
change in the management of blood donors. The bloodbanking
organizations are intensively searching for information
to enable the question to be precisely answered. I hope
that we will find a specific test for this condition before we make an irreversible decision.

F. Deinhardt, Munich:

Non-A, non-B is a major problem in New York. In countries
where ALT testing has been performed with blood donors
for a long time, all this anxiety has not happened. If I
myself would need a bloodtransfusion, only blood would pass
my body which was ALT-negative. I am delighted to notice
that the United States from a complete 'no' to this testing now are somewhere in the middle.

E&M Endocrinology and Metabolism

Progress in Research and Clinical Practice

Endocrinology and Metabolism
Progress in Research and Clinical Practice

Piero P. Foà
  Series Editor

Cohen and Foà (eds.): Hormone Resistance and Other Endocrine
  Paradoxes (Vol. 1)
Jovanovic (ed.): Controversies in Diabetes and Pregnancy (Vol. 2)
Cohen and Foà (eds.): The Brain as an Endocrine Organ (Vol. 3)
Ginsberg-Fellner and McEvoy (eds.): Autoimmunity and the
  Pathogenesis of Diabetes (Vol. 4)
Foà (ed.): Humoral Factors in the Regulation of Tissue Growth (Vol. 5)
Foà and Cohen (eds.): Ion Channels and Ion Pumps: Metabolic and Endocrine
  Relationships in Biology and Clinical Medicine (Vol. 6)